D0926688

Modern Medicine and Jewish Ethics

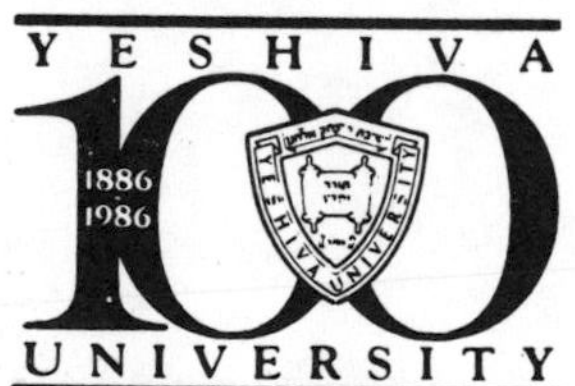
YESHIVA
1886
1986
UNIVERSITY

Modern Medicine and Jewish Ethics

by
Fred Rosner, M.D.

2nd REVISED AND AUGMENTED EDITION

KTAV PUBLISHING HOUSE, INC.
Hoboken, New Jersey

YESHIVA UNIVERSITY PRESS
NEW YORK
1991

Library of Congress Cataloging-in-Publication Data

Rosner, Fred.
Modern medicine and Jewish ethics.

Includes index.
1. Medical ethics. 2. Ethics, Jewish. I. Title.
[DNLM: 1. Ethics, Medical. 2. Judaism. 3. Religion and Medicine. W 50 R822m]
R724.R624 1986 174'.2 86-2910
ISBN 0-88125-091-0
ISBN 0-88125-102-X (pbk.)

MANUFACTURED IN THE UNITED STATES OF AMERICA

לז״נ
האשה הצנועה והצדקנית
אמי מורתי
שרה שיינדל רוזנר ע״ה
בת ר׳ מנחם מנדל חיים
נפ׳ כ״ט שבט תשמ״ה
ת נ צ ב ״ ה

In loving memory of
my revered mother
SARA ROSNER
who lived, died and was buried
in Petach Tikva, Israel,
the land she loved.

Contents

Foreword

by Sir Immanuel Jakobovits
Chief Rabbi of the British Commonwealth

Dr Fred Rosner is already well established as the leading medical writer on Jewish medical ethics. Numerous articles and several major books, culminating in his impressive translation of Julius Preuss' *Biblical and Talmudic Medicine* (New York, 1978), testified to his wide-ranging erudition and his prolific literary output in a field which now commands an ever-increasing interest among rabbis, doctors, patients, and enlightened lay readers alike.

To these enduring works, Dr Rosner has now added this volume on *Modern Medicine and Jewish Ethics*, which will no doubt also be hailed as another classic making a significant new contribution to the growing area in which medicine, ethics, and Jewish law converge.

This well-documented book covers the latest rabbinical and medical writings on subjects as old as abortion and euthanasia, and as new as smoking and genetic engineering. Indeed, the collection of these essays is almost encyclopedic in scope.

By thus making more widely available the insights of the Jewish tradition and the verdicts distilled from it in the latest authentic sources, Dr Rosner will further enhance, I hope, the impact of Judaism's teachings on the practice of medicine as well as the appreciation for the Jewish contribution to moral progress.

Sir Immanuel Jakobovits
Chief Rabbi

Preface to the First Edition

In 1972, I published a book of essays on Jewish medical ethics entitled *Modern Medicine and Jewish Law* (Bloch Publishing Company for Yeshiva University Press, New York, 216 pp). Several years later, in collaboration with Rabbi J. David Bleich, I published a popular and widely acclaimed book entitled *Jewish Bioethics* (Hebrew Publishing Company, New York, 1979, 424 pp). The field of medical ethics has progressed very rapidly since then because of major advances in biomedical technology and therapeutic procedures; hence the need for an up-to-date examination of the Jewish view on important bioethical issues.

The present book contains some material previously published in my two earlier books on Jewish medical ethics. Many of the chapters have been extensively revised and updated. Others did not appear in either of the above-mentioned books. The present work is not meant to be encyclopedic in scope but presents an in-depth Jewish analysis of twenty-six important topics in modern medical practice. It is my hope that publications such as this book will stimulate other writers and scholars to examine additional issues not specifically covered in this book such as mental health and Judaism.

I am deeply indebted to Dr. Alan Blum, editor of the *New York State Journal of Medicine* for permission to reprint my articles on euthanasia (Volume 67, pages 2499 to 2506), informing the patient (Volume 74, pages 1467 to 1469), best of physicians is destined for Gehenna (Volume 83, pages 970 to 972), definition of death (Volume 83, pages 973 to 978) and allocation of scarce medical resources (Volume 83, pages 353 to 358). I am also grateful to Rabbi Shalom Carmy, executive editor of *Tradition*, for permission to reprint my articles on abortion (Volume 10, pages 48 to 71), suicide (Volume 11, pages 25 to 40), autopsy (Volume 11, pages 43-63), who heals the sick? (Volume 12, pages 55 to 68) and contraception (Volume 13, pages 90 to 103); to Rabbi Alfred Cohen, editor of *The Journal of*

Halacha and Contemporary Society, for permission to reprint my articles on cigarette smoking (Number 4, pages 33 to 45) and priests *(kohanim)* studying medicine (Number 8, pages 48 to 61); to Reverend Harry C. Meserve, editor of *The Journal of Religion and Health* for permission to reprint my articles on the efficacy of prayer (Volume 14, pages 294 to 298), Tay-Sachs disease (Volume 15, pages 271 to 281), heroic measures to prolong dying (Volume 17, pages 8 to 18) and *in vitro* fertilization (Volume 22, pages 139 to 160); to Rabbi Robert Gordis, editor of *Judaism*, for permission to reprint my article on artificial insemination (Volume 19, pages 452 to 464); to Rabbi Pinchas Stolper for permission to reprint my article on organ transplantation from *Jewish Life* (Volume 37, pages 38 to 51); to Mrs. Shula Toledano, manager of the *Israel Journal of Medical Sciences* for permission to reprint my article on sex preselection (Volume 15, pages 784 to 787); and to Dr. H. Tristam Engelhardt Jr., editor of *The Journal of Medicine and Philosophy* for permission to reprint my article on the Jewish physician and biomedical ethics (Volume 8, pages 225 to 241).

I also owe a debt of gratitude to his excellency Sir Immanuel Jakobovits, Chief Rabbi of the British Commonwealth, for writing the foreword, to Rabbi Dr. J. David Bleich and Rabbi Dr. Moshe Tendler for rabbinic guidance and advice, to Mr. Samson Helfgott for technical assistance, and to Mrs. Sophie Falk and Mrs. Miriam Regenworm for secretarial help.

April 1985

Fred Rosner, M.D.
New York

Preface to the Second Edition

Five years have passed since the first edition of this book was published. Much has happened in the field of biomedical ethics. Hence, the need for a second edition. Several new chapters have been added, including an essay on the acquired immune deficiency syndrome (AIDS). A new chapter on the definition of death has been substituted for the old one. Several chapters from the first edition have been deleted or incorporated into other chapters so as not to increase the overall length of the book.

I am indebted to Rabbi Alfred Cohen, editor of the *Journal of Halacha and Contemporary Society*, for permission to reprint my articles on AIDS (Spring 1987 issue), dental emergencies on the Sabbath (Fall 1987 issue), skin grafting and skin banks (Spring 1988 issue), and the definition of death (Spring 1989 issue); to Rabbi Robert Gordis, editor of *Judaism*, for permission to reprint my article on Rabbi Moshe Feinstein and the treatment of the terminally ill (Spring 1988 issue); and to Ms. Jane Williamson, managing editor of the *Journal of the American Medical Women's Association*, for permission to reprint my article on maternal-fetal rights (May–June 1989 issue).

Since the first edition of this book was published, Britain's Chief Rabbi Immanuel Jakobovits, who wrote the foreword, was appointed by the Queen to the House of Lords. I am indebted to Lord Jakobovits not only for the foreword but for continuing encouragement and advice over many years. Similar rabbinic help and advice has also been kindly provided to me on an ongoing basis by my friends, colleagues, and teachers Rabbi Dr. Moshe D. Tendler and Rabbi Dr. J. David Bleich. I also thank Mrs. Annette Carbone and Mrs. Miriam Regenworm for secretarial assistance.

October 1989

Fred Rosner, M.D.
New York

Modern Medicine and Jewish Ethics

PART I
Physician and Patient

1

The Physician's License to Heal

Recent advances in biomedical technology and therapeutic procedures have generated a moral crisis in modern medicine. The vast strides made in medical science and technology have created options which only a few decades earlier would have been relegated to the realm of science fiction. Man, to a significant degree, now has the ability to exercise control not only over the ravages of disease but even over the very processes of life and death. With the unfolding of new discoveries and techniques, the scientific and intellectual communities have developed a keen awareness of the ethical issues which arise out of man's enhanced ability to control his destiny. In response to the concern for questions of this nature there has emerged the rapidly developing field of bioethics.

The first medical-ethical question from the Jewish standpoint is whether or not a person is allowed to become a physician and heal the sick. Does the practice of medicine by a mortal physician constitute an act of interference with the deliberate designs of Divine Providence? Does a physician play God when he practices medicine? This ethical question is based upon a scriptural passage in which God proclaims Himself to be the healer of the sick.

> *And he said: if thou wilt diligently hearken to the voice of the Lord thy God, and wilt do that which is right in His eyes, and wilt give ear to His commandments and keep all His statutes, I will put none of the diseases upon thee, which I have put upon the Egyptians, for I am the Lord that healeth thee.*[1]

The last phrase, *for I am the Lord that healeth thee*, literally translated from the original Hebrew means *for I am the Lord thy physician*. In fact, Rabbi Abraham Ibn Ezra, in his commentary, states that just as God "healed" the undrinkable waters at Marah for the Israelites, so too God will remove or heal all plagues on the earth and there will be no need for physicians. This perhaps is the basis for the Karaitic objection to human healing and medicine. The Karaites interpreted the above scriptural passage literally and totally rejected the permissibility of human healing. They vehemently objected to medicine and physicians and relied entirely on prayer for their healing, as stated in the Talmud: "man must ever pray not to become ill, for if he becomes so, it is demanded of him to show merit in order to be healed."[2]

Alternative interpretations of the above scriptural verse are possible. The Talmud asks: If we are told that God *will put none of the diseases upon thee*, what need is there for a cure?[3] Rabbi Yochanan answers that the verse means as follows: "If thou wilt hearken [to the voice of the Lord], I will not bring disease upon thee, but if thou wilt not, I will; yet even so, *I am the Lord that healeth thee*." Rabbi Baruch Halevi Epstein in his *Torah Temimah* explains that the intent of this biblical phrase is to show that the illness of the Egyptians was incurable, as it is written: *the boil of Egypt . . . wherefrom one cannot be healed*.[4] However, afflictions of the Israelites can be healed by God.

The father of all biblical commentators, Rabbi Solomon ben Isaac, known as *Rashi*, explains *for I am the Lord that healeth thee* to mean that God teaches the laws of the Torah in order to save man from these diseases. *Rashi* uses the analogy of a physician who tells his patient not to eat such and such a food lest it bring him into danger from disease. So too it is stated, continues *Rashi*, obedience to God *will be health to thy body and marrow to thy bones*.[5] In a similar vein, the extratalmudic collection of biblical interpretation known as the *Mechilta* asserts that the words of Torah are life as well as health, as it is written: *For they are life unto those that find them and health to all their flesh*.[6] Other commentators (*Sifsei Chachamim* and Rabbi Samson Raphael Hirsch, among others) extend this thought by propounding that the Divine Law restores health, and certainly prevents illness from occurring, thus serving as preventive medicine against all physical and social evil.

Rabbi Jacob ben Asher, known as the *Ba'al Haturim*, states that heavenly cure comes easily, whereas earthy or man-made cures come with difficulty. Finally, Rabbi Meir Leib ben Yechiel Michael, known as *Malbim*, in his commentary on the phrase *for I am the Lord that healeth thee* speaks of mental illness. He asserts that the laws of the Torah were given by God to Israel not like a master ordering his slave but like a physician ordering his patient. In the former case, the master benefits, not the slave. In the latter case, the patient and not the physician is healed from illness. Similarly, God's statutes are for our benefit, not His.

The multitude of interpretations of the scriptural phrase *for I am the Lord that healeth thee* indicates that this verse is not to be understood literally. There is no prohibition inherent in this verse against a mortal becoming a physician and healing the sick. In fact, specific permissibility and sanction for the physician to practice medicine is given in the Torah, as described below. The physician, however, must always recognize that God is the true healer of the sick and that a doctor is only an instrument of God in the ministrations to the sick.

Specific Divine license for a physician to heal is derived by the Rabbis from the biblical phrase *and heal he shall heal,*[7] which relates to compensation for personal injuries.

> *And if men quarrel and one smiteth the other with a stone or with his fist and he die not, but has to keep in bed . . . he must pay the loss entailed by absence from work and cause him to be thoroughly healed.*

The last phrase, translated literally, reads *and heal he shall heal.* The Talmud interprets this duplicate mention of healing as intended to teach us that authorization was granted by God to the physician to heal.[8] *Rashi* extends the words of the Talmud when he asserts "lest it be said that God smites and man heals." Thus he implies that a need exists for specific biblical sanctioning of human healing.

Many biblical commentators, including Rabbi Samson Raphael Hirsch and Rabbi Baruch Halevi Epstein *(Torah Temimah)*, echo the above talmudic teaching. That is, by the insistence or emphasis expressed in the double wording, the Bible uses the opportunity to oppose the erroneous idea that having recourse to medical aid shows lack of trust and confidence in Divine assistance. The Bible takes it for granted that medical therapy is used and actually demands it.

Other commentaries on the scriptural phrase *and heal he shall heal,* including those of the *Mechilta* and Rabbi Meir Leib ben Yechiel Michael *(Malbim)*, explain that the repetition of the word *heal* means that the patient must be repeatedly healed if the illness or injury recurs or becomes aggravated. In discussing the above case concerning personal injury, the Talmud also requires that where ulcers have grown on account of the wound and the wound breaks open again, the offender would still be liable to heal it (i.e., pay the medical expenses), even repeatedly.[9]

The most popular interpretation of *and heal he shall heal* is that compensation for the injury must be paid by the offender.[10] Such compensation consists of five items: the physician's fees and medical bills, payment for loss of time from work, the shame incurred by disfigurement, the pain suffered, and the physical damage produced. All agree, however, that human healing is sanctioned by this phrase of the Bible, if not explicitly, at least implicitly.

Rabbi Abraham Ibn Ezra seems to place a restriction on the permissibility for a physician to heal when he states that only external wounds can be healed by man. Internal wounds or ailments should be left to God. However, there is nearly universal acceptance that the sanctioning to the physician to heal is all-inclusive, encompassing all internal and external physical and mental illness. In fact, a commentary on the Talmud by *Tosafot* specifically states that it is permitted to heal not only man-induced wounds but even heavenly-induced sicknesses and afflictions, i.e., all illnesses.[11] The restrictive view of Ibn Ezra is also rejected by Rabbi Joseph Karo in his famous code of Jewish law.[12]

Although studying medicine is permissible in Jewish law, it is optional. However, once a person has become a physician, it is then obligatory upon him to heal the sick. The biblical mandate for the physician to heal is based upon two scriptural commandments. *And thou shalt restore it to him*[13] refers to the restoration of lost property. Moses Maimonides, in his *Commentary on the Mishnah*, states that "it is obligatory from the Torah for the physician to heal the sick, and this is included in the explanation of the scriptural phrase *and thou shalt restore it to him*, meaning to heal his body."[14]

Thus, Maimonides states that the law of restoration also includes the restoration of the health of one's fellowman. If a person has "lost his health" and the physician is able to restore it, he is obligated to do so. Rabbi Baruch Halevi Epstein *(Torah Temimah)*, in two separate places, asks why Maimonides totally omits the phrase *and heal he shall heal* as a warrant for the physician to heal.[15] Epstein offers an answer to his own question when he states that the verse in Exodus only grants permission for a physician to heal, whereas *and thou shalt restore it to him* makes it obligatory.

Maimonides' reasoning is probably based upon a key passage in the Talmud where it states: "whence do we know that one must save his neighbor from the loss of himself? From the verse *and thou shalt restore it to him.*"[16] Thus, not only if one is sick is a physician required but also if someone is attempting suicide, one must provide psychiatric or other competent assistance to save the person's life and health.

The second scriptural mandate for the physician to heal is based on the phrase *neither shalt thou stand idly by the blood of thy neighbor.*[17] The passage refers to the duties of human beings to their fellowmen and the moral principles which the sages expounded and applied to every phase of civil and criminal law. One example cited in the Talmud is the following:

> Whence do we know that if a man sees his neighbor drowning or mauled by beasts or attacked by robbers, he is bound to save him? From the verse *thou shalt not stand idly by the blood of thy neighbor.*[18]

Maimonides codifies the above talmudic passage in his code, where he states:

> Whoever is able to save another and does not save him transgresses the commandment *neither shalt thou stand idly by the blood of thy neighbor.* Similarly, if one sees another drowning in the sea, or being attacked by bandits, or being attacked by a wild animal and is able to rescue him . . . and does not rescue him . . . he transgresses the injunction *neither shalt thou stand idly by the blood of thy neighbor.*[19]

Such a case of drowning in the sea is considered as loss of one's body, and therefore, if one is obligated to save a whole body, one must certainly cure disease, which usually afflicts only one part of the body.

From the discussion so far, it seems evident that permission for the physician to heal is granted in the Bible from the phrase *and heal he shall heal.* Some scholars, notably Maimonides, claim that healing the sick is not only allowed but is actually obligatory. Rabbi Joseph Karo, in his code of Jewish law, combines both thoughts.

> The Torah gave permission to the physician to heal; moreover, this is a religious precept and it is included in the category of saving life; and if he withholds his services, it is considered as shedding blood.[20]

Rabbi David ben Shmuel Halevi, known as *Taz*, asks: If it is a religious precept to heal, why did the Torah have to grant specific permission for the physician to do so? His answer is that true healing lies only with God, but God gives the physician the wherewithal to heal by earthly or natural means. Once permission has been granted, then it is a commandment on the physician to heal. A similar thought is expressed by Rabbi Abraham Maskil Le'aytan, known as *Yad Avraham*, who states that permission is only granted if the physician heals with his heart toward heaven.

Rabbi Shabtai ben Meir HaKohen, known as *Sifsei Kohen*, offers an alternative reason for the Torah's granting permission to heal—that is, in order to avoid the physician saying, "Who needs this anguish? If I err, I will be considered as having spilled blood unintentionally." In a similar vein, Karo quotes Nachmanides, himself a physician, who says that without the warrant to treat, physicians might hesitate to treat patients for fear of fatal consequences, "in that there is an element of danger in every medical procedure; that which heals one may kill another."[21]

If one asks why God granted physicians license and even mandate to heal the sick, one can offer the following explanation. A cardinal principle of Judaism is that human life is of infinite value. The preservation of human life takes precedence over all commandments in the Bible except three: adultery, murder, and incest. Life's value is absolute and supreme. Thus an old man or woman, a mentally retarded person, a defective newborn, a dying cancer patient, and the like, all have the same right to life as you or I. In order to preserve a human life, the Sabbath and even the Day of Atonement may be desecrated, and all other rules and laws save the aforementioned three are suspended for the overriding consideration of saving a human life. He who saves one life is as if he saved a whole world.[22] Even a few moments of life are worthwhile. Judaism is a "right-to-life" religion. This obligation to save lives is an individual as well as a communal obligation. Certainly a physician, who has knowledge and expertise far beyond that of a layperson, is obligated to use his medical skills to heal the sick and thereby prolong and preserve life.

Notes

1. Exodus 15:26.
2. Shabbat 32a.
3. Sanhedrin 101a.
4. Deuteronomy 28:27.
5. Proverbs 3:8.
6. Proverbs 4:22.
7. Exodus 21:19.
8. Baba Kamma 85a.
9. Ibid.
10. *Rashi*, *Targum Onkelos*, Baba Kamma 85a, and others.
11. *Tosafot* to Baba Kamma 85a.
12. Karo, *Shulchan Aruch*, *Orach Chayim* 328:3.
13. Deuteronomy 22:2.
14. Maimonides, *Mishnah Commentary* on Nedarim 4:4.
15. *Torah Temimah* on Deuteronomy 22:2 and Exodus 21:19.
16. Sanhedrin 73a.
17. Leviticus 19:16.
18. Sanhedrin 73a.
19. Maimonides, *Mishneh Torah*, *Hilchot Rotze'ach* 1:14.
20. Karo, *Shulchan Aruch*, *Yoreh Deah* 336.
21. Karo, in his *Beth Yoseph* commentary on Jacob ben Asher's code of Jewish law known as *Tur*, *Yoreh Deah* 336.
22. Sanhedrin 37a.

2

The Patient's Obligation to Seek Healing

Does a sick person have the right to secure healing of his body, or should the illness run its course without interference? Should a person rely solely on Divine Providence for his physical as well as spiritual healing?

From the previous chapter, it is clear that the Torah gave specific sanction for the physician to heal and, according to some authorities, made it obligatory upon him to provide his medical skills to cure disease. It is not evident from the above, that the patient is permitted in Jewish law to seek human healing. Is an individual who asks a physician to treat him denying Divine Providence? Is such an individual transgressing the biblical teaching *For I am the Lord that healeth thee?*[1] Is a person's illness an affliction by God that serves as punishment for wrongdoing? And does such a person remove his atonement for sin by not accepting the suffering imposed by Divine judgment? Should there be, or is there, a distinction between heavenly afflictions and man-induced sickness in regard to the patient seeking medical aid? How does one define heavenly illness? What is cancer—God-induced (i.e., genetic) or man-induced (i.e., drugs, viruses, irradiation), or both? The number of such questions is endless, and lengthy prose could be written attempting to analyze them.

The patient's relationship to healing by a human physician is illustrated in a homiletical story in an ancient Jewish source about Rabbi Ishmael and Rabbi Akiba, who were walking through the streets of Jerusalem and met a sick man.[2] The ill person asked:

"Masters, tell me how I can be cured?" They answered: "Do thus and thus until you are cured." He said to them: "And who afflicted me?" "The Holy One, blessed be He," they replied. He said: "And you interfered in a matter which is not your concern. God afflicted you and you wish to heal?" The rabbis asked: "What is your vocation?" He responded: "I am a tiller of the soil. Here is the vine-cutter in my hand." They queried: "But who created the vineyard?" "The Holy One, blessed be He," he answered. "You interfered in this vineyard which is not yours? He created it and you cut away its fruits?" they asked. "Do you not see the vinecutter in my hands? Were I not to go out and plow and till and fertilize and weed, the vineyard would not produce any fruit," he explained. They said: "Fool, from your own work you have not learned what is written: *As for man his days are as grass?*[3] Just as the tree, if not weeded, fertilized, and ploughed will not grow and bring forth its fruits . . . so it is with the human body. The fertilizer is the medicine and the healing the means, and the tiller of the earth is the physician."

Some of these considerations are discussed in the Talmud, where it states that on going to be phlebotomized, a person should recite the following prayer:

> May it be Thy will, O Lord my God, that this operation may be a cure for me, and mayest Thou heal me, for Thou art a faithful healing God, and Thy healing is sure, since men have no power to heal but this is a habit with them.[4]

From this passage it would appear that conflicting viewpoints could emerge. The fact that the Talmud describes a patient going to a physician for an operative procedure can be interpreted to mean that certainly this is permissible. The only requirement is for the patient to recognize that the physician is acting as an agent of the Divine healer. In fact, *Rashi* explains the talmudic passage to mean that the afflicted person should have prayed for heavenly intervention rather than human healing and perhaps the bloodletting would not have been necessary.

On the other hand, the talmudic statement continues with an assertion by Abaye to the effect that a patient should not utter such a prayer because, in fact, the Torah gave specific consent for human healing in the phrase *and heal he shall heal.* Therefore, says Abaye, a patient should seek the help of a physician. A similar but not identical prayer is found in the codes of Jewish law of Maimonides and Rabbi Joseph Karo.[5]

A rather negative attitude to the question of the patient obtaining medical assistance is taken by Nachmanides, who, in his commentary on the scriptural phrase *and My soul shall not abhor you*[6] states that God will remove sickness from among the Israelites as He promised, *for I am the Lord that healeth thee.*[7] The righteous, continues Nachmanides, during the epochs of prophethood, even if they sinned and became ill, did not seek out physicians, only prophets. What therefore is the need for physicians if God promised to remove all sickness from man? To advise which foods and beverages to avoid in order not to get sick, answers Nachmanides, himself a physician. He explains the phrase *and heal he shall heal* to mean that the physician is allowed to practice medicine but the patient may not seek his healing but must turn to Divine Providence. Only people who do not believe in the healing powers of God turn to physicians for their cure, and for such individuals the Torah sanctions the physician to heal. The latter should not withhold his healing skills lest the patient die under his care, nor should he say that God alone heals.

Other than the Karaites, who strongly objected to physicians and medicines, Nachmanides seems to stand alone in his apparent prohibition for patients to seek medical aid. It is possible that he refers only to the righteous, who are free of illness because of their piety, and who do not require human healing. Perhaps the general populace, however, even devout believers in God, are allowed to seek human healing. Such an interpretation of Nachmanides' discussion is found in the commentary of Rabbi David ben Shmuel Halevi (popularly known as *Taz* or *Turei Zahav*) on Karo's code of Jewish law.[8] It may also be that Nachmanides refers only to heavenly illnesses, but for man-induced wounds and sicknesses healing may be sought.

Karo does not seem to make such a distinction when he states that "he who fasts and is able to tolerate the fast is called holy; but if not, such as if he is not healthy and strong, he is called a sinner."[9] It appears evident from this quotation that it is an obligation upon man to take all possible action to ensure a healthy body, and this includes the services of a physician. A less likely interpretation of Karo's statement is that if a person is able to tolerate sickness or pain, just as in the case of the fast, he should do so and not seek medical aid.

Another source that can be interpreted either in support of or against the permissibility for a patient to obtain human healing is the following story related in the Talmud.[10] Rabbi Yochanan once fell ill and Rabbi Chanina went to visit him, saying; "Are your sufferings welcome to you?" Rabbi Yochanan replied, "Neither they nor their reward," implying that one who lovingly accepts sufferings in this world will be greatly compensated in the world-to-come. Rabbi Chanina then said, "Give me your hand," which Rabbi Yochanan did, and he cured him. Why could not Rabbi Yochanan cure himself? asks the Talmud. The reply is, "Because the prisoner cannot free himself from jail," meaning the patient cannot cure himself. On the one hand, we see that Rabbi Yochanan required healing from Rabbi Chanina, and yet he did not use human healing, as he cured Rabbi Yochanan by touching his hand.

The strongest evidence from Jewish sources that gives the patient permission to seek treatment from a physician is found in Maimonides' *Mishneh Torah*. He states that a person should "set his heart that his body be healthy and strong in order that his soul be upright to know the Lord. For it is impossible for man to understand and comprehend the wisdoms [of the world] if he is hungry and ailing or if one of his limbs is aching."[11] He also recommends,[12] as does the Talmud,[13] that no wise person should reside in a city that does not possess a physician. Maimonides' position is further stated as follows:

> Since when the body is healthy and sound [one treads] in the ways of the Lord, it being impossible to understand or know anything of the knowledge of the Creator when one is sick, it is obligatory upon man to avoid things which are detrimental to the body and acclimate himself to things which heal and fortify it.[14]

There are numerous talmudic citations which support the position that not only allows but requires the patient to seek medical aid when sick. We are told that he who is in pain should go to a physician.[15] Further, if one is bitten by a snake, one may call a physician even if it means desecrating the Sabbath, because all restrictions are set aside in the case of possible danger to human life.[16] Similarly, if one's eye becomes afflicted on the Sabbath, one may prepare and apply medication thereto, even on the Sabbath.[17] When Rabbi Judah the Prince, compiler of the Mishnah, contracted an eye disease, his physician, Samuel Yarchina'ah, cured it by placing a vial of chemicals under the rabbi's pillow so that the powerful vapors would penetrate the eye.[18] The Talmud also speaks of another physician curing a patient.[19] Finally, in a case of bodily injury where the offender says to the victim that he will bring a physician who will heal for no fee, the victim can object and say, "A physician who heals for nothing is worth nothing."[20] If the offender offers to bring a physician from far away, the victim may say, "My eye will be blind before he arrives." If the injured person says to the offender, "Give me the money and I will cure myself," the latter can retort, "You might neglect yourself and remain a cripple." From these and other talmudic passages, it seems evident that an individual is undoubtedly permitted and probably required to seek medical attention when he is ill.

Further support for this contention is mentioned by Britain's Chief Rabbi Immanuel Jakobovits, who cites the fifteenth-century philosopher Isaac Arama's work *Akedat Yitzchak.*[21] Rabbi Arama proves from biblical narratives, such as the Patriarchs' efforts to save themselves when in danger, and biblical legislation, such as the duty to construct parapets around roofs for the prevention of accidents,[22] that man must not rely on miracles or Providence alone, but must himself do whatever he can to maintain his life and health.

Rabbi Chayim Azulai, an eighteenth-century commentator on Karo's code of Jewish law, writing under the pen name of *Birké Yoseph,* summarized Jewish thought and practice relating to our question. His views are cited by Jakobovits as follows:

> Nowadays one must not rely on miracles, and the sick man is duty bound to conduct himself in accordance with the natural order by calling on a physician to heal him. In fact, to depart from the general practice by claiming greater merit than the many saints [in previous] generations, who were cured by physicians, is almost sinful on account of both the implied arrogance and the reliance on miracles when there is danger to life. . . . Hence, one should adopt the ways of all men and be healed by physicians.

One might arrive at the same conclusion if one were to literally interpret the pentateuchal admonition *Take ye therefore good heed unto yourselves.*[23] Thus, it is clear that the patient is obligated to care for his health and life. Man does not have full title over his body and life. He is charged with dignifying and preserving his life. He must eat and drink and sustain himself and must seek healing when he is ill.

Finally, the Jewish attitude toward the physician and his r
art, as well as the patient's responsibility to seek medic

beautifully depicted by Ben Sira, who perceived in the physician an instrument of Providence.[24]

Honor a physician before need of him,
Him also hath God apportioned.
From God a physician getteth wisdom
And from a king he shall receive gifts.
The skill of a physician shall lift up his head
And he shall stand before nobles.
God bringeth out medicines from the earth
And let a prudent man not refuse them.
Was not water made sweet with wood
For to acquaint every man with His power?
And He gave man understanding
To glory in His might.
By them doth the physician assuage pain
And likewise the apothecary maketh a confection,
That His work may not fail
Nor health from among the sons of men.
My son, in sickness be not negligent,
Pray unto God, for He will heal.
Free from iniquity, and from respect of persons,
And from all transgressions, cleanse thy heart.
Offer a sweet savor as a memorial
And fatness estimated according to thy substance.
And to the physician also give a place,
And he shall not remove, for there is need of him likewise,
For there is a time when in his hand is good success.
For he too will supplicate unto God
That He will prosper to him the treatment
And the healing, for the sake of his living.
He that sinneth against his Maker
Will behave himself proudly against a physician.[25]

Notes

1. Exodus 15:26.
2. J. D. Eisenstein, *Otzar Midrashim* (New York, 1915), vol. 2, pp. 580–581.
3. Psalms 103:15.
4. Berachot 60a.
5. Maimonides, *Mishneh Torah, Hilchot Berachot* 10:21; Karo, *Shulchan Aruch, Orach Chayim* 230:4.
6. Leviticus 26:11.
7. Exodus 15:26.
8. *Taz* on *Shulchan Aruch, Yoreh Deah* 336:1.
9. Karo, *Shulchan Aruch, Orach Chayim* 571.
10. Berachot 5b.
11. Maimonides, *Mishneh Torah, Hilchot Deot* 3:3.
12. Ibid. 4:23.
13. Sanhedrin 17b.
14. Maimonides, *Mishneh Torah, Hilchot Deot* 4:1.
15. Baba Kamma 46b.
16. Yoma 83b.
17. Avodah Zarah 28b.
18. Baba Metzia 85b.
19. Ketubot 75a.
20. Baba Kamma 85a.
21. I. Jakobovits, *Jewish Medical Ethics*, (New York: Bloch, 1975), pp. 2–6.
22. Deuteronomy 22:8.
23. Ibid. 4:15.
24. H. Friedenwald, *The Jews and Medicine* (Baltimore: Johns Hopkins Press, 1944), vol. 1, pp. 6–7.
25. Ecclesiasticus, chap. 38.

3

The Best of Physicians Is Destined for Gehenna

Judaism has always held the physician in high esteem. Ancient and medieval Jewish writings are replete with expressions of admiration and praise for the "faithful physician."[1] Therefore, it is not surprising that the at-first-glance derogatory talmudic statement "the best of physicians is destined for Gehenna"[2] has generated extensive discussion and commentary throughout the centuries.

The Hebrew epigram *tov sheberofim legehinnom* is variously translated as "the best among physicians is destined to Gehinnom,"[3] "the best among physicians is destined for Gehenna,"[4] "the best of physicians is fit for Gehenna,"[5] "the best among doctors is for Gehenna,"[6] "the best of doctors are destined for Gehenna,"[7] "to hell with the best of physicians,"[8] and "the best physician is destined to go to hell."[9]

Jakobovits points out that the Talmud does not comment on this epigram at all, which is as significant as it is unusual. Probably the earliest commentary on the mishnaic assertion that "the best physicians are destined for Gehenna" is that of Rabbi Solomon ben Isaac, popularly known as *Rashi* (1040–1105), who says that the reasons are because a physician "is not afraid of illness, and tells the patient to eat food fit for healthy people, and does not subdue his heart before God, and sometimes causes the death of people, and is able to heal the poor [free] but does not do so."[10] Physicians were thus censured for their overconfidence in their craft, which results in their trusting in it, and their haughtiness before God, instead of trusting in Him. They are further blamed for commercializing their profession, to the extent that they sometimes fail or refuse to attend the poor,[11] which may indirectly cause the latter's death.[12] Furthermore, according to *Rashi*, physicians may err in their treatment regimens and thus cause the death of patients. A descendant of *Rashi*, Rabbi Isaac Sen, known as *Tosafot Ri Hazaken*, simply states that physicians "cause the death of the patient."

Another talmudic passage states that "seven have no portion in the world-to-come [if they do not conduct their affairs with the utmost caution and sincerity], viz., a scribe, a writer, the best of doctors, a city judge, a diviner, a communal official and a butcher."[13]

Rabbi Joshua Falk, in his commentary *Binyan Yehoshua* on this tractate, cites the aforementioned *Rashi* verbatim and then adds that he is critical of physicians because the physician treats the patient on the basis of his own knowledge and understanding and does not ask other physicians to join him in his deliberations. In monetary matters the sages state that it is proper to include in the deliberations all those rabbis who understand the case under consideration.[14] If that is the case where money is at stake, how much more so when someone's life is at stake. To save one life one should consult with the whole world, if necessary. Falk continues by stating that there are many well-known and widely disseminated explanations of the phrase "the best of doctors is destined for Gehenna" and concludes, "May the Lord save us from their hands." Preuss points out that Falk is only saying what Diodorus asserted about the famous Egyptian physicians: "We wish that we should not have need for any one of them."[15]

Rabbi Menachem ben Solomon Meiri, known simply as *Mei'ri* (1249–1316), in his talmudic commentary, opines that "the best of physicians is destined for Gehenna" because "many times he sheds blood because he gives up and does not try hard enough in his medical art [to heal the patient]; or sometimes he doesn't know the cause of the patient's illness or how to treat it and considers himself to be an expert."

According to Kalonymus ben Kalonymus (1286–1328), a Provençal writer and philosopher, in his ethical treatise *Even Bochan* ("The Touchstone"), the epigram "physicians are fit only for Gehenna" refers not to genuine physicians but to quacks because "their art is lying and deception; all their boasting is empty falsehood; their hearts are turned away from God; and their hands are covered with blood."[16]

Friedenwald states that an interesting explanation of this difficult sentence is to be found in Rabbi Solomon Ibn Verga's *Shevet Yehud-*

dah in the course of a discussion between Pope Martin V and Don Samuel Abrabalia and Don Salomo ha-Levi, ambassadors of the Spanish Jews to Rome in 1418. The latter, in answering, said: " 'The best physician is fit for Gehenna' signifies that he should always see Gehenna opened before him should he cause the death of anyone whose health had been entrusted to him. As a consequence he must carefully consider [the treatment] and apply all his thought to it. It is well therefore that he should be mindful that he is destined for Gehenna if he does not give sufficient thought to his patients."[17] Ibn Verga was a physician who lived in Seville in the second half of the fifteenth century.

Also in the fifteenth century, Rabbi Simon Duran (1361–1444), in his Responsa, believed the mishnaic epigram sought to castigate only those physicians who maintained their own views in the presence of greater experts and who relied on their own experiments.[18] A similar explanation was given by the talmudist Rabbi Samuel Edels, known as *Maharsha* (1555–1631), who states that the condemning judgment of going to hell applies to the physician who considers himself to be the best and most expert among physicians and that there is none like him.[19] He relies excessively on his own expertise because of his haughtiness. Sometimes he errs in his understanding of the nature or constitution of a specific patient and causes the patient's death with remedies that are harmful to that patient. Rather, he should consult with other physicians because it is a matter of life and death.

In the following century, Rabbi Jonathan Eybeschutz (1690–1764), in his famous *Kereti Upeleti*, related the dictum to his theory that the Divine sanction of healing applies only to external injuries, whereas attempts to cure internal diseases were deprecated.[20] His contemporary Rabbi Isaac Lampronti (1678–1756), in his renowned *Pachad Yitzchok*, suggested that the condemnation was aimed at surgeons "because they vary the instructions of the wise [diagnosticians], and, in particular, they exceed, or fall short of, the proper measure when letting blood, according to their limited intelligence, thus killing their patients; and many times have I seen . . . such evil."

The famous Mishnah commentator Rabbi Yom Tov Lippman Heller (1578–1654), known as *Tosafot Yom Tov*, and the two prominent commentators on the Jerusalem Talmud, Rabbi Moses Margoliot, known as *Pne Moshe* (d. 1781), and Rabbi David Fraenkel, known as *Korban Ha'edah* (1707–1762), all cite the previously mentioned *Rashi* verbatim.[21] Rabbi Eleazar Fleckeles (1754–1826), in his work

Teshuvah Meyahavah, reiterates the interpretation that physicians who are overly confident in their own skills and who profess that "good" (Heb. *tov)* or the "best" emanates from them rather than God are the ones to whom the epigram "the best of physicians is destined for Gehenna" is addressed.[22]

In Jacob ibn Habib's famous *Eyn Yaakov*, one finds the commentary of Rabbi Hanokh Zundel ben Joseph (d. 1867), known as *Etz Yoseph*, on the famous epigram about physicians and Gehenna. *Etz Joseph* asserts the following:

> It appears to me that this statement is not derogatory toward the physician. On the contrary, it is a compliment to an expert physician. . . . He who thinks of himself as the most expert physician is destined for Gehenna because through his haughtiness he relies on his imperfect knowledge and does not consult with his colleagues. . . . also because of his conceit he does not even consider the possibility of his being in error and does not delve adequately into medical books before he administers medicinal remedies. He is, therefore, not sufficiently acquainted with their side effects and does not administer them slowly as is required for dangerously ill patients.
>
> The text of the Mishnah does not say that the doctor is evil or will definitely go to hell. Rather, it states "to Gehenna," which implies that it is in a state of readiness and that by his actions he might go to Gehenna. However, if he conducts himself properly [and consults with colleagues and refers the patient to experts when appropriate] he will, on the contrary, be rewarded and praised [and share in the world-to-come].

Rabbi Israel Lipschutz, known as *Tiferet Yisrael* (1792–1860), in his Mishnah commentary has nearly identical language as *Etz Yoseph* but also cites a long story to illustrate the meaning of the famous epigram.[23]

Another view is that the dictum of the Mishnah is not directed against healing as such but against the "advanced" views held by physicians in those days.[24] Zimmels suggests that the dictum might have been originally an ancient proverb censuring physicians for counteracting heavenly decrees.[25] Friedenwald offers a kabbalistic philosophical interpretation of the Mishnah by the great Rabbi Loeb of Prague: Gehenna stands for the material world, which according to the doctrine of the kabbalists is nothing but the negation of real existence, the spiritual. The physician or, in other words, the naturalist, who knows only the material world, will end in Gehenna, in "nonexistence." In the original form of the saying about the physician and the netherworld, the point made was that even the most skilled physician cannot save himself from death, and it read accordingly, "The best of physicians has to descend to the dwelling of the netherworld."[26]

Both Friedenwald and Jakobovits seem to be convinced that the association of physicians with hell, in its original form, was nothing but a pun, based on the assonance of *rophim*, meaning "physicians," and *r'pho'im*, meaning "the dwellers of the netherworld."[27] Several examples from Scriptures are cited by Friedenwald and Jakobovits to show how easily *rophim* and *r'pho'im* were confused.

Friedenwald also cites a personal communication from H. Malter, who wrote:

> The ancient rabbis had foreseen that a time will come when there will be no more rabbis; doctors will replace them. Only doctors and no rabbis will reign; doctors who will cure the eyes, and leave the heart and soul sick, and in a burst of passion and jealousy they scolded these doctors, saying, "the best of the doctors should go to hell."

A novel interpretation of the epigram of the Mishnah "the best of physicians is destined for Gehenna," using the numerical value of the word "best" (the Hebrew word *tov* has the numerical value 17), is that of Rabbi Meir of Przemyslan in his *Margenitha di R. Meir.* The most important part of the daily prayer service is the recitation of the Eighteen (now 19) Benedictions *(Shemoneh Esreh* in Hebrew), known simply as *Tefillah*, or "prayer." The eighth benediction is a petition for healing for all who are ill, strength for all who are feeble, and relief for all who suffer pain.[28] The benediction begins with the phrase. "Heal us, O Lord, and we shall be healed," and concludes with the phrase "Blessed art Thou, O Lord, who healest the sick of Thy people Israel." According to Rabbi Meir of Przemyslan, "the best of physicians is destined for Gehenna" refers to those physicians who only believe in seventeen of the eighteen benedictions in that they do not recognize that God is the true Healer of the ill. Although these physicians may recite all eighteen benedictions, if their trust in themselves and conceit in their own medical skills preclude their acceptance of the eighth benediction, which acknowledges God as the trustworthy and merciful Healer, such physicians are considered as "the best" (Heb. *tov)* and are destined for Gehenna.

A recent writer offers yet other interpretations of the dictum of the Mishnah.[29] He states that all knowledge is divided into two types: precise, objective, and scientific knowledge, and humanistic, philosophic, and historical knowledge. Medicine is a combination of both precise and imprecise knowledge. A human being is also composed of two parts, a physical body and a spiritual soul, which complement and supplement each other. Manipulation of either body or soul, of necessity, affects the other. On the other hand, no two human beings are alike either in physical features or in body temperaments. If a person is ill, the remedy to cure him may not be the same as the remedy for another individual with a similar illness. Host factors vary from patient to patient. There is thus room for wide variation in efficacy and toxicity of every therapeutic regimen employed by a physician. Therefore, how easy it is for even the best of physicians to unwittingly harm a patient by any given treatment. This is the meaning of "the best of physicians is destined for Gehenna."

Another explanation offered by the same writer is the following: Since medicine was traditionally considered to be a praiseworthy profession, many Jewish scholars studied and practiced medicine. The sages were concerned lest large numbers of the best minds in Israel forsake the study of the Torah to pursue careers in medicine. Hence, perhaps, to discourage this trend, the sages enunciated the dictum "the best of physicians is destined for Gehenna."

Preuss adds that there is no dearth of other explanations of the famous epigram.[30] In fact, he states that an entire book on the subject was written in 1724 by Reinecke. Two authors, Buxtorf and Schenkel, cited by Preuss, interpret the dictum to mean a general deprecation of physicians, whereas another author (Israëls) considers it a vote of censure of physicians who follow Greek philosophy. Finally, Preuss quotes Landau, who states that the phrase refers to the sect of Essenes.

Based on many of these interpretations, Jakobovits concludes that "to hell with the best of the physicians" was never understood as a denunciation of the conscientious practitioner.[31] Physicians are among a group of communal servants who have heavy public responsibilities and are warned against the danger of negligence or error. The talmudic epigram with its curse is thus limited to physicians who are overly confident in their craft, or are guilty of commercializing their profession, or lie and deceive as do quacks, or who fail to acknowledge God as the true Healer of the sick, or who fail to consult with colleagues or medical texts when appropriate, or who perform surgery without heeding proper advice from diagnosticians, or who fail to heal the poor and thus indirectly cause their death, or who fail to try hard enough to heal their patients, or who consider themselves to be the best in their field, or who otherwise fail to conduct themselves in an ethical and professional manner.

May the Lord remove all sickness from this world and heal all those who need physical or spiritual healing. In the meantime, may every physician practice his art with the approach cited in the morning prayers: "Heal us, O Lord, and we shall be healed; save us, and we shall be saved; for Thou art our praise."[32]

Notes

1. F. Rosner, trans., *Julius Preuss' Biblical and Talmudic Medicine* (New York: Hebrew Publishing Co, 1978), pp. 23–26; H. Friedenwald, *The Jews and Medicine* (Baltimore: Johns Hopkins Press, 1944), vol. 1, pp. 11–13; I. Jakobovits, *Jewish Medical Ethics* (New York: Bloch, 1959), pp. 202–204.
2. Kiddushin 4:14.
3. H. J. Zimmels, *Magicians, Theologians and Doctors* (London: E. Goldston & Son, 1952), p. 170.
4. H. Danby, trans., *The Mishnah* (London: Oxford University Press, 1933).
5. Friedenwald, loc. cit.
6. P. Blackman, *Mishnayot: Order Nashim*, (New York: Judaica Press, 1965), vol. 3, p. 482.
7. I. Epstein, ed., *The Babylonian Talmud: Tractate Kiddushin*, trans. H. Feldman (London: Soncino Press, 1936), vol. 4, p. 423.
8. Jakobovits, loc. cit.
9. Rosner, loc. cit.
10. See *Rashi*'s commentary on Kiddushin 82a.
11. Friedenwald, loc. cit.
12. Rosner, loc. cit.
13. Avot de Rabbi Nathan 36:5.
14. Sanhedrin 7b.
15. Rosner, op. cit., p. 26.
16. Friedenwald, op cit., p. 74.
17. Ibn Verga, *Shevet Yehudah*, chap. 41.
18. Duran, Responsa *Tashbatz*, pt. 3, no. 82.
19. Commentary of *Maharsha* on Kiddushin 82a.
20. Eybeschutz, *Kereti Upeleti, Yoreh Deah*, no. 188; Zimmels, loc. cit.
21. See their comments to Kiddushin 41a.
22. Fleckeles, *Teshuvah Meyahavah*, sec. 3, no. 336.
23. See *Tiferet Yisrael* to Kiddushin 4:14.
24. Rosner, op. cit., pp. 23–26.
25. Zimmels, op. cit., p. 170.
26. Friedenwald, op. cit., vol. 1, pp. 11–13.
27. Ibid. and Jakobovits, loc. cit.
28. J. H. Hertz, *The Authorized Daily Prayer Book*, rev. (New York: Bloch, 1959), p. 141.
29. Y. A. Shapiro, in *Halachah Urefuah*, 2 (1981): 335–339.
30. Rosner, op. cit., pp. 23–26.
31. Jakobovits, op. cit., pp. 202–204.
32. Hertz, loc. cit.

4

Priests Studying and Practicing Medicine

Introduction

The question as to whether or not a priest *(kohen)* in modern times is permitted to study and practice medicine has been debated in the rabbinic responsa literature for over a century. Very little on this subject has been written in English, although brief summaries by Jakobovits and Bleich are available.[1] The present essay reviews the controversy of priests as medical students and physicians, and attempts to objectively present the varying viewpoints.

Ban Against Priestly Defilement

> *And the Lord said unto Moses; Speak unto the priests the sons of Aaron, and say unto them: There shall none defile himself for the dead among his people; except for his kin that is near unto him, for his mother, and for his father, and for his son, and for his daughter, and for his brother, and for his sister a virgin.*[2]

Based upon this biblical admonition, Jewish law, as codified by Moses Maimonides, states that if a priest defiles himself for a dead body other than that of any of the six relatives expressly stated in the Bible, or that of his wife, and there are witnesses to testify to this effect and due warning has been given him, he is subject to the penalty of flagellation, as it is written: *there shall none defile himself for the dead among his people.*[3]

Similarly, Joseph Karo's code rules that a *kohen* is forewarned not to defile himself through a corpse nor through any of the defilements that emanate from it nor through a burial stone nor through a tombstone.[4] Hence, it seems clear from Maimonides and Karo that priests are forbidden to come into contact with a dead body except in the case of the death of a close relative because they would thereby become ritually defiled.

On the other hand, Abraham Ibn Daud, popularly known as *Ravad*, states that "priests nowadays are already ritually defiled by the dead; furthermore, they are not charged with the guilt of defilement, and he who wishes to charge them has the onus of adducing evidence to prove the charge."[5]

The reasoning behind *Ravad*'s position is that since, in the absence of the ashes of the red heifer, there is no means nowadays to effect purification of a priest ritually defiled through corpse contact, the priest remains in a permanent state of impurity. Additional contact with a corpse does not add to this state of impurity.

In a lengthy responsum, Rabbi Shmuel Huebner analyzes the talmudic discussion upon which *Ravad*'s opinion is based[6] and lists the three possible interpretations.[7] Some authorities, such as Rabbis Judah Rozanes, Isaac Samuel Reggio, and Akiba Eger, maintain that, according to *Ravad*, there exists no prohibition whatsoever against a priest coming into contact with a corpse if he has indeed previously become ritually impure.[8] Other authorities are of the opinion that *Ravad*'s position is that defilement by corpse contact is not today considered to be a biblical offense but is still rabbinically prohibited.[9] Yet others, such as Rabbis Ezekiel Landau, Moses Schreiber, Moshe Zvi Fuchs, and Yehudah Leib Zirelson, interpret *Ravad* to mean that the offense, while still biblically forbidden, is nowadays not subject to the penalty of flagellation.[10] Landau apparently changed his opinion in that he first agreed with Rozanes that nowadays there is no prohibition at all for a priest who is already defiled from defiling himself through corpse contact. Landau's change of heart is claimed by Schreiber to have occurred following a lengthy meeting in Prague between Landau and Rabbi Nathan Adler.

Whatever the correct interpretation of *Ravad*'s opinion, it is and remains a minority view opposed by most early and present-day authorities, who maintain that each additional act of defilement is a separate transgression.

Priests as Medical Students

The most recent, erudite discussion on the subject of priests as medical students is that of Rabbi J. David Bleich,[11] who points out that the question was first answered by the Italian scholar Isaac Samuel Reggio in 1854 in regard to a priest whose livelihood was at stake because he had been appointed by the king to inspect corpses to verify the signs of death and then to arrange for burial.[12] Reggio permitted the priest to maintain his job for several reasons, one of which is Reggio's interpretation of *Ravad* that nowadays there is no prohibition at all for a priest to come into contact with a corpse since all priests are already defiled and there exists no method today to purify them. In 1868, Rabbi Tzvi Benjamin Auerbach charged Reggio with "a patent falsehood" for allowing the priest to defile himself on the strength of *Ravad*'s opinion.[13] Most more recent responsa support Auerbach's position (see below).

The second reason for Reggio's permissive ruling is based on the talmudic statement that a priest may defile himself by leaving the land of Israel "for monetary reasons, to save a life, to sanctify the new moon, to intercalate the year, to save his field from a gentile, to study Torah, and to marry a woman."[14] Therefore, states Reggio, the priest whose livelihood depends on touching corpses is permitted to do so. Bleich points out that the editor of *Kerem Chemed* correctly called attention to the fact that the Talmud cites cases of acts without which financial losses would be incurred. However, that does not give a priest the right to plan his livelihood if he knows in advance that he will have to defile himself by corpse contact. Furthermore, states Bleich, the Talmud only permits a priest to avoid a monetary loss by moving out of Israel, which is only a rabbinic prohibition, but not to defile himself by touching a corpse, which is a biblical prohibition.

A third reason which Reggio offers for permitting a priest to become defiled is that Reggio believes that all the warnings to priests against defilement cited in Leviticus relate only to laws applicable when there is a Temple. Since there is no Temple and no sacrifices and no method of purification, the priests no longer have to avoid defilement. Bleich states that such reasoning is contrary to Maimonides' explicit statement in *Hilchot Nezirut* that priests are forewarned against defilement even in our own times. Bleich points out other mistakes in Reggio's reasoning and bemoans the fact that Reggio's erroneous conclusions were compounded by Rabbi Tzvi Hakohen Sherashefsky, who repeated them thirty years later.[15]

Sherashefsky added that "nowadays our priests are only considered to be true priests for rabbinical but not biblical matters because priests today do not inspect signs of leprosy nor declare lepers clean," to which Bleich comments: "is the inspection of leprosy signs nullified because of the absence of priests who can prove their true pedigree?" It should be noted that Reggio was never accepted by rabbinic scholars as a halachic authority.

Bleich also dismisses the suggestion that priests are allowed to study medicine because they will later save lives, pointing out that Rabbi Ezekiel Landau specifically forbids this on the grounds that there is no patient immediately at hand *(lefanenu)* whose life is to be saved and there are nonpriests (i.e., Israelites and Levites) who can study medicine and save lives without transgressing this prohibition.[16] Bleich also dismisses the suggestion of Rabbi Abraham Preiss that priests are permitted to study anatomy if they wear gloves because only rabbinic defilement is involved and it is set aside for the *mitzvah* (commandment) of healing.[17] Bleich, quoting Rabbi Moshe Feinstein,[18] states that there is no obligation for a priest to study medicine and discusses this point in great detail.

Finally, Bleich discusses the suggestion of Rabbi Shlomo Goren that a priest should wear on his body a metal object which became defiled by corpse contact.[19] Goren's reasoning is based on Maimonides, who states that the talmudic expression "the sword is equal in uncleanness to the corpse"[20] means that metal utensils which touch a corpse incur seven-day uncleanness.[21] The commentary of *Tosafot* states that a priest is only forbidden to become defiled by corpse contact but not by contact with metal utensils, which themselves are defiled by corpse contact. Hence, suggests Goren, any simultaneous contact by a priest wearing a defiled metal object does not constitute a punishable transgression. Bleich agrees that only if a priest incurs seven-day uncleanness by corpse contact can he not become simultaneously defiled by contact with another corpse. However, even that is forbidden according to Maimonides.[22] The wearing of a ritually defiled object does not remove the prohibition of his becoming defiled by simultaneous corpse contact, and hence it is forbidden.

Rabbi Mordechai Hakohen cites Rabbi Ben Zion Uziel, who allows anatomical dissection of human cadavers for the sake of studying medicine, provided it is done with dignity and respect and that all parts of the body, including the minutest portions, are buried.[23] One of the reasons for this permissive ruling is the later saving of lives *(piku'ach nefesh)* by the physician after he completes his medical training. Based on this reasoning, Hakohen allows a priest who is strongly desirous of studying medicine and whose entire motivation is to heal the sick and to save lives to attend medical school even if that includes ritual defilement of that priest by corpse contact.

A similar permissive ruling had already been enunciated several decades earlier by Rabbi Chaim Hirschenson, who quotes Rabbi Bernard Revel and Rabbi Elyakim Goldberg, both of whom prohibit a priest from studying medicine.[24] Nevertheless, says Hirschenson, "my opinion is that nowadays he who can find a permissive ruling according to the Torah for those things for which the people have a strong craving is obligated to do so." However, he continues, one should not rely solely on the opinion of *Ravad*, which is a minority view. He then devotes twenty-three pages of responsum to a lengthy analysis of the question and concludes that priests throughout the generations have been and continue to be careful not to ritually defile themselves. Nevertheless, if a priest has a very strong desire to study medicine he is allowed to do so, because most if not all corpses nowadays are non-Jews and, according to many authorities, do not defile, and also because such a priest-physician would later save lives. Like Reggio, Hakohen and Hirschenson are not considered by rabbinic scholars to be halachic authorities on this matter.

Rabbi Feinstein strongly rejects the opinion of Hirschenson and Hakohen and states that only if one already is a physician is one obligated to heal and to save lives.[25] However, one is not obligated to study medicine to become a physician anymore than one is obligated to conduct a lot of business to become rich in order to give charity. Feinstein disapproves of this viewpoint, stating that "it is foolish and vain and should not be articulated by any intelligent person." Feinstein also strongly denounces priests who rely on this opinion and attend medical school, and says:

> It is clear to me that if the priests who study medicine and ritually defile themselves through contact with corpses would really wish to know the true law in this regard, they would know who to ask . . . rather, they are not at all concerned about this prohibition and delude themselves . . . by claiming to have found [a lenient ruling in] some pamphlet upon which they rely.

Feinstein concludes:

> . . . it is absolutely clear that it is prohibited for a priest to ritually defile himself through contact with a corpse and this fact is well known throughout the world. Therefore, it is abso-

lutely clear that even if the most learned rabbis in the world would be lenient [and say otherwise], one should not listen to them. . . .

. . . it is prohibited for priests to study medicine in medical schools in countries where it is necessary to have contact with corpses. One should not point to some of our ancient Sages who were both priests and physicians and were able to learn all of medical science by oral teachings without any observations on or physical contact with corpses. In our times, this is impossible and therefore it is prohibited.

Rabbi Yekuthiel Yehudah Greenwald also voices the view of most authorities:

It is totally prohibited for a priest to study medicine because in our times, before he completes his studies, he must know the parts of the human body, including the veins and internal organs and anatomy. Medical students take home for study portions of the flesh of organs from corpses. It is an absolute prohibition for a priest to ritually defile himself even by touching a gentile corpse. Often without knowing it, they even dissect Jewish or apostate corpses.[26]

Greenwald cites the lenient rulings of Reggio and Sherashefsky and others and states that most rabbinic authorities are strongly opposed to these lenient rulings, which are based on misinterpretations of *Ravad* (see above). Furthermore, *Ravad* is a single opinion and Jewish law always follows the majority view. Greenwald cites rabbinic responsa which point out the gross errors and lack of substance in these lenient rulings and asserts that "their words fly in the air," that is to say, are of no consequence.

Loss of Privileges for Priests Who Attend Medical School

The practical consequences for a priest who disobeys the prohibition against ritual defilement by corpse contact are cited in Karo's *Shulchan Aruch.*[27] Such a priest may not recite the priestly benediction nor be called first to the Torah reading until he repents and undertakes to henceforth avoid contact with corpses. Based on Karo's statement, Rabbis Moses Schreiber, Abraham Schreiber, Abraham Zvi Hirsh Eisenstadt, and others rule that a priest who defies the prohibition against ritual defilement loses his priestly privileges.[28] Rabbi David Hoffman asserts that a priest–medical student should not be honored in the synagogue by being called up to the Torah until he ceases and desists from further contact with corpses; otherwise his conduct would be erroneously viewed as being rabbinically sanctioned.[29] The rabbi must so inform his *gabbai* or sexton. If the rabbi's recommendation is likely to be ignored, he may remain silent so that the offense is unwitting rather than deliberate.

Rabbi Yehudah Assad states that a priest would not intentionally disobey the prohibition against ritual defilement and that a priest–medical student either erroneously believes the prohibition not to include corpse contact with non-Jews or else erroneously assumes that the later saving of lives allows him to disregard the prohibition.[30] Hence, continues Assad, one is obligated to speak softly to this medical student and to show him the *Shulchan Aruch* (Code of Jewish Law) to correct his misconceptions. If he fails to repent by making a solemn declaration to henceforth avoid any corpse contact, he is not to be accorded the usual synagogue privileges of a priest cited above. Rabbi Abraham Schreiber requires the priest to take a noncancellable vow to henceforth avoid ritual defilement by corpse contact before the honors and privileges of the priestly office are restored to him.[31]

Priests as Practicing Physicians

Once a priest has become a physician, the questions then arise as to whether or not he is permitted to practice medicine, to treat the terminally ill *(gosses)*, and/or to visit and treat noncritically ill patients in a hospital where corpses are frequently present. Rabbi Joseph Karo prohibits a priest to enter a house where there is a dying person,[32] whereas Rabbi Moses Isserles permits it.[33] Based on Karo's ruling, Rabbi Jacob ben Samuel prohibits a priestly physician to defile himself on behalf of a dying person.[34] Jakobovits asserts that Isserles means that Karo's ruling does not apply to physicians.[35] Thus, many authorities sanction medical visits by priestly physicians to terminally ill patients.[36] Some authorities limit this permissibility to the situation where no other physician is available.[37] If there is another, nonpriestly physician, permission to the priestly physician depends on whether the patient specifically requests the priestly physician's care, and on the rabbinic argument as to whether biblical laws are permanently suspended *(dechuyah)* or only temporarily waived *(hutrah)* for the saving of a life.

Rabbinic authorities also state that if the patient has already been pronounced dead, the priestly physician should assist in the resuscitative efforts because of the possibility, however remote, of restoring the patient's life.[38] Many authorities quote the famous question by the commentary of *Tosafot*[39] as to how Elijah the Prophet, who was also a priest, was permitted to revive a dead boy by direct physical contact.[40] The reply given is that Elijah knew the successful outcome of his efforts because they were divinely instructed. Hence, the boy was not really dead, since the resuscitation efforts were successful.

Other references concerning the permissibility for a priestly physician to practice medicine are cited by Jakobovits, Bleich, Steinberg, and others.[41]

Priests as Patients in a Hospital

Is a priest, irrespective of whether or not he is a physician, permitted to enter a hospital for medical treatment? Does it matter whether or not the medical condition requiring treatment is serious? Rabbi Sholom Mordechai Schwadron permits such treatment in a hospital even for a nonserious illness.[42] Rabbi Samuel Engel also permits hospital treatment for a priest, provided the mortuary is not attached to the main hospital building.[43] Rabbi M. Arak allows such treatment for a serious illness in which there may be danger to life even if such treatment can safely be given at home.[44]

Rabbi Mordechai Breisch distinguishes between hospitals where most patients and hence corpses are Gentiles and hospitals where most patients are Jews.[45] Since most hospitals today fall in the former category, Breisch gives a lenient ruling allowing priests to seek treatment in a hospital. Breisch also discusses the question of whether the pregnant wife of a priest can give birth to a baby in a hospital because of the prohibition against defiling the priestly infant.[46] He rules in the affirmative even if most patients and corpses in that hospital are Jews. Rabbi Shlomo Zalman Auerbach, however, recommends that such infants be sent home as soon as medically possible, preferably after twenty-four hours.[47]

Hospital Employment for a Priest

Is it permitted for a priest to accept and maintain employment in a hospital? Rabbi Shlomo Kluger allows male priests to serve as nurses in hospitals to earn their livelihood even if dead bodies are housed there from time to time.[48] The reasoning cited by Rabbi Eliezer Waldenberg for this lenient ruling is that at the time the priest enters the hospital, he does so legitimately, assuming there are no corpses there at the time.[49] If a patient later dies in the hospital, the male nurse is allowed to remain to care for the seriously ill patients to whom he is assigned.

Rabbi Eliezer Chayim Deitsch allows priests to serve as chaplains in a hospital to visit the sick and recite the *viduy*, or confession prayer, with dying patients.[50]

On the other hand, Rabbi Moshe Feinstein permits a priest to work in a hospital if he can leave the hospital when a death occurs and if most patients are non-Jews.[51] From the practical and pragmatic standpoint, Feinstein thus allows priests to secure and maintain hospital employment. The explanation of Rabbi Feinstein's ruling provided by Rabbi Moshe Tendler is the fact that in Jewish law modern hospitals are considered as a series of compartments, each being a discrete unit with reference to the laws of containing ritual defilement (*ohel hamet*).[52] If an object which ritually defiles, such as a dead body, is inside a closed room, the ritual defilement is contained within the room (*chotzetz mipney hatumah*). Even if a deceased individual is being transported through a corridor to the elevator, the corpse does not ritually defile people and objects in rooms which open into that corridor if the doors to these rooms are closed, since Jewish law deems the corridor and the elevator to be the sites through which the ritual defilement exits (*sof tumah latzet*). A priest employee in the hospital is, therefore, advised to keep the door to his room closed. This analysis does not apply when the place of hospital employment of the priest is the mortuary or pathology laboratory of a large metropolitan hospital with a large Jewish population.

Non-physician Priests Visiting the Sick

Is a non-physician priest allowed to visit patients in the hospital to fulfill the commandment of *bikur cholim?* This question was reviewed at length by Rabbi S. Arieli, who concludes in favor of permitting such visits unless it is definitely known that a dead person is there at the time.[53] He confirms rulings of others.[54] Rabbi Feinstein also answers the question in the affirmative because of "great need," such as emotional pain and anguish.[55] He thus permits such visits to a parent or child or spouse or to one's wife's relatives because we assume that most patients are non-Jews and any corpses or parts thereof in the hospital at any given time are those of non-Jews and do not impart ritual defilement by being in the same room or building with a Jew. If possible, one should inquire whether a Jewish corpse is there, but if it cannot be ascertained with ease, one may assume that there is none there. Other authorities who allow priests to visit patients in hospitals also advise the priest to inquire in advance whether or not there are any Jewish corpses there at the time.[56]

Perhaps in part because of the impracticality of the above suggestion, some authorities oppose such visits by priests to patients in hospitals for fear that large, modern hospitals contain not only corpses but preserved human organs or embryos which ritually defile priests.[57]

Priests on an Airplane with a Corpse

Rabbi Feinstein permits a priest to travel on an airplane in which a Jewish corpse in the baggage compartment is being transported to Israel for burial, since the entire plane is made of metal other than the six types of metal specified in the Torah which transmit ritual defilement, viz., gold, silver, copper, iron, tin, and lead.[58] Since the plane is made primarily of other types of metal, such as aluminum and magnesium, it does not transmit defilement. The presence of insulating layers or wall coverings also serves to contain the defilement within the baggage compartment.[59]

Conclusion

Priests are commanded to avoid ritual defilement through corpse contact. Since anatomical dissection of humans is part of the medical curriculum, it is prohibited for priests to attend medical school as students. Lenient rulings have been enunciated by some rabbis to allow priests to become physicians. The reasons offered include the assumption that the ban against priestly defilement is not applicable nowadays, the later saving of lives by the priestly physicians, the extenuating circumstances of the need to make a livelihood, and the strong desire to become a physician. All these reasons are dismissed by the most respected rabbinic authorities, who maintain not only that priests are prohibited from attending medical school but that their priestly privileges are revoked if they defy the ban.

Once a priest has become a physician, many authorities sanction medical visits to critically or terminally ill patients and even to nonseriously ill patients. Priests are allowed to enter a hospital for care if they are patients and may also visit close relatives who are ill in a hospital, such as a parent or child or spouse. If possible, they should inquire in advance whether or not there are any Jewish corpses there at the time.

Notes

1. I. Jakobovits, *Jewish Medical Ethics* (New York: Bloch, 1959), pp. 238–243; idem, "May a *Kohen* Study Medicine?" *Tradition* (1962): 262–264; idem, *Jewish Law Faces Modern Problems* (New York: Yeshiva University Press, 1965), pp. 61–63; idem, *Journal of a Rabbi* (New York: Living Books, 1966), p. 172: J. D. Bleich, *Judaism and Healing* (New York: Ktav, 1981), pp. 37–42.

2. Leviticus 21:1–3.

3. Maimonides, *Mishneh Torah, Hilchot Avel* 3:1.

4. Karo, *Shulchan Aruch, Yoreh Deah* 369:1.

5. *Ravad's* gloss on Maimonides' *Hilchot Nezirut* 5:15.

6. Nazir 42b.

7. S. Huebner, *Hadarom* (New York), Elul 5721, pp. 17–28.

8. Rozanes, *Mishneh Lemelech* commentary on Maimonides' *Hilchot Avel* 3:1; Reggio, *Kerem Chemed*, vol. 8 (1854); Eger, Responsa *R. Akiba Eger, Mahadura Tinyana*, no. 18.

9. M. M. Schneierson, Responsa *Tzemach Tzedek*, no. 238; *Yeshu'ot Yaakov, Orach Chayim* 343:2 (cited by Bleich, loc. cit.).

10. Landau, *Dagul Me-Revavah, Yoreh Deah* 372:2; Schreiber, Responsa *Chatam Sofer, Yoreh Deah*, no. 338, and *Orach Chayim*, no. 23; Fuchs, Responsa *Yad Ramah*, no. 128; Zirelson, Responsa *Gevul Yehudah, Yoreh Deah*, no. 31.

11. J. D. Bleich, in *Torah She Ba'al Peh* (Jerusalem: Mossad Harav Kook, 5742 1982), pp. 84–94; and in *Halachah Urefuah* (5743/1983): 199–210.

12. Reggio, loc. cit.

13. Auerbach, Responsa *Nachal Eshkol*, introduction.

14. Avel Rabati 4:25.

15. Sherashefsky, in *Hamelitz*, 5644, fol. 1.

16. Landau, Responsa *Nodah Biyehudah, Mahadura Tinyana, Yoreh Deah*, no. 210.

17. Preiss, *Mishnah Avraham* commentary on *Sefer Chasidim*, pt. 2, p. 283.

18. Feinstein, in *Noam* vol 8 (5728): p 9, and Responsa *Iggrot Moshe, Yoreh Deah*, pt. 3, no. 155.

19. Goren, unpublished responsum dated 2 Adar 2, 5741 (copy kindly provided to me by Rabbi Moshe David Tendler).

20. Nazir 54b, based on Numbers 19:16.

21. Maimonides, *Mishneh Torah, Hilchot Tumat Met* 5:3.

22. Ibid., *Hilchot Avel* 2:15.

23. Hakohen, in *Torah She Be'al Peh* 6 (5724/1964): 74–81; also in *Sinai* 14, nos. 1–2 (Tishri–Chesvan 5724): 40–46 and *Machanayim*, no. 123 (Kislev 5730), pp. 120–129; Uziel, Responsa *Mishpetei Uziel* 1:28.

24. Hirschenson, *Malki Bakodesh*, pt. 3, no. 5, pp. 9–12 and 153–176;

Revel, in *Yagdil Torah.* 8 (5676): 85–90; Goldberg, in ibid., pp. 19–21, 135–141, and 256–259.

25. Feinstein, loc. cit.

26. Greenwald, *Kol Bo Al Avelut*, sec. 5:22, pp. 81–84.

27. *Orach Chayim* 128:41.

28. M. Schreiber, Responsa *Chatam Sofer, Yoreh Deah*, no. 358; A. Schreiber, Responsa *Ketav Sofer. Orach Chayim*, no. 16; Eisenstadt, *Pitchei Teshuvah, Yoreh Deah*, no. 370:1; see also authorities cited by A. Steinberg in *Sefer Assia* (Jerusalem, 5736), p. 311: *Shevet Miyehudah*, pt. 1, chap. 13:7 ff.; *Harefuah VeHaya'adut*, chap. 21; *Hadarom*, Elul 5721; *Hakinus Hashishi Le Torah She Be'al Peh* (Mossad Harav Kook), p. 75; *Machanayim*, no. 123, p. 120.

29. Hoffman, Responsa *Melamed Leho'il, Orach Chayim*, no. 31.

30. Assad, Responsa *Yehuda Ya'aleh*, no. 47.

31. Schreiber, loc. cit.

32. Karo, *Shulchan Aruch, Yoreh Deah* 370:1.

33. Isserles, *Ramah* on *Shulchan Aruch*, *Yoreh Deah* 370:1.

34. Jacob ben Samuel, Responsa *Bet Yakov*, no. 130.

35. Jakobovits, *Jewish Medical Ethics*, pp. 238–243.

36. Z. H. Eisentadt, *Pitchei Teshuvah* and *Nachalat Zvi* on *Yoreh Deah*, no. 370:1; Z. H. Chayes, *Darchei Hahora'ah*, no. 1; D. Tirni, *Ikrey Dinim, Yoreh Deah*, no. 35:32; E. Y. Waldenberg, Responsa *Tzitz Eliezer, Ramat Rachel*, sec. 28, par. 3.

37. Schreiber, Responsa *Chatam Sofer, Yoreh Deah* 358; A. Steinberg, Responsa *Machazeh Avraham*, pt. 2, *Yoreh Deah*, no. 19.

38. Eisenstadt, loc. cit.; Waldenberg, loc. cit.

39. Baba Metzia 114b.

40. I Kings 17:17 ff.

41. Jakobovits, *Jewish Medical Ethics*, pp. 238–243; Bleich, *Judaism and Healing*, pp. 37–42; Steinberg, *Sefer Assia* (Jerusalem, 5736), p. 312.

42. Schwadron, Responsa *Maharsham*, pt. 2, no. 233.

43. Engel, Responsa *Maharash Engel*, pt. 3, no. 27.

44. Arak, *Vayelakket Yoseph* (5672), vol. 14, no. 74.

45. Breisch, Responsa *Chelkat Yaakov*, pt. 1, no. 27.

46. Ibid., no. 28, referring to Karo, *Shulchan Aruch, Yoreh Deah* 373.

47. cited by A. Steinberg in *Sefer Leb Abraham* (Jerusalem), vol. 1, chap. 21, n. 10.

48. Kluger, Responsa *Tuv Ta'am Vada'at*, vol. 3, pt. 2, no. 212.

49. Waldenberg, Responsa *Tzitz Eliezer*, vol. 4, sec. 4:9.

50. Deitsch, Responsa *Duda'ey Hasadeh*, no. 100.

51. Feinstein, Responsa *Iggrot Moshe, Yoreh Deah* vol. 1, no. 241.

52. M. D. Tendler, personal communication, May 11, 1984.

53. Arieli, in *Noam*, vol. 2, pp. 55 ff.

54. Greenwald, *Kol Bo Al Avelut*, sec. 1:5, p. 19.

55. Feinstein, Responsa *Iggrot Moshe, Yoreh Deah*, vol. 2, no. 166.

56. S. J. Tabak, Responsa *Teshurat Shay*, no. 559.

57. J. Meskin, Responsa *Even Yaakov*, nos. 47–51; see also the authorities cited by A. Steinberg, in *Sefer Assia* (Jerusalem, 5741), vol. 2, p. 15.: *She'arim Hametzuyanim Behalachah*, no. 202:6; Responsa *Shevet Halevi, Yoreh Deah*, no. 205; and *Kol Bo Al Avelut*, p. 19.

58. Feinstein, Responsa *Iggrot Moshe, Yoreh Deah*, vol. 2, no. 164.

59. Tendler, personal communication, May 11, 1984.

5

Visiting the Sick

Introduction

Visiting the sick in Judaism is not just the paying of a social call. Historically, there were no hospitals in biblical and talmudic times, and hence a person who visited a sick friend or relative had to provide for the physical and emotional needs of the patient.

In addition to cheering the patient up and encouraging him to get better, the visitor would cook and clean and perform other tasks for the patient, as needed. Furthermore, Jewish law requires that the visitor pray for the recovery of the patient, either in the latter's presence or not. These three activities are all essential components of what is known as *bikkur cholim*, or visiting the sick, and are applicable to this very day.

History and Importance of Visiting the Sick

It is a duty incumbent upon everyone to visit the sick. God visits the sick, and we must emulate Him. How do we know this? Scripture states: *Ye shall walk after the Lord your God.*[1] Is it possible to walk after God? The answer is that we should try to emulate His attributes. Just as He visited the sick, so, too, we should visit the sick.[2] When did God visit the sick? He visited the Patriarch Abraham after the latter's circumcision, as it is written: *and the Lord appeared unto him.*[3] God blesses bridegrooms, adorns brides, visits the sick, buries the dead, and recites the blessing for mourners.[4] It is also written: *and thou shalt show them the way they must walk,*[5] which the sages interpret to refer to the duty of visiting the sick.[6] There is a difference of opinion among the sages as to whether the duty of visiting the sick is of biblical or rabbinic origin.

Another example in the Bible of visiting the sick is when the prophet Isaiah visited King Hezekiah when the latter was ill.[7] The conversation between the two is vividly described in the Talmud[8] and concerns the fact that Hezekiah had never married and was admonished by Isaiah for not having fulfilled the commandment of procreation. The end of the story is a happy one in that Hezekiah did penitence and was cured of his illness and lived another fifteen years.

Numerous instances of sages visiting their sick colleagues are found in the Talmud. Rabbi Yosei ben Kisma was ill, and Rabbi Chanina ben Teradion went to visit him.[9] Rabbi Yannai ben Ishmael was sick, and Rabbi Ishmael ben Zirud and others called to inquire about him.[10] Comforting mourners, visiting the sick, and the practice of loving-kindness bring welfare into the world.[11]

The importance of visiting the sick is further underscored by the following talmudic passage:

> Rabbi Chelbo once fell ill. Thereupon Rabbi Kahana went and proclaimed: "Rabbi Chelbo is sick." But none visited him. He rebuked them [i.e., the sages], saying: "Did it not once happen that one of Rabbi Akiba's disciples fell sick and the sages did not visit him?" So Rabbi Akiba himself entered [the disciple's house] to visit him and, because they swept and sprinkled the grounds before him,[12] he recovered. "My master," said the disciple, "you have revived me." Whereupon, Rabbi Akiba propounded: He who does not visit the sick is like a shedder of blood.[13]

Thus, helping to take care of the needs of a sick patient may save his life or certainly contribute to the restoration of his health. The concept of being guilty of shedding blood if one does not help one's ill fellowman is based on the biblical injunction: *neither shalt thou stand idly by the blood of thy neighbor.*[14] Maimonides codifies the talmudic passage which requires one to save one's fellowman if one can[15] as follows:

> Whoever is able to save another, and does not save him, transgresses the commandment *neither shalt thou stand idly by thy neighbor.* Similarly, if one sees another drowning in the sea, or being attacked by bandits or by a wild animal and is able to rescue him . . . transgresses the injunction *neither shalt thou stand idly by the blood of thy neighbor.*[16]

In addition to taking care of the physical and emotional needs of the patient, the second major purpose of visiting the sick is for the caller to pray on the patient's behalf. If one visits the sick on the Sabbath, one should say: "It is the Sabbath, when one must not cry out, and recovery will come soon."[17] Others say: "May the Sabbath have compassion."[18] Yet others say: "May God have compassion upon you and upon the sick of Israel."[19] Today, we recite special prayers for the sick in the synagogue and even give the patient an additional name as a supplication to God to heal him.

When not in the patient's presence, one should only pray in Hebrew, since the ministering angels only understand Hebrew. In the patient's presence, one can pray in any language, since God Himself ministers to the sick,[20] and the Divine Presence rests upon the patient's bed. For the same reason, one should not sit on the patient's bed. Although this may seem primitive and even mythical, we have here a reflection of the desire of the sages to emphasize the closeness of God to the patient, a point which is brought home by necessitating Hebrew in other situations while allowing any language in the presence of the patient.

Rab says: "He who visits the sick will be delivered from the punishments of Gehenna."[21] Visits to the sick are considered among the most meritorious acts of true charity. The Talmud lists visiting the sick among those things the fruit of which man eats in this world while the principal remains for him in the world-to-come.[22] For other good deeds, the reward is only in the world-to-come. The importance of this obligation is recited daily in the morning prayers by observant Jews.

Procedures Regarding Visiting the Sick

There is no limit to the visiting of the sick.[23] Rabbi Joseph says this means that the reward is unlimited. Abaye says it means that even a prominent person must visit a simple person. Raba says it means that there is no limit to the frequency of such visits, even one hundred a day.[24] For the sake of good neighborly relations, one should also visit non-Jewish patients.

One talmudic sage asserts that he who visits the sick takes away one-sixtieth of his illness. If so, let sixty people visit and the patient will be cured? The answer is that each visitor removes one-sixtieth of the remaining illness.[25] Rav Huna says that a visitor only reduces the patient's illness by one-sixtieth if he loves the patient like himself.[26] Some sages allow even an enemy to visit his sick neighbor. Others feel it might cause anguish to the patient and hence should be avoided. Yet others state that an enemy may visit if he secures permission in advance from the sick patient.

One should not receive financial remuneration for visiting the sick[27] either because one would thus be demeaning the visit[28] or because one should not receive payment for fulfilling a Divine commandment.[29]

One should not visit the sick during the first three hours or the last three hours of the day lest he misjudge the patient's status and not pray for him and not care for him. In the morning, the patient looks better and feels better than he really is, and in the evening the reverse is true.[30] The modern physician is well aware of the accuracy of this statement. Fever is usually lower in the morning and higher in the evening in a patient with a febrile illness.

One should not visit patients with illnesses of the bowel (diarrhea), eye diseases, or headaches; the first because of embarrassment and the latter two because speech is harmful to them.[31] One can readily understand that a patient with diarrhea might be embarrassed in the presence of a visitor. There seems to be no rational medical reason, however, why speech is harmful to patients with eye diseases or headaches. Perhaps such patients would rather lie quietly without speaking because speech is uncomfortable for them, but there is no known medical detriment to their speaking, if they so desire. Mar Samuel said that one should not visit a patient until his fever has subsided.[32] Close relatives and friends usually visit first, and more distant relatives and acquaintances only visit after three days. If the illness occurred suddenly, all may visit simultaneously.[33]

There is a difference of opinion among the codes of Jewish law and rabbinic responsa as to the obligation of visiting people ill with contagious diseases. The prevailing view is that no one is obligated to endanger his life to fulfill the precept of visiting the sick. Today, one can protect oneself from contracting a contagious disease by avoiding direct contact with the patient and by taking other precautionary steps as dictated by the medical circumstances.

Rabbi Chanina once fell ill. Rabbi Yochanan went to visit him. He said: "How do you feel?" He replied: "How grievous are my sufferings!" He said: "But surely the reward for them is also great!" He said: "I want neither them nor their reward!"[34]

Rabbi Simeon ben Yochai used to visit the sick. He once met a man who was swollen and afflicted with intestinal disease uttering blasphemies against God. Said Rabbi Simeon: "Worthless one! Pray rather for mercy for yourself." Said the patient: "May God remove these sufferings from me and place them upon you."[35]

Recovery from Illness

Rabbi Zera was once ill. Rabbi Abbahu went to visit him and made a vow, saying: "If Rabbi Zera recovers, I will make a feast for the rabbis." He recovered, so he made a feast.[36]

When a person recovers from a serious illness, he has to recite a special prayer of thanksgiving (*birchat ha-gomel*). Rabbi Judah was ill and recovered. Rabbi Channa of Baghdad and other sages went to visit him. They said: "Blessed is God, who gave you back to us." Rabbi Judah answered "amen" and was absolved of reciting the *birchat ha-gomel.*[37]

There may not be a precise non-Jewish equivalent of the *birchat ha-gomel*, but it seems logical that any God-fearing person, Jew or non-Jew, would offer some kind of thanks to the Lord upon recovering from a serious illness or operation. The format of the thanks, however, may vary from the recitation of a prayer of thanksgiving to the donation of money to charity.

Sick-Visiting Societies

Already in the Bible, we find municipally regulated care of the poor whereby the provision for the needy is not left to the "good hearts" of the wealthy. This public care of the poor seems to have been built into a firm legal system in the Talmud. In many times, already during the period of the Temple, there existed a town brotherhood, known as *chever ha'ir*, whose function was to collect and distribute funds to the poor. Brotherhoods (or societies) also concerned themselves with other charitable deeds, mainly the burial of the dead and the visiting of the sick. Such a society is explicitly mentioned in the Talmud.[38] It is also related that Abimi, a member of a sick-visiting society, used to visit the sick.[39]

Notes

1. Deuteronomy 13:5.
2. Sotah 14a.
3. Genesis 18:1.
4. Genesis Rabbah 8:13.
5. Exodus 18:20.
6. Baba Kamma 100a and Baba Metzia 30b.
7. Isaiah 38:1.
8. Berachot 10a.
9. Avodah Zarah 18a.
10. Ibid. 30a.
11. Avot deRabbi Natan 30:1.
12. Rabbi Jacob ben Asher, known as *Rosh*, interprets this to mean that Rabbi Akiba, finding the room neglected, gave the necessary orders to sweep and sprinkle the ground.
13. Nedarim 40a.
14. Leviticus 19:16.
15. Sanhedrin 73a.
16. Maimonides, *Mishneh Torah*, *Hilchot Rotze'ach* 1:14.
17. Shabbat 12a.
18. Ibid.
19. Ibid. 12b.
20. Psalms 41:4.
21. Nedarim 40a.
22. Shabbat 127a.
23. Nedarim 39b.
24. Ibid.
25. Ibid.
26. Leviticus Rabbah 34:1.
27. Nedarim 39a.
28. Commentary of *Rosh* on Nedarim 39a.
29. Commentary of *Tosafot* on Nedarim 39a.
30. Nedarim 40a.
31. Ibid. 41a.
32. Ibid.
33. Jerusalem Talmud, Peah 3:17.
34. Song of Songs Rabbah 2:16:2.
35. Avot deRabbi Natan 4:1.
36. Berachot 46a.
37. Ibid. 54b.
38. Moed Katan 27b.
39. Genesis Rabbah 13:16.

6

AIDS: A Jewish View

Introduction

The acquired immunodeficiency syndrome (AIDS) has been described as this century's greatest health peril. Thousands have already died from the disease and there is no cure in sight. The emotional toll on patients with AIDS, their families, and their caregivers needs to be actively and aggressively addressed. The public hysteria should be alleviated by a well planned, coordinated, and implemented educational program involving not only health professionals but the mass media and press, which have in part fueled the public fear about AIDS. Prudent practices in health care and private industry workplaces have been suggested and should be followed. Governmental involvement in terms of increased AIDS treatment and research funding is sorely needed. Finally, public policy decisions need to be made with compassion and understanding and the conviction that this disease can be tamed and eventually overcome by a concerted effort of all parties concerned.

Homosexuality and Drug Abuse in Judaism

Ninety percent of all patients with AIDS are homosexuals or intravenous drug abusers. The Torah labels homosexual intercourse as an abomination[1] and ordains capital punishment for both transgressors,[2] though minors under thirteen years of age are exempt from this as from any other penalty.[3] This biblical directive is codified by Maimonides:

In the case of a man who lies with a male, or causes a male to have connection with him, once sexual contact has been initiated, the rule is as follows: If both are adults, they are punishable by stoning, as it is said, *Thou shalt not lie with a male*, i.e., whether he is the active or the passive participant in the act.[4]

The prohibition of homosexuality proper is omitted from the *Shulchan Aruch*, which omission reflects the virtual absence of homosexuality among Jews rather than any difference of views on the criminality of these acts.[5] The Torah only refers to incidents involving homosexuality in regard to the sinful city of Sodom[6] and in regard to the conduct of a group of Benjaminites in Gibeah, leading to a disastrous civil war.[7] Isolated cases are also described in the Talmud.[8]

Rabbi Jakobovits cites rabbinic sources for the strict ban on homosexuality that is included among the seven commandments of the sons of Noah: they state that it is an unnatural perversion debasing the dignity of man, frustrating the procreative purpose of sex, and damaging family life.[9] He concludes that Jewish law rejects the view that homosexuality is merely a disease or morally neutral.

Rabbi Barry Freundel has posited that Jewish law views the homosexual or drug addict as no different than a Sabbath desecrator or an adulterer.[10] He has no greater or lesser rights or obligations and deserves no special treatment or concessions. The term "homosexual," says Freundel, is inappropriate. We should refer to this individual as a person engaged in homosexual activity. The term is not a noun but an adjective. The Jewish community should, therefore, deal with the practitioner of homosexuality as a full-fledged Jew, albeit a sinner; he should be counseled and treated and be the concern of outreach and proper education.

The use of consciousness-expanding drugs such as LSD or other addictive substances is generally considered to be proscribed by the halachah. According to Rabbi Moshe Feinstein, the harmful effects of marijuana are among the reasons for prohibiting its use.[11] The same can be said about smoking in Judaism.[12] Certainly the abuse of narcotics and other substances by the intravenous and other routes is detrimental to one's health and, therefore, prohibited in Judaism, for the Torah instructs us not to intentionally place ourselves in danger: *Take heed to thyself, and take care of thy life*[13] and *take good care of your lives*.[14] The avoidance of danger is exemplified in the biblical commandment to make a parapet for one's roof so that no one fall therefrom.[15] Hence, the smoking of marijuana and the abuse of intravenous narcotics, which constitute a danger and hazard to life, are considered pernicious habits and should be prohibited. The subterfuge of "it is no concern of others if I endanger myself" is specifically disallowed by Maimonides[16] and the *Shulchan Aruch.*[17]

Jewish Legal Questions Relating to AIDS

Not only is the intentional endangerment of one's health or life by the use of intravenous drugs prohibited in Jewish law, but wounding oneself without fatal intent is also disallowed in the Talmud[18] and the codes of Maimonides[19] and Rav Joseph Karo.[20] Since most patients with AIDS are homosexuals and/or drug addicts, they are considered sinners, thereby raising a variety of Jewish legal questions. Should a Jewish drug addict who develops AIDS as a result of sinful activity be treated any differently than any other patient? Should the Jewish homosexual who develops AIDS as a result of "abominable" behavior be treated? Does Judaism teach compassion for all who suffer illness irrespective of whether or not the illness is the result of practices which Judaism abhors and prohibits? Should every effort be made to heal these patients or at least alleviate their pain and suffering? Is a physician or nurse or other health worker obligated to treat a patient with AIDS or other contagious disease if there is a risk that he may contract the illness from the patient? Should the Jewish community expend resources for AIDS research and treatment, since most such patients are sinners? Would not the resources be better allocated if spent for the health of law-abiding citizens? Can patients with AIDS be counted in a quorum of ten men (*minyan*)? Can they serve as cantors or Torah readers? Should they be given honors in the synagogue? Can a *kohen* with AIDS go up to the *duchan* and offer the priestly blessing? Can a patient with AIDS serve as a witness in a Jewish legal proceeding? Is a patient with AIDS to be given all the usual burial rites? Is mourning to be observed for such a patient? These and other halachic questions pertaining not only to AIDS patients but to sinners in general were addressed in two separate discourses delivered by Rabbi Hershel Schacter and Rabbi Moshe Tendler, both senior faculty members at Yeshiva University. The following discussion is based in part on those discourses.

Obligation of the Physician to Heal a Sinner

The physician's license to heal is based on the biblical phrase *and heal he shall heal,*[21] from which the talmudic sages deduce that divine authorization is given to the human physician to heal.[22] In his biblical commentary, Rabbi Moses Nachmanides, known as *Ramban*, states that since the physician may inadvertently harm his patient, divine permissibility to heal was necessary to absolve the physician of responsibility for any poor medical outcome, provided he was not negligent. Other commentaries assert that since sickness is Divinely inflicted as punishment for sin, Divine permission to heal is required to allow a human physician to intervene and provide healing.

Maimonides expands the permissibility for the human physician to heal into an obligation or mandate based on the biblical commandment for restoring a lost object to its rightful owner[23]—if a physician is able to restore a patient's lost health, he is obligated to do so. If a patient dies as a result of a physician's refusal to heal him, the physician is guilty of shedding blood for having stood idly by.[24] A detailed discussion of the physician's obligation to heal in Judaism can be found elsewhere.[25]

God cherishes the life of every human being and therefore requires all biblical and rabbinic commandments except idolatry, incest, and murder to be waived in order to save the life of a person in danger (*piku'ach nefesh*). The Sabbath must be desecrated to save a human life.[26] But is the desecration of the Sabbath allowed and/or mandated to save the life of a sinner who is guilty of a crime such as homosexuality for which the death penalty might be imposed?

The Talmud[27] permits the killing of a pursuer (*rodef*) to prevent him from killing the person he is pursuing; the one who kills him has no sin because the pursuer is considered to be legally (halachically) like a dead man (*gavra ketila*). For the same reason, one may *not* desecrate the Sabbath to save the life of the pursuer if a building collapses on him and his life is in danger. The same is true of a person sentenced to death by the court (Bet Din) in that one may not desecrate the Sabbath on his behalf if his life is in danger because he, too, is halachically considered like a dead man. However, a sinner who has not been sentenced by the Bet Din is considered as a live human being. As a result, although he is a transgressor, all biblical and rabbinic commandments must be suspended to save his life. Therefore, it seems clear that patients with AIDS should be treated medically and psychosocially no differently than other patients, and physicians and other medical personnel are obligated to heal patients with AIDS. The Talmud clearly states that every life is worth saving without distinction as to whether the person whose life is in danger is a criminal or a transgressor or a law-abiding citizen.[28] In fact, the Talmud requires that one expend money from one's own pocket to provide whatever is necessary to save another's life.

Some contemporary writers raise the issue of the difference between a provocative sinner (*mumar lehachis*) and a lustful sinner (*mumar lete'avon*).[29] The Talmud rules that a provocative sinner is not to be helped but actually hindered (*moridin velo ma'alin*).[30] The commentary of *Rashi* there and the code of Maimonides interpret a provocative sinner to refer to one who habitually and willfully sins.[31] On the other hand, one who only occasionally sins out of lust or appetite is considered like one whose life and property are to be protected and carefully treated.[32] It would seem therefore that physicians and other health personnel have an obligation to care for patients with AIDS no differently than for other patients.

Danger to Medical Personnel Treating Patients with AIDS

Jewish law requires that if one sees his neighbor drowning or mauled by beasts or attacked by robbers, he is bound to save him.[33] Elsewhere the *Shulchan Aruch* rules that if one observes a ship sinking with Jews on board, or a river flooding over its banks thereby endangering lives, or a pursued person whose life is in danger, one is obligated to desecrate the Sabbath to save them.[34] The commentaries of *Mishnah Berurah* and *Pitchei Teshuvah* add that if doing so involves danger for the rescuer, he is not obligated to endanger his life because his life takes precedence over that of his fellow man.[35] If there is only a doubtful risk (*sofek sakanah*) for the rescuer, he should carefully evaluate the small risk or the potential danger to himself and act accordingly.

What should a physician do if his patient is suffering from a contagious disease which the physician might contract? Is the physician allowed to refuse to treat the patient because of the risk or the fear by the physician of contracting the disease? What if the risk is very small? What is the definition of *sofek sakanah?* If there is a 50 percent chance of the physician contracting the disease from his patient, halachah would certainly agree that such odds are more than doubtful and the physician would not be obligated to care for that patient without taking precautionary measures to protect himself. If he wishes to do so in spite of the risk, his act is considered to be a pious act (*midat chasidut*) by some writers, and folly (*chasid shoteh*) by others.[36] But if the risk is very remote, the physician must care for that patient because *the Lord preserveth the simple-*

tons.[37] This phrase is invoked in the Talmud in relation to the remote danger of conception in a minor child[38] and is discussed in great detail by Rabbi Moshe Feinstein in a lengthy responsum concerning the use of a contraceptive device by a woman in whom pregnancy would constitute a danger to her life.[39] Contraception, states Rabbi Feinstein, is permissible for *sofek sakanah* but not where the risk is extremely small. Rabbi Shneur Zalman of Lublin and Rabbi Chayim Ozer Grodzensky respectively discuss whether the above biblical phrase is invoked for a minor risk (less than 50 percent) or only for a very remote and rare risk.[40]

Rabbi Yitzchok Zilberstein discusses the case of a female physician in her first trimester of pregnancy who is called to see a seriously ill patient with rubella (German measles).[41] The physician is at 50 percent risk of acquiring rubella and possibly giving birth to a seriously defective baby (blind, deaf, or mentally retarded) or she may abort or have a stillbirth. Although there are no fetal indications in halachah which would allow abortion, Rabbi Zilberstein posits that halachah considers miscarriage to be a situation of *pikuach nefesh* and rules therefore that the female physician is not obligated to care for a patient with rubella.

The question as to whether or not a person is obligated to subject himself to a risk in order to save another person's life is discussed in great detail in several recent articles[42] and briefly summarized by Professor A. S. Abraham in an article on human experimentation.[43] The matter is related to the well-known difference of opinion recorded in the two Talmuds. The Jerusalem Talmud posits that a person is obligated to potentially endanger his life (*sofek sakanah*) to save the life of his fellow man from certain danger (*vadai sakanah*).[44] This position is supported by Rabbi Meir Hacohen[45] as ciated by Rav Yosef[46] and by Rav Karo himself.[47] On the other hand, the Babylonian Talmud voices the opinion that a person is not obligated to endanger his life to save that of another even if the risk is small (*sofek sakanah*).[48] The ruling from the Jerusalem Talmud is omitted from the Codes of *Rif*, *Rambam*, *Rosh*, *Tur*, and *Ramo*.

The prevailing opinion among the various rabbinic sources seems to be the one cited by the *Radvaz:*[49] If there is great danger to the rescuer, he is not allowed to attempt to save his fellow man; if he nevertheless does so, he is called a pious fool; if the danger to the rescuer is small and the danger to his fellow man very great, the rescuer is allowed but not obligated to attempt the rescue, and if he does so his act is called an act of loving-kindness (*midat chasidut*). If there is no risk at all to the rescuer or if the risk is very small or remote, he is obligated to try to save his fellow man. If he refuses to do so, he is guilty of transgressing the commandment *thou shalt not stand idly by the blood of thy fellow man.*[50] This approach is also adopted by recent rabbinic decisors including Rabbi Moshe Feinstein and Rabbi Eliezer Yehudah Waldenberg.[51] Since the risk to physicians and other health personnel in caring for AIDS patients is infinitessimally small (less than a fraction of 1 percent), it follows that a physician is obligated under Jewish law to care for such patients.

The same logic is used to allow but not require healthy people to donate a kidney to save the life of a close relative dying of kidney failure. Most rabbis, including Rabbi Ovadiah Yosef, Rabbi Jacob Weiss, and Rabbi Eliezer Waldenberg, support this halachic position.[52]

Visiting Patients with Infectious Diseases such as AIDS

It is a duty incumbent upon everyone to visit the sick, for God visits the sick[53] and we must emulate Him.[54] Rabbi Jakobovits points out that the question whether the duty to visit the sick extends to visiting patients suffering from an infectious or contagious disease was already answered with a qualified affirmative by the *Ramo* against the view of some later authorities who questioned the need to expose oneself to the hazard of contagion in the fulfillment of this precept.[55] *Ramo* holds that there is no distinction in respect of visiting the sick between ordinary and infectious diseases, with the sole exception of leprosy.[56] A recent reexamination of this question, continues Rabbi Jakobovits, leads one to the conclusion, based on several talmudic narratives,[57] that the ruling of *Ramo* applies only to an infection which would not endanger the life of the visitor even if he caught it, but that one is not required to risk one's life merely for the sake of fulfilling the rabbinic precept of visiting the sick, nor can anyone be compelled to serve such patients. Elsewhere Rabbi Jakobovits asserts that in practice, the view of *Ramo* did not prevail, and approval was expressed for the custom not to assign visitations of plague-stricken patients to anyone except specially appointed persons who were highly paid for their perilous work.[58] Rabbi Jakobovits also cites the seventeenth-century records of the Portuguese Congregation in Hamburg, which indicate that even the communal doctors and nurses were exempt from the obligation to attend to infectious cases and that the required services were rendered by volunteers entitled to special remuneration.[59]

Rabbi Jekuthiel Jehudah Greenwald states that if there is hope of healing the patient from his illness, one is obligated to visit and serve him even if there is a risk of contracting the disease, because, according to the Jerusalem Talmud, one is obligated to accept a small risk in order to save one's fellow man from a definite danger.[60] However, if there is no chance of saving the patient, one should not endanger one's own life by visiting the patient.[61]

The Talmud states that those sent to perform a religious duty do not suffer harm (*shiluchei mitzvah aynon nizakin*).[62] This rule is also codified in Jewish law but only where there is no danger involved for the person performing the precept.[63] Where there is prevalent danger (*hezekey matzui*), the rule may not apply and the person may be foolhardy to risk his life to perform the precept (*chasid shoteh*). However, if the risk is infinitessimally small, such as one in a thousand or less, the person should fulfill the precept.

The risk of contracting AIDS by visiting or touching the patient seems to be nil. No case of AIDS has yet been contracted by casual contact with an AIDS patient. The virus is only transmitted through the blood and by sexual contact. Hence, physicians are obligated to care for patients with AIDS and everyone is obligated to visit patients sick with AIDS. The only precaution one need take is to avoid sticking oneself with a needle used to draw blood from or give an injection to an AIDS patient.

Allocation of Resources for AIDS Research and Treatment

Some people claim that governmental and societal resources should not be devoted to AIDS research because the disease is self-inflicted. This approach is obviously invalid, because some patients acquire AIDS through no fault of their own, i.e., through blood transfusions as in hemophiliacs, or transplacentally as in infants born of AIDS mothers. Even if a disease occurs only in sinners, society is still obligated to expend resources to try and conquer the disease, and physicians are obligated to heal patients suffering from that disease. The Talmud clearly states that every life is worth saving without distinction as to whether the person whose life is in danger is a criminal or a law-abiding citizen.[64]

The problem of the allocation of the resources of society when money for health care and medical research is limited is discussed in greater detail elsewhere.[65] Similarly, physicians have to allocate their time and energy among their various patients, raising halachic questions such as the permissibility (or prohibition) for a physician to leave one patient to care for another, much sicker patient. This topic, however, is beyond the scope of this essay.

Can Patients with AIDS Be Counted as Part of a Minyan?

May patients with AIDS who are homosexuals and/or drug addicts be counted as part of a quorum of ten men (*minyan*)? The *Shulchan Aruch* states that a sinner who transgresses the decrees of the Jewish community or who commits a biblical or rabbinic transgression can be counted as part of a *minyan* as long as he has not been excommunicated.[66] Even if he is excommunicated and cannot be counted as part of a *minyan*, a sinner is allowed to pray in the synagogue unless the congregants strongly object.[67] The *Mishnah Berurah* cites the *Pri Megadim*, who says that this rule applies only if the sinner is one who sins occasionally out of lust or appetite (*mumar le-te'avon*), but a provocative sinner (*mumar le-hachis*) or one who worships idols or who publicly desecrates the Sabbath is judged like a non-Jew and cannot be counted for a *minyan*.[68]

Rabbi Yechiel Weinberg quotes earlier Hungarian rabbis who say that today no Jew is excommunicated and, therefore, all Jews, even sinners, can be counted as part of a *minyan*.[69] However, he continues, other rabbis say that if a person is worthy of being excommunicated by virtue of transgressions he has committed, he cannot be counted as part of a *minyan* even though he is not actually excommunicated. The clarification of this rabbinic disagreement is important, for homosexuality is a sin for which the transgressor is worthy of being excommunicated. Nevertheless, this responsum of Rabbi Weinberg is difficult to understand in view of the clear statement in *Shulchan Aruch* that unless the sinner is actually excommunicated, he may be counted as part of a *minyan*.

Can Patients with AIDS Lead Synagogue Services?

The question has been raised as to whether or not a patient with AIDS can lead services in the synagogue as a cantor (*shaliach tzibur*) or Torah reader. Jewish law requires that the cantor be worthy, be free of sins, and not have a bad name even when he was younger.[70] Moreover, he should be humble and desired by the congregants, have a sweet voice, and study Torah regularly. Rabbi Moshe Isserles asserts that if someone transgresses unintentionally (*beshogeg*) and repents, he is allowed to serve as a *shaliach tzibur*, but not if he sinned intentionally (*bemayzid*) because he had a bad name before he repented.[71] The *Mishnah Berurah* cites *Magen Avraham*, who quotes many rabbinic decisors that even if one sinned intentionally, he can serve as a *shaliach tzibur* if he repents.[72] However, on fast-days and on the High Holy Days, one should not appoint him as a cantor, although once appointed he should not be removed.

For the High Holy Days, one should seek out a cantor who is most worthy, most learned in Torah, has performed many meritorious deeds, is married, and is over thirty years of age.[73] The *Mishnah Berurah* adds that the cantor and the one who blows the *shofar* should have fully repented from their sins, although one who begins as a cantor or *shofar* blower should not be removed.[74] It thus seems that if an AIDS patient has repented for his sins, including the sin of homosexuality, and if he meets the above qualifications and is acceptable to the congregation, it is permissible to have him lead synagogue services or blow the *shofar* or read from the Torah.

Should a Kohen with AIDS Recite the Priestly Blessing?

Is it permissible for a *kohen* to offer the priestly benediction (go up to the *duchan*) if he has AIDS related to homosexuality or drug addiction? The *Shulchan Aruch* states that if a *kohen* kills someone even unintentionally he should not offer the priestly blessing even if he repents.[75] *Ramo* adds, in the name of many rabbinic decisors: "If he repents, he is allowed to recite the priestly blessing, and this is the practice which one should follow."

The *Shulchan Aruch* also asserts that if the *kohen* is an apostate he should not recite the priestly blessing, although some rabbis allow him to do so if he repents.[76] If a *kohen* is intoxicated, he should not recite the priestly blessing.[77] So, too, if he marries a divorced woman.[78]

However, continues Rav Karo, if none of the above circumstances which prevent a *kohen* from reciting the priestly blessing are present, even if he is not careful about the observance of other commandments, he is allowed to recite the blessing.[79] The *Mishnah Berurah* explains that such commandments include even serious prohibitions such as forbidden sexual relationships (*arayot*).[80] It would appear, therefore, that a *kohen* with AIDS is permitted to offer the priestly benediction. *Mishnah Berurah*, quoting the *Zohar*, adds that if the *kohen* is despised by the congregation, he should not recite the priestly blessing.[81] The reason why even a *kohen* who has sinned is allowed to offer the priestly blessing is that one should not prevent him from performing the positive commandment of blessing the people, thus adding to his sins by not allowing him to fulfill this and other commandments.[82]

Someone might ask: what good is his blessing if he is a sinner? The answer is that the *kohen* only recites the words but the actual blessing comes from God, as it is written: *and I will bless them.*[83]

Should a Patient with AIDS Be Honored in the Synagogue?

The Talmud states that it is prohibited to flatter the wicked in this world because it encourages them to believe that they are not doing anything wrong.[84] Furthermore, if a homosexual AIDS patient is honored in the synagogue by being called up to the Torah, people may be misled into thinking that his behavior is acceptable. Thus honoring a sinner might constitute transgression of the negative precept of *not placing a stumbling block before the blind.*[85] The same question arises when a person who publicly violates biblical commandments is honored at a testimonial dinner. Is not the bestowing of such an honor prohibited because it misleads the sinner and the public into believing that the person's violations are being condoned?

Rabbi Feinstein discusses the case of a very philanthropic and charitable Jewish physician who performs many deeds of loving-kindness but is married to a non-Jewish woman.[86] Ordinarily, one should not give this physician any honors in the synagogue because of "the stumbling block that is being placed before the blind" in that such honors might mislead him into believing that his marriage to a non-Jew is not wrong. However, if the honor might lead the sinner to repent, or if one tells him that what he is doing is wrong, it is permissible to give him the honor. In the case under discussion, Rav Feinstein concludes that it is permissible to have the physician open and close the holy ark and remove and subsequently return the Torah to the ark because all the congregants know that he is being honored because of his philanthropy and good deeds, thus the honor does not represent acquiescence to his wrongdoing. Furthermore, the public is in need of his services (*rabim tzerichim loh*) because of his expertise as a physician, and he may, therefore, be accorded the aforementioned honor.

However, the *Chatam Sofer* rules that one should not call a sinner to the Torah for a portion of the Torah reading (*aliyah*) because of the aforementioned possibility of misleading the sinner and/or the public into believing that the sin is being condoned.[87]

Can a Patient with AIDS Serve as a Witness?

Maimonides lists ten classes of individuals who are ineligible to attest or testify before a Jewish court: women, slaves, minors, the mentally deficient, deaf-mutes, the blind, transgressors, the contemptible, relatives, and interested parties.[88] Transgressors are ineligible as witnesses by biblical law, for it is written: *Put not thy hand with the wicked to be an unrighteous witness*,[89] which is interpreted as "accept not the wicked as a witness."[90] Maimonides then enumerates the various types of transgressors, including those who are liable to be flogged, thieves, robbers, tricksters, gamblers, usurers, as well as idlers and vagabonds who are suspected of spending their leisure time in criminal activity.[91]

How should one classify the transgressions of homosexuality and drug addiction, the most common risk factors for the development of AIDS? Those who sin unintentionally are eligible to serve as witnesses, but AIDS patients who are homosexuals know what they are doing. Perhaps such patients can be considered to lack self-control over their strong desire; Jewish law states that a person who sins under compulsion is divinely exempted from punishment (*onus rachamanah patrey*). Support for this position can be found in the talmudic commentary known as *Tosafot*,[92] which quotes the passage stating that one who is suspected of adultery is nevertheless eligible as a witness.[93]

Burial, Funeral Rites, and Mourning for an AIDS Patient

Two cases known to this writer involved AIDS patients who died, where the members of the burial society (*chevra kadisha*) refused to perform the ritual purification of the deceased (*taharah*) because of their fear of contracting AIDS. It is now known that one cannot acquire AIDS by casual contact and their fear was unfounded. However, the problem arises with deceased individuals who had a real contagious disease vis-à-vis the ritual purification for the dead. If the members of the burial society can take precautions such as wearing masks, gloves, and gowns, they should do so. If they cannot or will not do so out of fear, they are not obligated to perform the *taharah* because the latter is only a custom and not a law.[94]

Are the laws of mourning (*avelut*) to be observed for a homosexual patient who died of AIDS? Jewish law states that there is no mourning for those who cast off the yoke of commandments and act like apostates.[95] However, if they repent, mourning is observed for them.

Rabbi Abraham Sofer distinguishes between a sinner who suffers for weeks, months, or years before his death and one who dies suddenly. The former probably repented, the latter did not. Therefore, AIDS patients who suffer for variable periods of time before their death should probably be mourned on the assumption that they repented.[96]

It is certainly not proper to honor an AIDS patient after death by naming a school or playground after him. The Talmud interprets the biblical phrase, *But the name of the wicked shall rot,*[97] to mean that rottenness enters their names in that none name their children after them.[98] If it is public knowledge that the AIDS patient was a sinner, he should not be honored after death by having a person or thing named after him. It is also a punishment for the wicked not to honor them after death.

Use of the Mikvah by Women Fearful of Contracting AIDS

The Talmud states that if wine or olive sap falls into a ritual bath or ritualarium (*mikvah*) and changes its color, it becomes invalid.[99] Based on this ruling, some rabbis prohibit the addition of chlorine to a *mikvah* because the color of the water is changed to green. As a result of this prohibition, some women are afraid of using such a *mikvah* for fear of contracting AIDS from the water used by other women whose husbands may have AIDS. However, this fear is totally unfounded, since AIDS cannot be transmitted through water but only by sexual contact or through blood or blood products. Secondly, most rabbis do not prohibit the use of chlorine, because only a minute amount is used to provide antisepsis of the *mikvah* water. (Sufficient chlorine to make the water change color to green would be intolerable to humans and produce serious eye irritation and skin burning. The greenish color of some *mikva'ot* is due to the green or blue tiles lining the *mikvah.*) Furthermore, the rabbis who prohibit the use of chlorine because of the problem of the change in the appearance (*shinuy mareh*) of the water can offer the solution of using chlorine crystals rather than liquid chlorine. The addition of solids such as foods or chemicals, states the talmudic commentary called *Mishnah Acharonah*, does not invalidate a *mikvah* even if the color of the water is thereby changed.[100]

Circumcision of a Baby with AIDS

The AIDS virus can be transmitted through the placenta from an AIDS-suffering women, usually a drug addict or sexual partner of an AIDS man, to her unborn fetus. AIDS in newborns or infants is a rare but well-recognized disorder. Is it permissible or mandatory to perform a ritual circumcision (*brit milah*) on such a male infant on the eighth day of life? Must it be postponed until the child recovers from the illness? But there is no cure for AIDS! How does one perform the *metzitzah*, or sucking, which is part of the ritual circumcision? May *metzitzah* be omitted in cases of AIDS?

In a lengthy article, Dr. Abraham Steinberg discusses medical-halachic considerations in the performance of *brit milah*.[101] He reviews the reasons for this Divine commandment and the various medical conditions for which the circumcision may or must be postponed. Steinberg cites numerous rabbinic responsa which address these issues. The rules on these matters can be found in the classic codes of Maimonides and Rav Joseph Karo.[102]

If an infant has a generalized illness from which he is not expected to recover, but the physicians state that circumcision would not in any way endanger the infant nor add to the illness, *brit milah* should be performed, preferably on the eighth day.[103] Some rabbis rule that a baby who cannot live for twelve months should be circumcised on a weekday but not on the Sabbath.[104] The *Chatam Sofer* gave a similar ruling in the case of a baby who was not expected to live three months.[105]

On the other hand, Rabbi Bakshi-Doron refused to allow a baby with spina bifida and paraplegia to be circumcised in spite of the medical testimony that the baby had no feeling in the lower half of his body and would not be harmed medically by a *brit milah*.[106] This rabbi and others rule that circumcision should be postponed in any baby with a generalized illness "until it recovers." Most infants with AIDS are critically ill, and circumcision is usually medically and therefore halachically contraindicated.

Conclusion

At the same time that we condemn homosexuality as an immoral act characterized in the Torah as an abomination, we are nevertheless duty bound to defend the basic rights to which homosexuals are entitled. The Torah teaches that even one who is tried, convicted, and executed for a capital crime is still entitled to the respect due to any human being created in the image of God. Thus, his corpse may not go unburied overnight.[107] The plight of Jewish AIDS victims doomed to almost certain death should arouse our compassion.

In Judaism, the value of human life is infinite. Whether a person is a homosexual or not, we are obligated to give him proper care if he is sick, charity if he is needy, food if he is hungry, and a burial after death. If he breaks a law of the Torah, he will be punished according to the transgression. Even if AIDS is a punishment by God for the sin of homosexuality, Jewish tradition teaches us that such a Divine affliction may serve as an atonement for that sin or the patient may repent while ill, making the AIDS victim even more deserving of our mercy and loving-kindness as a fellow Jew.

The compassion of Jewish law in requiring treatment for AIDS patients, however, should not be confused with acquiescence to the behavior of homosexuals who develop AIDS. Under no circumstances does Judaism condone homosexuality, which we characterize as an abomination. Nevertheless, the patient with AIDS should be treated and his life saved. To stand idly by and see the homosexual die without trying to help him is prohibited.[108] Evil should be banned, but the evildoers should be helped to repent.[109]

Notes

1. Leviticus 18:22.
2. Ibid. 20:13.
3. Sanhedrin 54a.
4. *Mishneh Torah, Hilchot Issurei Biah* 1:14.
5. I. Jakobovits, *Encyclopedia Judaica* (Jerusalem: Keter, 1972), vol. 8, cols. 961–962.
6. Genesis 19:5.
7. Judges 19:20.
8. Sotah 13b and Jerusalem Talmud, Sanhedrin 6:6, 23c.
9. Sanhedrin 57b–58a.
10. "Homosexuality and Judaism," *Journal of Halacha and Contemporary Society* 2 (Spring 1986): 70–87.
11. Responsa *Iggrot Moshe, Yoreh Deah*, vol. 3, no. 35.
12. Below, pp. 391–403.
13. Deuteronomy 4:9.
14. Ibid. 4:15.
15. Ibid. 22:8.
16. *Mishneh Torah, Hilchot Rotze'ach* 11:4 ff.
17. *Shulchan Aruch, Choshen Mishpat* 427 and *Yoreh Deah* 116.
18. Baba Kamma 91b.
19. *Mishneh Torah, Hilchot Chovel Umazik* 5:1.
20. *Shulchan Aruch, Choshen Mishpat* 420:31 and *Orach Chayim* 571.
21. Exodus 21:19.
22. Baba Kamma 85a.
23. Deuteronomy 22:2.
24. *Mishneh Torah, Hilchot Rotze'ach* 1:14.
25. Rosner, *Modern Medicine and Jewish Ethics*, pp. 7–13.
26. *Shulchan Aruch, Orach Chayim* 328:2.
27. Sanhedrin 27b.
28. Ibid. 73a.
29. D. Novak, personal communication.
30. Avodah Zarah 26b.
31. *Mishneh Torah, Hilchot Rotze'ach* 10:12.
32. Commentary of *Tosafot*, Avodah Zarah 26b s.v. *ani;* Maimonides' *Mishnah Commentary* on Nedarim 4:4; *Shulchan Aruch, Choshen Mishpat* 425:5.
33. Sanhedrin 73a, *Shulchan Aruch, Choshen Mishpat* 426:1, *Orach Chayim* 329:8.
34. *Shulchan Aruch, Orach Chayim* 329:8.
35. *Mishnah Berurah* 329:19; *Pitchei Teshuvah, Choshen Mishpat* 426:2.
36. *Mishnah Berurah* 328.
37. Psalms 116:6.

38. Yebamot 12b.

39. Responsa *Iggrot Moshe, Even Haezer*, no. 63.

40. *Torat Chesed, Even Haezer*, no. 44; *Achiezer*, part 1, no. 23.

41. Y. Zilberstein, *Assia* 11, no. 11 (Nissan 5746/May 1986): 5–11.

42. M. Hershler, *Halacha Urefuah* 2 (1981): 52–57; M.Y. Sloshitz, ibid 3 (1983): 158–163; A. Metzger, *Harefuah Le'or HaHalachah*, 4 (1985): 10–34; A. S. Abraham, *Hamayan*, Nissan 5742, pp. 31 ff.

43. A. S. Abraham, *Assia* 5 (1986): 18–23.

44. *Terumot*, end of chap. 8, according to *Ha'amek She'elah, She'iltot* 147:1.

45. Known as *Hagahot Maimuniyot*.

46. *Keseph Mishneh* Commentary of *Hilchot Rotze'ach* 1:14.

47. *Bet Yoseph, Tur Shulchan Aruch, Choshen Mishpat* 426.

48. Sanhedrin 73a, according to *Agudat Aizov, Derushim*, fol. 3b, and *Hashmatot*, fol. 38b.

49. *Radvaz*, pt. 5 (p. 2 in *Leshonot HaRambam*, sec. 1, 582); *Radvaz*, pt. 3, no. 627, and *Sheiltot Radvaz* 1:52.

50. Leviticus 19:16.

51. Responsa *Iggrot Moshe, Yoreh Deah*, pt. 2. no. 174:4; Responsa *Tzitz Eliezer*, vol. 10, no. 25:7.

52. O. Yosef, *Halachah Urefuah* 3 (1983): 61–63; J. J. Weiss, Responsa *Minchat Yitzchok*, pt. 6, no. 103:2; Responsa *Tzitz Eliezer*, vol. 10, no. 25:7. See also M. Meiselman, *Halachah Urefuah*, 2 (1981): 114–121; M. Hershler, ibid. 2 (1981): 122–127.

53. Genesis 18:1.

54. Sotah 14a.

55. I. Jakobovits, *Journal of a Rabbi* (New York, Living Books, 1966). p. 156.

56. Responsa *Ramo*, no. 9 (end).

57. Nedarim 39b, Berachot 22b, and *Rashi* on Shabbat 30a.

58. I. Jakobovits, *Jewish Medical Ethics* (New York, Bloch, 1959), pp. 108–109.

59. J. Cassuto, *Jahrbuch der Jeudisch-Literarischen Gesellschaft* 10 (1912): 252 and 280 (in minutes dated 1664 and 1666).

60. J. J. Greenwald, *Kol Bo Al Avelut* (New York/Jerusalem, Feldheim), p. 17.

61. *Mishneh Torah, Hilchot Shemirat Hanefesh* 1:7.

62. Pesachim 8b.

63. *Turei Zahav (Taz)* on *Shulchan Aruch, Orach Chayim* 455:3.

64. Sanhedrin 73a.

65. Below, pp. 375–390.

66. *Shulchan Aruch, Orach Chayim* 55:11.

67. Ibid. 55:12.

68. *Mishnah Berurah* 55:11:46.

69. Responsa *Seridei Aish*, pt. 2, no. 6.

70. *Shulchan Aruch, Orach Chayim* 53:4.
71. *Ramo* on *Orach Chayim* 53:5.
72. *Mishnah Berurah* 53:5:22.
73. *Ramo* on *Orach Chayim* 581:1.
74. *Mishnah Berurah* 581:1:11.
75. *Shulchan Aruch, Orach Chayim* 128:35.
76. Ibid. 128:37.
77. Ibid. 128:38.
78. Ibid. 128:40.
79. Ibid. 128:39.
80. *Mishnah Berurah* 128:39:143.
81. Ibid. 128:10:37.
82. *Hasagot of Ramah* (Jerusalem, 5744 solidus 1984), *Hilchot Nesiyat Kapayim* 18:6.
83. Numbers 6:27.
84. Sotah 41b.
85. Leviticus 19:14.
86. Responsa *Iggrot Moshe, Orach Chayim*, pt. 2, no. 51.
87. Responsa *Chatam Sofer, Orach Chayim*, no. 15.
88. *Mishneh Torah, Hilchot Eydut* 9:1.
89. Exodus 23:1.
90. *Mishneh Torah, Hilchot Eydut* 10:1.
91. Ibid. 10:2–5.
92. *Tosafot* on Sanhedrin 9b, s.v. *liretzono.*
93. Sanhedrin 26b.
94. *Chochmat Adam*, beginning of the customs of the *chevra kadisha.*
95. *Shulchan Aruch, Yoreh Deah* 345:5.
96. Responsa *Ketav Sofer, Yoreh Deah*, no. 171.
97. Proverbs 10:7.
98. Yoma 38b.
99. Mikva'ot 7:3.
100. Ibid.
101. A. Steinberg, *Assia* (5743 solidus 1983): 207–228.
102. *Mishneh Torah, Hilchot Milah* 1:1 ff; *Shulchan Aruch, Yoreh Deah* 260 ff.
103. Responsa *Minchat Yitzchok*, vol. 5, no. 11.
104. Responsa *Maharam Schick, Yoreh Deah*, no. 243.
105. Responsa *Chatam Sofer*, no. 64.
106. E. Bakshi-Doron, *Halachah Urefuah* 2 (1981): 268–272.
107. Deuteronomy 21:23.
108. Leviticus 19:16.
109. Psalms 104:35.

PART II
The Beginning of Life

7

Contraception

Introduction

Controversy surrounding the problems associated with contraception is by no means on the decline. On the contrary, a veritable recent flood of books and articles in the medical and lay press, as well as innumerable programs on the mass communication media devoted to family planning, contraceptive practice, and birth control, attest to the widespread and increasing interest in this subject. Introduction of the pill in the early 1960s revolutionized many people's thinking toward birth control and has had a major impact on the overall picture of world population limitation.

It is beyond the scope of this essay to provide the reader with a comprehensive discussion of the various contraceptive methods, their effectiveness or lack thereof, the physiological mechanisms involved, and the possible side effects that may be encountered. For such information the reader is referred to the standard textbooks of obstetrics and gynecology. Suffice it simply to enumerate the major methods employed: the condom, *coitus interruptus*, the diaphragm and cervical caps, chemical contraceptives, the safe period or rhythm method, oral contraceptives, and the intrauterine devices. Sterilization and abortion should also be mentioned, as well as a variety of minor methods, such as douching, sponges and tampons, scrotal hyperthermia and *coitus reservatus* and *saxonicus*.

Moral Aspects of Contraception

The morality (or immorality) of contraception boils down to a two-sided argument. On the one hand, many people claim that there is no moral difference between preventing the natural process of conception by contraception and preventing the natural process of obesity by diet or pills. On the other hand, traditional Judaic-Christian teaching maintains that by the mind and will of God there is an objective standard of right and wrong in the universe, and that men are possessed with the rational faculty to choose one or the other. Thus, if the Torah considers any interference with the act of procreation as morally wrong, then such interference is legally prohibited in Jewish law. The commandment of *be fruitful and multiply*[1] interdicts the indiscriminate use of contraceptives.

The argument that contraceptive chemicals may kill a fertilized ovum (i.e., a potential person) is more germane to a treatise on abortion and will not be discussed here. Furthermore, such an argument is not applicable to most modern methods of contraception, including the pill and intrauterine devices. The problem of eugenics and population control is as much a moral dilemma as it is a matter of social ethics.

The economic argument for contraception emphasizes that parents should only have the number of children they can support in an adequate fashion. This argument possesses its greatest strength and appeal when it is applied to large families with below-average income. That some good may be derived from contraception employed for economical reasons does not, however, make such a practice morally right. In order that all children in a family be provided with adequate food, clothing, shelter, and education, contraception may be no more morally justified than robbery by the parents to provide for the needs of the children. Robbery and contraception are both immoral, although both might achieve a desirable outcome. The solution to the economic argument for contraception is a better organization of society, with sufficient work and distribution of wealth for all.

Medical indications for the use of contraceptive devices and methods are many and include diseases wherein pregnancy would result in a marked deterioration of the mother's health or even threaten her life. Such conditions are rheumatic heart disease, tuberculosis, certain kidney diseases, severe diabetes, and others. However, to masquerade behind a medical indication, particularly psychiatric illness, where none exists, or where the risks are minimal, is certainly immoral.

It is sometimes asserted that the stability, or even the preservation, of a marriage depends upon the practice of contraception. Reasons may include the desire of a wife to continue working after marriage, the lure of a professional career, unwillingness to give up an active social life, and reluctance to financially drain the marriage by having children. Such reasons, purely of convenience, for the use of contraceptives, are certainly immoral.

Catholic Attitude Toward Contraception

The most thorough, scholarly, objective analysis of Catholic doctrine on birth control throughout history is the work of John T. Noonan, Jr.[2] This book traces the development of the church's position on contraception, and analyzes the historical situations that influenced various church decisions over the centuries from the year 50 C.E. until 1965.

The traditional Catholic viewpoint is to prohibit all forms of contraception, except the rhythm method. This position is based upon the doctrine that the primary purpose of marriage is procreation, not companionship. Any method of birth control which violates the "natural law" is thus prohibited. Birth control by natural means, that is, using the rhythm method or abstinence, is not considered a violation of the "natural law."

Recent pronouncements by several Popes have reaffirmed the traditional Catholic teaching on this matter. In his famous 1930 Encyclical *Casti Connubii* ("On Christian Marriage"), Pope Pius XI solemnly restated the condemnation of contraception, but gave his approval to the rhythm method. This approval was repeated by Pope Pius XII in 1951 when he said:

> We affirm the legitimacy and, at the same time, the limits—in truth very wide—of a regulation of offspring which, unlike so-called "birth control," is compatible with the law of God. One may even hope that science will succeed in providing this licit [rhythm] method with a sufficiency basis.[3]

In a second address in 1951 the Pope elaborated on the conditions under which Catholics may use the rhythm method and be exempt from the duty of procreation and parenthood. Examples are "serious reasons, such as those often provided in the so-called indications of the medical, eugenical, economic and social order."[4] In an address to hematologists in 1958, Pope Pius XII approved the use of oral contraceptives for the treatment of disease, but condemned their use for birth control.

In 1966, a papal commission, appointed two years earlier to

reexamine the church's position on marriage and the family, submitted its report to Pope Paul VI. There were both minority and majority reports. The former recommended continued adherence to the traditional beliefs, whereas the latter urged changes in past teachings to allow chemical and mechanical contraceptives. In July 1968, in his Encyclical *Humane Vitae*, the Pope rejected the majority report and condemned the use of techniques other than abstinence or the rhythm method. Dissent within the Catholic hierarchy was considerable, with progressive views being voiced by Catholic theologians and laymen alike.

Protestant Views on Contraception

Protestant churches are virtually unanimous in their endorsement of birth control, as enunciated in the 1961 statement of the National Council of Churches, the federation of thirty-two major Protestant denominations. Such an endorsement stems from the view that the basic purposes of marriage include not only procreation but also the "nourishment of the mutual love and companionship of husband and wife and their service to society."[5]

Jewish Attitude Toward Contraception

The most extensive study of the principles of Judaism concerning contraception, based on a wealth of primary sources, is that of David Feldman.[6] In his book, Rabbi Feldman examines the relevant precepts of the Talmud, codes, commentaries, and rabbinic responsa. Feldman's work is so exhaustive that recent articles on the subject add very little to the overall picture.

A brief discussion of the biblical commandment *be fruitful and multiply*, as decreed first to Adam and Eve,[7] and later to Noah and his sons,[8] and to Jacob,[9] seems appropriate. The importance of this commandment is stated in the Talmud:[10]

> Rabbi Eliezer stated: He who does not engage in propagation of the race is as though he sheds blood; for it is said, *Whoso sheddeth man's blood by man shall his blood be shed;*[11] and this is immediately followed by the text *And you, be ye fruitful and multiply.*[12] Rabbi Jacob said: As though he has diminished the Divine Image; since it is said, *For in the image of God made He man,*[13] and this is immediately followed by *And you, be ye*

fruitful and multiply.[14] Ben Azzai said: As though he sheds blood *and* diminishes the Divine Image.

The explanation of the commandment is provided by the *Mishnah,*[15] where it states:

> A man shall not abstain from the performance of the duty of the propagation of the race unless he already has children. [As to the number], Bet Shammai ruled: two males, and Bet Hillel ruled: A male and a female, as it is written, *male and female created He them.*[16]

It is beyond the scope of the present essay to delve in depth into the rabbinic ramifications of the commandment of procreation. Suffice it to say that the moral obligation, if not the commandment of propagating the race still rests upon the husband when he already has two children. The role of the woman in procreation is described by Feldman and summarized in a quotation from the fourteenth-century talmudic commentary of Rabbi Nissim (known as *Chiddushei Ran):*

> . . . even though she is not personally commanded concerning procreation, she performs a *mitzvah* [meritorious act] in getting married because she thereby assists her husband in the fulfillment of his *mitzvah* [religious duty] of *be fruitful and multiply.*[17]

In a Jewish marriage, over and above the question of procreation, there exist the conjugal rights of the wife, technically termed *onah.* Thus, nonprocreative intercourse, such as occurs if the wife is too young to bear children, or is barren, or is pregnant, or postmenopausal, or following a hysterectomy, is not only allowed but required. Improper emission of seed *(hashchatat zera)* is not involved, or is canceled out so long as the intercourse is in the manner of procreation. Not only are such sexual activities permitted, but they are in fact required by biblical law.[18] "Marriage and marital relations are both independent of procreation, achieving the many desiderata spoken of in talmudic, responsa and mystic literatures."[19] Such goals include fulfilling the wife's desire, physical release of the husband's sexual pressures, and the maintenance of marital harmony and domestic peace.

A lengthy chapter in Feldman's book is devoted to a discussion of the legitimacy of sexual pleasure in Judaism. He quotes Nachmanides, who said that "sexual intercourse is holy and pure when carried on properly, in the proper time and with the proper intentions. No one should claim that it is ugly or unseemly. God forbid!" In a similar vein, Rabbi Jacob Emden is cited as having said: "to us the sexual act is worthy, good and beneficial even to the soul. No other human activity compares with it; when performed with pure and clean intention it is certainly holy. There is nothing impure or defective about it, rather much exaltation."

Thus, whereas Christian teaching promulgates that procreation is the sole purpose of marriage and sexual intercourse, Judaism teaches not only that procreation need not result from sex, but that mutual pleasure is sufficient reason for the sex act.

There are at least six methods of contraception mentioned in the Bible and Talmud. The first of these is *coitus interruptus*, which is unequivocally prohibited, as stated by Maimonides:

> It is forbidden to expend semen to no purpose. Consequently, a man should not thresh within and ejaculate without. . . . As for masturbators, not only do they commit a strictly forbidden act, but they are also excommunicated. Concerning them it is written, *Your hands are full of blood*,[20] and it is regarded as equivalent to killing a human being.[21]

A similar prohibition is found in *Asheri* (Rabbi Jacob ben Asher), known as *Rosh*,[22] and in Karo's code[23] as well as in other codes of Jewish law.

The scriptural source upon which is based the prohibition of improper emission of seed is not clear, although many consider the act of Er and Onan to be the classic case of *coitus interruptus*.[24] The Talmud, however, views the act of Er and Onan as unnatural intercourse.[25] Er wanted to preserve his wife's beauty by preventing her from becoming pregnant, and Onan sought to frustrate the levirate law. Therefore, argues Feldman, if this was Onan's sin, no clear biblical prohibition of improper emission of seed can be derived from the story of Onan, because the circumstances of the levirate marriage are special, and allow for no more than an intimation *(remez)* of the evil of this method of contraception.

Other possible biblical sources outlawing emission of seed for naught have been suggested. The Decalogue's commandment against adultery is said to have wider application, perhaps to immorality in general. The generation destroyed by the great flood is thought to have been liquidated because of the sin of improper emission of seed. Others say that this cardinal sin is implied in the commandment of *be fruitful and multiply*. Finally, states Feldman,[26] the injunction against incest,[27] literally, "immorality with one's own flesh" *(ish ish el kol sh'er b'saro)*, includes improper emission of seed.

Whether this offense is considered homicide or only immoral as self-defilement is also a matter of argumentation. The *Zohar* apparently espouses both reasons. Bringing forth semen in vain would also be prohibited if a man were to use a condom during intercourse, even if the sex act were performed in the natural way. Procurement of sperm for medical reasons (i.e., not in vain) is permitted under certain circumstances, such as sterility testing. Abstinence as a contraceptive method is prohibited as a double destruction of seed. Not only is the seed prevented from fulfilling its function of procreation, but it also fails to fulfill the commandment of *onah*, the wife's conjugal rights.

Since the commandment of procreation in Judaism rests primarily on the man, any contraceptive method employed by him, such as *coitus interruptus*, the condom, or abstinence, would be strictly prohibited because of the Onanite nature of these methods. Even in situations where contraception is permitted by Jewish law, such as for situations in which pregnancy might endanger the life of the mother, these methods are not allowable.

The Talmud discusses four methods and techniques employed by the woman to prevent conception: the safe period, twisting movements following cohabitation, an oral contraceptive, and the use of an absorbent material during intercouse.

The period of fertility of a woman is mentioned in the Talmud as follows:[28]

> Rabbi Isaac . . . stated: A woman conceives only immediately before her menstrual period, for it is said, *Behold, I was brought forth in iniquity*.[29] But Rabbi Yochanan stated: A woman conceives only immediately after her ritual immersion, for it is said, *And in cleansing did my mother conceive me*.[30]

Feldman cites rabbinic responsa that call attention to cycles of fertility and sterility as a possible method of contraception. He concludes that there is no impropriety in the use of this method when birth control is required, such as in situations of hazard to the mother. However, by its use, the commandment of procreation and the wife's conjugal rights *(onah)* are both frustrated. Furthermore, the unreliability of this method makes it unacceptable in cases of danger to life.

An ancient method of contraception is when the woman makes violent and twisting movements following cohabitation in order to spill her husand's seed. This method is described in the Talmud by Rabbi Jose, who is of the opinion that "a woman who plays harlot turns over in order to prevent conception."[31] The Talmud further entitles a woman to receive her marriage settlement (*ketubah*) if the husband imposes a vow on her to produce violent movements immediately after intercourse to avoid conception.[32]

Throughout the centuries, numerous recipes have been recommended for oral contraception, from Pliny the Elder's parsley and mint, to Dioscorides' willow leaves in water; from Soranes' opapanix, with cyrenaiac sap, to the marjoram, parsley, and thyme of medieval Germany. In the Talmud, there are at least two discussions of a "cup of roots," or sterility potion. First we find the following:

> Judith, the wife of Rabbi Chiyya, having suffered agonizing pains of childbirth, changed her clothes [on recovery] and appeared [in her disguise] before Rabbi Chiyya. She asked: "Is a woman commanded to propagate the race?" He replied: "No." And relying on this decision [lit. she went], she drank a sterilizing potion.[33]

Elsewhere the Talmud states that a potion of roots may be imbibed on the Sabbath because it is a cure for jaundice and gonorrhea.[34] However, the imbiber may become impotent thereby. Thus, a woman may drink a sterilizing (i.e., contraceptive) potion as a cure for jaundice. A smaller dose recommended to treat gonorrhea does not produce permanent sterility. The ingredients of this "cup of roots" are enumerated by Rabbi Yochanan and include Alexandrian gum, liquid alum, and garden crocus, powdered and mixed with beer (for jaundice) or wine (for gonorrhea).[35] The *Tosefta* specifically states that a man is not allowed to drink any potion in order not to be fertile, because he is commanded to propagate the race, whereas a woman is permitted to drink the potion in order not to conceive.[36]

The latter ruling is codified by both Maimonides and Karo unconditionally.[37] Later rabbis, however, stipulate that there must be some medical indication, as in the case of Rabbi Chiyya's wife, to allow the use of the potion of roots. Furthermore, as pointed out by

Feldman, "the bulk of the legal discussion surrounding the cup of roots is based on the crucial assumption that the sterilizing effect of this potion is permanent," thus raising the problem of castration, an act prohibited by Jewish law.[38]

The oral contraceptive pill of today seems to embody within itself the talmudic cup of roots. It allows intercourse to proceed in a natural and unimpeded manner, thus allowing fulfillment of the wife's conjugal rights. Furthermore, whereas the effect of the cup of roots is permanent, the effect of the pill is temporary, thereby setting aside the question of castration. No improper emission of seed is involved in the use of the pill.[39] However, without medical indication it appears as if the oral contraceptives should not be employed prior to the fulfillment of the commandment of procreation (i.e., at least two children). Furthermore, the question of the safety of the pill is both of medical and Jewish legal concern. Certainly, women in whom medical contraindications make the use of oral contraceptives dangerous would be prohibited by Jewish law from taking them. Other deleterious side effects must also be taken into consideration. However, at the moment, the pill seems to be the least objectionable method of birth control in Jewish law.

Virtually all rabbinic rulings on the subject of contraception are based upon a key talmudic statement which has been called "The *Beraita* of the Three Women."[40]

> Rabbi Bebai recited before Rabbi Nachman: Three [categories of] women may [or must] use an absorbent [Heb. *moch*] in their marital intercourse [to prevent conception]: a minor, a pregnant woman, and a nursing woman. The minor, because [otherwise] she might become pregnant and as a result might die. A pregnant woman because [otherwise] she might cause her fetus to become a *sandal* [a flat fish-shaped abortion due to superfetation]. A nursing woman, because [otherwise] she might have to wean her child prematurely [owing to her second conception], and he would die. And what is a minor? From the age of eleven years and one day until the age of twelve years and one day. One who is under or over this age [when conception is not possible or where pregnancy involves no fatal outcome, respectively] carries on her marital intercourse in the usual manner. This is the opinion of Rabbi Meir. But the sages say: The one as well as the other carries on her marital intercourse in the usual manner, and mercy be vouchsafed from Heaven [to save her from danger], for Scripture says, *The Lord preserveth the simple.*[41]

The nature and the status of the absorbent (or *moch*) in talmudic law is explored in an entire chapter of Feldman's book. Subsequent chapters are devoted to an in-depth consideration of the three categories of women in the *beraita* and the many levels of debate concerning the meaning of the *beraita*.

Does the *beraita* allow or require the three women to use the absorbent? Rashi states that Rabbi Meir means "may use" and the sages mean "may not," whereas Rabbenu Tam reports that Rabbi Meir means "must" and the sages mean "must not but may." A second level of debate is concerned with whether the absorbent is to be used before (i.e., during) or after coitus? The outcome of the argumentation in the interpretation of the *beraita* is summarized by Rabbi Immanuel Jakobovits, as follows:[42]

> . . . several authorities assume that this dispute applies only to these particular cases [i.e., three women] where the danger of a conception is in any event rather remote; hence, they infer that, in cases of a more definite threat to the mother's life arising from a pregnancy, there would be no objection at all to the use of contraceptives. Others hold that the three women are mentioned to illustrate the attitude to cases of resultant danger to life in general; while yet others regard the entire sanction as limited to these three women only.[43]

Jakobovits, Feldman, and others express surprise at the omission of reference to the pivotal *beraita* by the major codes of Jewish law, Maimonides and Karo. Even the codes which mention the *beraita* (*Asheri* and *Alfasi*) only relay it verbatim without deriving any legal ruling therefrom. To perhaps compensate for this silence, there is available an enormous rabbinic responsa literature dealing with contraception. The most lenient or permissive view is that of sixteenth-century Rabbi Solomon Luria, who allows the wife to apply a tampon before intercourse if a conception and pregnancy would prove dangerous. Many subsequent writers, including Rabbis Solomon Zalman of Posen, Simchah Bunem Sofer, Mordechai Horowitz, Chayim Ozer Grodzinsky, Sholem Mordechai Schwadron, David Hoffmann, and others, agree with Luria.[44] On the other hand, there is a school of nonpermissivists who do not allow any impediment to natural intercourse. The chief proponents of this school are Rabbis Akiba Eger, Jacob Ettlinger, and Moses Schreiber.[45]

For situations of pregnancy hazard, the pessary or diaphragm is allowed by numerous authorities, including Rabbis Joshua Baumol,

Sholom Mordechai Schwadron, Chayim Sofer, and Moshe Feinstein.[46] The reason is that the normal coital act is not interfered with. This is not the case with the condom, which constitutes an improper interference and is strictly prohibited. Chemical spermicides and douches are other contraceptive methods which leave the sex act alone and are thus permitted by many responsa writers, but only in a case of danger to the mother from pregnancy. Whether spermicides are preferable to the use of a diaphragm, or vice versa, is a matter of debate. On the one hand, the occlusive diaphragm does in fact constitute a mechanical barrier. On the other hand, "spermicides destroy the seed immediately upon its entry into the canal."[47]

As to the intrauterine contraceptive devices, recent medical evidence seems to indicate that these produce contraception by inhibiting proper implantation of the fertilized ovum in the wall of the uterus. If this is so, then their abortifacient action would prohibit their use, as it is akin to abortion.

Recently, Rabbi Feinstein has written that if pregnancy would constitute a danger to a woman's life, she may use a diaphragm or oral contraceptive pills. If all other methods fail or cannot be used, surgical sterilization of the woman is permitted to prevent conception, especially if she and her husband have already had two or more children.[48] Rabbi Eliezer Waldenberg also states that the diaphragm is preferable to oral contraception for a woman in whom pregnancy is medically contraindicated.[49] Rabbi Ben Zion Uziel asserts that a woman with heart disease is allowed to use contraception, especially if she already has children.[50]

Numerous statements about contraception are found in the responsa of Rabbi Isaac Weisz, who rules that in general it is prohibited to use contraceptive methods unless there is a threat to the mother's life, in which case oral contraception is the preferred method.[51] If pills cannot be used, she may employ other methods but should select the simplest and most effective. The pill may also be used to avoid extreme pain of childbirth. Spermicidal jellies or foams are also acceptable contraceptive methods where pregnancy would constitute a serious health hazard to the mother, including blindness and mental illness. Contraception is not allowed, according to Rabbi Uziel, for financial or social reasons or for the sake of convenience or because of the fear that the baby may be born with mental deficiency. Where indicated to preserve the health or life of the mother, temporary contraception is preferable to permanent contraception. All these permissive rulings, concludes Uziel, are for one-year periods and must be reviewed annually with a reappraisal of the medical and psychiatric status of the woman.

Recent review articles on contraception in Jewish sources are those of Moshe Halevi Steinberg and Abraham Steinberg.[52] The latter article is profusely annotated and discusses in detail family planning in Jewish law, demography of Jews, the commandment of *be fruitful and multiply*, and the prohibition of destroying human seed. Another recent review of family planning and contraception by Aviner presents in-depth discussions of both the medical and Jewish legal aspects.[53] The author contrasts the "strict" rulings of Weisz with the "in between" rulings of Feinstein and the "lenient" rulings of Waldenberg. Aviner also claims that it is permissible to use contraception to space one's children for valid reasons, such as the preservation of domestic tranquillity and/or the difficulty or inability to raise several small children at once. Certainly for physical or mental danger to the mother that a pregnancy might produce, it is permitted (and even mandated) that she use contraception. The methods in order of preference are the pill, the intrauterine device, spermicidal jellies or foams, and the diaphragm.

Rabbi Immanuel Jakobovits has capsulized the voluminous rabbinic literature on contraception by saying that leading rabbis

> broadly agree that contraceptive precautions should be taken only on medical grounds. Where the danger resulting from a pregnancy is not acute, sanction for certain types of contraceptive devices will more readily be given for a limited period, usually of two years, and if the precept of procreation [i.e., the birth of a son and a daughter] has already been fulfilled.
>
> In a recent volume of Responsa [Feldman's *Birth Control in Jewish Law*] the various methods of birth control have been graded, from the most to the least favored, according to their degree of direct interference with the generative act and organs, as follows: 1) oral contraceptives ("the pill") and intra-uterine devices (IUD), provided they do not have an abortifacient effect, to be used so long as there is some sound medical indication; 2) female sterilization, if the danger of a pregnancy is permanent; 3) postcoital removal of semen by tampon or douche; 4) cervical rubber cap to close the mouth of the uterus; 5) spermicides; 6) tampon or diaphragm inserted before coitus; 7) IUD, if the effect is to abort the impregnated egg; and 8) male condom, to be used only in extreme cases of acute danger and if other means are unavailable or unacceptable.[54]

Conclusion

The Jewish attitude toward contraception by any method is a nonpermissive one if no medical or psychiatric threat to the mother or child exists. The duty of procreation, which is primarily a commandment on men, coupled with the wife's conjugal rights in Jewish law, militates against the use of the condom, *coitus interruptus*, or abstinence under any circumstances. Where pregnancy hazard exists, and where rabbinic sanction for the use of birth control is obtained, a hierarchy of acceptability emerges from the talmudic and rabbinic sources. Most acceptable are contraceptive means that least interfere with the natural sex act and least interfere with the full mobility of the sperm and its natural course. "Oral contraception by pill enjoys preferred status as the least objectionable method of birth control".[55] Since many different factors must be brought to bear on the final decision, it is suggested that competent rabbinic opinion be sought to adjudicate any given case, such opinion to be based upon expert medical testimony.

Notes

1. Genesis 1:28.
2. J. T. Noonan, Jr., *Contraception: A History of Its Treatment by the Catholic Theologians and Canonists*, (Cambridge, Mass.: Harvard University Press, 1966).
3. A. Guttmacher, *Birth Control and Love*, 2d ed. (London: Macmillan Co., 1969), pp. 141–168.
4. Ibid.
5. Ibid.
6. D. Feldman, *Birth Control in Jewish Law* (New York: New York University Press, 1968).
7. Genesis 1:28.
8. Ibid. 9:1 and 7.
9. Ibid. 35:11.
10. Yevamot 63b.
11. Genesis 9:6.
12. Ibid. 9:7.
13. Ibid. 9:6.
14. Ibid. 9:7.
15. Yevamot 6:6.
16. Genesis 1:27 and 5:2.
17. *Chiddushei Ran* on Kiddushin 41a.
18. Based on Exodus 21:10.
19. Feldman, op. cit., p. 60 . . ..
20. Isaiah 1:15.
21. Maimonides, *Mishneh Torah, Hilchot Issurei Biyah* 21:18.
22. *Teshuvot HaRosh* 33:3.
23. Karo, *Shulchan Aruch, Even Ha'ezer* 23:5.
24. Genesis 38:7–10.
25. Yevamot 34b.
26. Feldman, op. cit., p. 113.
27. Leviticus 18:6.
28. Niddah 31b.
29. Psalms 51:7.
30. Ibid.
31. Ketubot 37a.
32. Ibid. 72a.
33. Yevamot 65b.
34. Shabbat 109b–110b.
35. Ibid. 110a.
36. Yevamot 8:2.
37. Maimonides, *Mishneh Torah, Hilchot Issurei Biyah* 12:12, Karo, *Shulchan Aruch, Even Ha'ezer* 5:12.
38. Feldman, op. cit., p. 244.

39. M. Feinstein, Responsa *Iggrot Moshe*, vol. 1, *Even Ha'ezer*, no. 65, and E. Y. Waldenberg, Responsa *Tzitz Eliezer*, vol. 9, no. 51, Talmud, *Shabbat* 110b–111a, based upon the biblical phrase *that which has its stones bruised or crushed or broken or cut, ye shall not offer unto the Lord; neither shall ye do thus in your land* (Lev. 22:24).

40. Yevamot 12b.

41. Psalms 116:6.

42. I. Jakobovits, *Jewish Medical Ethics*, 2d. ed. (New York: Bloch, 1975), p. 389.

43. Luria, *Yam Shel Shelomoh*, Yevamot 1:8.

44. Solomon of Posen, Responsa *Chemdat Shlomo*, *Even Ha'ezer* 46; Sofer, Responsa *Shevet Sofer*, *Even Ha'ezer* 2; Horowitz, Responsa *Mattei Levy*, vol. 2, no. 31. Grodzinsky, Responsa *Achiezer*, *Even Ha'ezer* 23. Schwadron, Responsa *Maharsham*, vol. 1, no. 58. Hoffman, Responsa *Melamed Leho'il*, *Even Ha'ezer*, no. 18.

45. Egar, Responsa *Akiba Eger*, no. 71; Ettlinger, Responsa *Binyan Tziyon*, no. 137; Schreiber, Responsa *Chatam Sofer*, *Yoreh Deah*, no. 172.

46. Baumol, Responsa *Emek Halacha*, no. 66; Schwadron, Responsa *Maharsham*, Vol. 1, no. 58; Sofer, Responsa *Machaneh Chayim*, *Even Ha'ezer*, no. 53; Feinstein, Responsa *Iggrot Moshe*, vol. 1, *Even Ha'ezer*, no. 63 and Vol. 2, no. 12.

47. Waldenberg, Responsa *Tzitz Eliezer*, Vol. 9 no. 51:2–3.

48. M. Feinstein, "Women in Whom Pregnancy Is Dangerous to Life," in *Halachah Urefuah* (M. Hershler, edit.) Jerusalem, Regensberg Inst. Vol. 1, 1980, pp. 328-331.

49. Waldenberg, Responsa *Tzitz Eliezer*, Vol. 10, Sect. 25 Part 10.

50. Uziel, Responsa *Mishpetei Uziel*, Vol. 3. *Choshen Mishpat* no. 51.

51. Weisz, Responsa *Minchat Yitzchak*, Vol. 1 no. 100:3 and 115; Vol. 3 25:5 and 26:1–3, Vol. 4 no. 120; Vol. 5 no. 100–103; Vol. 6 no. 144.

52. M. H. Steinberg, "The Law About Methods Used to Prevent Conception," *Assia* 4 (1983): p. 161–166, A. Steinberg, "The General Jewish View on Contraception," in *Assia*, Jerusalem, Rubin Mass, Vol. 4, 1983, pp. 139–160.

53. S. C. Aviner, "Family Planning and Contraception," in *Assia*, Jerusalem, Rubin Mass, Vol. 4, 1983, pp. 167–181.

54. I. Jakobovits, "Medicine and Judaism—an Overview," in *Assia*. Jerusalem, Rubin Mass, 1983. pp. 289–310.

55. Feldman, op. cit., p. 248.

8

Artificial Insemination

Definition and Introduction

Artificial insemination is the instrumental deposition of semen into the female genital tract without sexual intercourse. There are two types of insemination, and they are frequently referred to by their abbreviations, which are, respectively, AIH (artificial insemination, husband) and AID (artificial insemination, donor). One can also use a mixture of semen obtained from husband and donor. Results of artificial insemination employing the husband's semen are good if the indication for the procedure is an anatomical defect, but fair to poor if there is moderate infertility in the male. Women can conceive two or more times from donor insemination.[1]

Artificial insemination has been practiced in animals for many years, primarily to increase the usefulness of the best male animals. For example, a single prize bull can provide enough semen to inseminate and impregnate five hundred cows. In the human, John Hunter is known to have artificially inseminated a woman in London in 1790, although earlier accounts are described, while in the United States, J. Marion Sims is credited with the first insemination in 1866. Today, there are an estimated 250,000 people in this country who are the offspring of such inseminations, thousands of which are performed annually.

These days, there is much writing—books, articles, reviews, and monographs—in the medical and lay press concerning this subject from the moral, legal, religious, medical, psychological, sociological, genetic, and other standpoints. The present paper deals primarily with the Jewish religious viewpoint.

Since many moral, legal, and religious problems may arise from artificial insemination, one might well ask why a barren couple should not simplify matters and adopt a baby? The psychological stress on women who consider themselves adulteresses following AID would be bypassed if adoption were resorted to, and, similarly, the emotional strains on some husbands, perhaps due to feelings of inadequate masculinity, might vanish if an adopted child, rather than one conceived from AID, became part of the family.

There are, however, numerous reasons why a woman prefers to carry and give birth to her own child. First, her emotional craving to be pregnant is fulfilled; she has proven her femininity. Second, both the husband and the wife are part of the conception, the antenatal care, the whole pregnancy, and the delivery, whereas an adopted child is usually not granted until it is several months old. Third, the child physically resembles the siblings, and the father, too, if AIH is resorted to; with an adopted child this resemblance is impossible. Fourth, the adopted child's new parents always fear the appearance of the real mother, a fear which does not exist with a child born following artificial insemination. Finally, since two-thirds of the adopted infants are born to unwed mothers and the other third are unwanted babies, the genetic background of these children may be poor and less desirable to the couple wishing to acquire a child, whereas semen from donors is frequently obtained from college and graduate students.

Around the major parties who may be involved in artificial insemination, namely the husband, the wife, the child, the physician, the donor, and the donor's wife, any number of legal questions may arise. Can the husband sue for divorce on the grounds of adultery following AID if he can prove that he is sterile? Can the physician and/or donor also be implicated as having participated in the adultery? Would the question of adultery vanish if the husband made the injection? Is the doctor responsible if a defective child is born? Is the doctor guilty of perjury when he signs the birth certificate, since he knows that the true father is not the one named on the birth certificate? Is the child considered legitimate? What are his rights concerning inheritance, support, and custody? Can he sue for the donor's estate? Can the mother sue the donor for support of the child? Can the donor sue for custody of the child? Should the husband legally adopt the child when his wife gives birth? How do adoption laws apply here, if at all? If insemination is performed without the woman's consent, is it considered rape? If so, by whom—the physician, the donor, or the husband?

Jewish Viewpoint

ANCIENT SOURCES

Before entering into Jewish legal discussions in the rabbinic responsa literature dealing with artificial insemination, it might be useful to cite three major ancient sources in the Talmud and the codes of Jewish law upon which these discussions are based. They are a passage in the Babylonian Talmud, a pronouncement in the thirteenth century by Rabbi Peretz ben Elijah of Corbeil, and the midrashic legend of Ben Sira.

In the Talmud we find:

> Ben Zoma was asked: May a high priest marry a maiden who has become pregnant [yet who claims she is still a virgin]? Do we take into consideration Samuel's statement, for Samuel said: I can have repeated sexual connections without [causing] bleeding [i.e., without the woman losing her virginity], or is the case of Samuel rare? He replied: The case of Samuel is rare, but we do consider [the possibility] that she may have conceived in a bath [into which a male has discharged semen].[2]

From this fifth-century talmudic passage we see that generation *sine concubito* was recognized as possible by the sages of old. Though Rabbi Judah Rozanes of Constantinople, the renowned commentator on Maimonides' *Mishneh Torah*, expresses doubt that impregnation through bathing in water into which a man had previously discharged semen can occur,[3] many authorities, including Rabbi Chaim Joseph David Azulai, Rabbi Jonathan Eybeschutz, and Rabbi Jacob Ettlinger, differ with him and interpret the talmudic passage literally.[4] Others, however, agree with Rabbi Rozanes.[5]

The second major ancient source indicating the possibility of pregnancy without sexual intercourse is by Rabbi Peretz ben Elijah of Corbeil in his work *Hagahot Smak*, who states:

> . . . a woman may lie on her husband's sheets but should be careful not to lie on sheets upon which another man slept lest she become impregnated from his sperm. Why are we not afraid that she become pregnant from her husband's sperm and the child will be conceived of a *niddah* [menstruating female]? The answer is that since there is no forbidden intercourse, the child is completely legitimate [lit. kosher] even from the sperm of another, just as Ben Sira was legitimate. However, we are

concerned about the sperm of another man because the child may eventually marry his sister.[6]

Several things emerge from this statement. First, generation *sine concubito* was recognized. Second, the offspring is considered legitimate. Third, no prohibition is mentioned concerning cohabitation of the woman with her husband afterwards, even if she has become pregnant from another. The only reason for her to avoid contact with the linen upon which another has lain is to prevent incest at a later date, i.e., the child marrying its own sibling. Finally, only forbidden intercourse would make her forbidden to her husband, whether or not she has lost her virginity, and irrespective of whether or not her male partner has emitted sperm into her genital tract during the forbidden sexual act.

The third ancient source for artificial insemination is the legend of Ben Sira, first mentioned by Rabbi Jacob Molin Segal (1365–1427) in his work entitled *Likutei Maharil*. This midrashic legend relates that Ben Sira was conceived without sexual intercourse by the prophet Jeremiah's daughter, in a bath, the father having been Jeremiah himself, who, coerced by a group of wicked men, emitted semen into the water.[7] The legend has since been quoted many times in medical literature[8] as well as in nearly all of the rabbinic responsa dealing with artificial insemination.

Some authorities, notably Rabbi David Gans,[9] deny the legend of Ben Sira's birth having followed a conception *sine concubito*. Rabbi Gans claims that he could not find the legend of Ben Sira in either the Talmud or the Midrash, and quotes Rabbi Solomon Ibn Verga, who says that Ben Sira was the son of the daughter of Joshua ben Jehozadak, the high priest mentioned in the book of Ezra.[10]

RECENT RULINGS

Since there is a vast rabbinic literature which addresses itself to the question of artificial insemination, and since the problem is so complex from the Jewish legal viewpoint, it seems desirable to subdivide the discussion into the major questions involved. Some of these are: Is the woman prohibited to her husband following an artificial insemination? Is it considered an act of adultery? What is the status of the child? Is the child a *mamzer* (illegitimate)? Is artificial insemination permitted at all? Is it permissible to use the sperm of the husband, or a donor, or a gentile? Does the donor fulfill the commandment of procreation? Is the offspring considered the child of the donor? Is the woman considered to be the pregnant or nursing wife of another and prohibited to marry again for a certain interval if her husband should die or divorce her? Is the husband permitted to provide his sperm for analysis and subsequent insemination if it is found suitable? How should one obtain the sperm from husband or donor? If artificial insemination is permitted, may it be performed during the woman's unclean period (menstruation and the ritual cleansing period thereafter)?

Is the woman prohibited to her husband following AID? The question obviously does not apply to AIH since the problem of possible adultery arises only with the semen of a man other than the husband. The case in the Talmud of the high priest marrying a pregnant maiden who claims to be a virgin, as cited above, concludes that Samuel's capacity to impregnate a woman without producing bleeding or loss of virginity is extremely rare. Thus, the maiden is permitted to marry the high priest, as she is deemed trustworthy when she claims to be a virgin despite having been impregnated in a bath into which a man had previously discharged semen. It would seem from this talmudic passage that only the act of sexual intercourse makes a maiden ineligible to marry a high priest.

The analogy between these situations can, however, be invalidated. The case of a high priest requires only that the girl's virginity be preserved to comply with the biblical commandment *but a virgin [betulah] of his own people shall he take to wife.*[11] Thus, if she becomes pregnant *sine concubito* or if she cohabits with a man without her virginity being lost, as in the case of Samuel, she is still permitted to a high priest. However, to prohibit a woman to her husband requires only a sexual union between the woman and another (*be'ulat ba'al*), as enunciated in Deuteronomy 22:22. Therefore, even without the loss of virginity, she is considered an adulteress.

The question remains: Does AID constitute an adulterous act or not? Rabbi Judah Rozanes states that even without loss of virginity the sexual act makes a maiden prohibited to marry a high priest.[12]

Rabbi Chananel ben Chusiel (11th cent.), in his commentary on the Talmud, interprets the discussion of the maiden and the high priest entirely differently. He states that the whole question revolves around the requirement of the pregnant maiden to bring a sacrifice to purify herself from the ritual impurity of birth. Does the biblical phrase *if a woman conceive seed and bear a man child, then she shall be unclean for seven days*[13] apply only to a woman who has become pregnant as a result of sexual intercourse, or is it also applicable for conception *sine concubito?* This, says Rabbi Chananel, is the major question discussed in the Talmud, and the problem of the maiden's permissibility to a high priest is only coincidental.

Thus, whether or not we subscribe to Rabbi Chananel's interpretation of the talmudic passage, it seems difficult, if not impossible, from this source to resolve the question as to whether AID constitutes an act of adultery which would prohibit the woman to her husband.

We then turn to another ancient source, namely the pronouncement of Rabbi Peretz ben Elijah of Corbeil, who doubts the feasibility of conception *sine concubito* and specifically states that a married woman who becomes impregnated in a bathhouse is not forbidden to her husband because there has been no prohibited intercourse involved.

In our times, Rabbi Ben Zion Uziel also states that no adultery or incest can occur unless there is a physical union of man and woman.[14] Rabbi Moses Feinstein agrees that without an act of sexual intercourse, the woman is not prohibited to her husband even if she has been inseminated with the semen of another without the husband's consent. The law of an adulteress, says Rabbi Feinstein, applies only for the sexual act and is involved even if there is no emission of sperm or even if the act is performed in an unnatural manner, i.e., sodomy.[15] Other authorities, such as Rabbi Sholom Mordecai Schwadron, Rabbi Yehoshua Baumol, and Rabbi Aaron Wolkin, also permit the woman to her husband if no sexual contact has occurred between her and the donor of the semen.[16]

Others disagree vehemently. Rabbi Judah Leib Zirelsohn looks upon AID as adultery, plain and simple.[17] The same view is held by Rabbi Abraham Lurie of South Africa and Rabbi Ovadya Hedaya.[18] Rabbi Eliezer Yehuda Waldenberg of Jerusalem is of the opinion that AID is akin to adultery and cites numerous rabbinic responsa to support his viewpoint.[19] He dismisses the talmudic passage and the pronouncement of Rabbi Peretz ben Elijah, stating that in both instances impregnation of the woman occurred passively and as an accident. On the other hand, AID entails the active participation of woman, physician, and donor and thus constitutes a prohibited act. The husband, continues Rabbi Waldenberg, is entitled to divorce his wife on these grounds, and she forfeits the monetary settlement written into the marriage contract (*ketubah*).

What is the status of the child? Is it illegitimate (mamzer)? Here there is marked difference of opinion in the rabbinic literature. Rabbis Zirelsohn, Lurie, Hedaya, Mordecai Jacob Breisch,[20] and others consider the child to be a *mamzer*, while Rabbi Waldenberg and others consider the child a questionable or possible *mamzer* (lit. *sofek mamzer*). On the other hand, Rabbis Uziel, Weinberg, Feinstein, Baumohl, Wolkin, Joseph Saul Nathanson, Manachem Kirshbaum, Raphael Pladi, Abraham Y. Neemrok, and Shlomo Zalman Auerbach, as well as others are of the opinion that the child is perfectly legitimate and not a *mamzer.*[21]

Is artificial insemination from a donor permissible? The previous questions dealt with the result of AID, but the question as to whether AID is permitted at all has not yet been definitively answered. Rabbi Waldenberg categorically prohibits it as an utter abomination, and cites Rashi's comment on a talmudic passage. Rashi interprets the biblical phrase *to be a God unto thee and to thy seed after thee*[22] to mean that God favors only those whose genealogy (i.e., paternity) is known.[23] The phrase in the Talmud itself reads "to distinguish between the seed of the first [husband] and the seed of the second." Thus, Rabbi Waldenberg prohibits AID because the genealogy of the child is unknown. Another reason given by Rabbi Waldenberg and in many other responsa is "lest he marry his sister," as mentioned in the Talmud. Therefore, avoidance of possible incest would interdict AID. A third reason for prohibiting it is that after the "proxy" father's death, his other children may "steal" the portion of inheritance belonging to the child produced by AID. Alternatively, the child may wrongly receive inheritance from his mother's husband upon the latter's death. Therefore, the question of stealing an inheritance makes AID forbidden.

Even if the donor's identity is known, continues Rabbi Waldenberg, AID is still prohibited, one reason being that the scriptural phrase *And thou shalt not lie carnally with thy neighbor's wife to defile thyself with her*[24] includes the prohibition of having one's semen enter another's wife even without the sexual act. There is, generally, strong rabbinic opinion, including that of Jakobovits, that AID should be condemned as "an act of hideousness" or "an abomination" or "human stud farming." Although, technically, AID does not produce an illegitimate offspring, according to most viewpoints, it should be outlawed lest it pave the way to increased promiscuity. Only under situations of extreme need does rabbinic opinion, as stated by Schwadron and Baumol, permit AID.

Does the donor fulfill the commandment of procreation? Is the child considered the child of the donor? Again, there are differing viewpoints on this problem. The specific question is asked by Rabbi Moshe of Brisk in his commentary on Karo's code as follows:

> . . . one may raise the question, in the case of a woman who became pregnant in a bathhouse, whether the father has fulfilled [the precept] of *be fruitful and multiply* [Gen. 1:28, 9:1, and 9:7] and if the child is considered his son in all respects. And in the *Likutei Maharil* we find that Ben Sira was the son of Jeremiah, who washed in the bathhouse, because Sira numerically equals Jeremiah" [i.e., the arithmetical sum of the Hebrew letters of the name Sira is identical with that of Jeremiah].[24]

Another commentary on Karo's code, that of Rabbi Samuel ben Uri, answers that the child is considered the man's son in all respects.[25] He bases his answer on the pronouncement of Rabbi Peretz ben Elijah (*Hagahot Smak*) quoted above. Rabbi Rozanes quotes both Rabbi Moshe of Brisk and Rabbi Samuel ben Uri and states that he agrees with them. Others, such as Rabbis Jacob ben Samuel, Yisroel Zev Mintzberg, Simon ben Zemach Duran, and Jacob Ettlinger, also subscribe to this viewpoint.[26] Some, such as Rabbis Jacob Emden[27] and Moshe Schick, disagree, and claim that although the child is considered the son of the donor, the donor has not fulfilled the precept of procreation because there has been no sexual act involved. Yet others, such as Rabbis Hedaya and Moshe Ayreh Leb Shapiro, state that the child is not his nor has he fulfilled the commandment of procreation.[28]

One might argue that if the case of impregnation in the bathhouse, where there was no intent on the part of the true father to impregnate the woman, results in a child considered to be his son in all respects and he has fulfilled the commandment of procreation (according to most authorities), then certainly *a fortiori* the same results should pertain to AID, where at least the doctor and the woman intentionally seek a pregnancy. This argument can be countered by the fact that anonymous donors provide their sperm to semen banks without intention as to their use for a specific woman, but on the other hand, there is the intent on the part of the donor that his sperm be utilized for the purpose of artificial insemination. Thus, the argument of intent seems to have little if any validity or applicability to the problem under discussion.

Following AID, is the woman considered to be the pregnant or nursing wife of another? Should the woman's husband die or divorce her following AID, is she allowed to remarry while she is still pregnant or, following delivery, while she is still nursing? A talmudic pronouncement states that a man should not marry the pregnant wife of another or the nursing wife of another, even though she has been divorced or widowed, until after the child is born or until she stops nursing, respectively.[29] Three reasons are given. First, we are concerned lest the woman conceive again while she is pregnant, thus making it impossible to identify which part of the child is the offspring of the first husband and which is the offspring of the second. Whether a woman can conceive by two different men and produce one child has been stated as fact by some[30] and denied by others.[31] Second, there may be danger to the fetus from abdominal pressure from sexual relations with the new husband, who might not be as careful to avoid harming the unborn fetus as would the true father. Third, if the woman conceives during the nursing period, her milk would become turbid and the nursing baby might die of starvation.

This rule has been codified by Maimonides, who states:

> And the sages also ordained that a man not marry the pregnant wife of another or the nursing wife of another, even though [in the former case] the owner of the seed which made her pregnant is known—lest the fetus be harmed during intercourse because he is not careful with the child of another. And [in the case of] a nursing woman lest her milk become turbid and he does not pay attention to heal the milk with things which improve turbid milk.[32]

Rabbi Jacob ben Asher and Rabbi Joseph Karo in their codes also state that "the sages decreed that a person should not marry nor betroth the pregnant wife of another or the nursing wife of another."[33]

With this discussion as background, Rabbi Waldenberg ponders whether the decree against a man marrying the pregnant or nursing wife of another is applicable to the husband whose wife has undergone AID. He concludes in the affirmative, and the new husband must, as a result, abstain from cohabitation with his wife until after she stops nursing. Some rabbis, such as Malchiel Zvi Halevy Tanenbaum,[34] Zirelsohn, and Uziel, agree with Waldenberg, whereas others, such as Chayim Joseph David Azulay,[35] are in doubt whether the decree applies to AID.

Artificial insemination using the husband's semen. Using the husband's sperm to inseminate the woman would eliminate many of the objections raised regarding AID, such as possible adultery, the offspring possibly marrying a sibling, "stealing" of an inheritance, and licentiousness, among others. Is then AIH permissible? Difference of opinion exists on this question in the responsa literature. Rabbis Feinstein, Schwadron, Wolkin, Zvi Pesach Frank, and others state that AIH is permissible.[36] Others, such as Rabbis Tannenbaum and Waldenberg, frown upon it, stating it is permissible only in extreme situations. The rabbis who normally forbid AIH claim that Rabbi Elijah ben Peretz's pronouncement allowing a woman to lie on sheets upon which her husband has lain (and possibly emitted sperm) is because impregnation in that situation is extremely rare. However, AIH commonly leads to pregnancy. Furthermore, in the case described by Rabbi Elijah, pregnancy occurred passively and by accident, whereas in AIH the physician, the donor, and the woman are active participants. Furthermore, claim the rabbis who object to AIH, if AIH were permitted, the physician might be tempted to add foreign semen to that of the husband in order to facilitate conception, thus performing AID, which is certainly prohibited. Even the rabbis who permit AIH would prohibit the use of a mixture of the husband's and another man's sperm. Thus, Rabbi Feinstein states that such an admixture of semens is a trick to overcome the weakness of the husband's sperm and is, therefore, considered like AID and is not AIH. Rabbis Waldenberg, Henkin, and others agree. One must be sure that only the husband's sperm is employed and only trustworthy physicians must be sought.

Insemination while the woman is ritually unclean (niddah). If we follow the permissive ruling regarding AIH, then the question arises as to whether it is allowed to perform artificial insemination on a woman during the period of her ritual uncleanliness.

Rabbi Abraham Isaiah Karelitz, known as the *Chazon Ish*, in the book *Haish Vechazyono*, relates that he was asked about a woman who had very short menstrual cycles, so that her fertile periods always occurred during her counting of the "seven clean days." Physicians recommended that AIH be performed during this period prior to the woman's *tevilah* (ritual immersion for purification), and Rabbi Karelitz answered that she should abbreviate her unclean period to four days but that she should not be inseminated while ritually unclean prior to *tevilah*.

Rabbis Schwadron, Waldenberg, Hedaya, Tannenbaum, and others permit AIH but not while the woman is ritually unclean, whereas

Rabbis Feinstein, Wolkin, Auerbach, and others permit AIH even during this period if no other way proves successful.

An additional requirement before AIH can be performed is an interval of time after the wedding during which pregnancy has been attempted in the usual manner of cohabitation, but without results. This interval must be ten years, according to Rabbi Jacob Yitzchak Weiss,[37] five years in the opinion of Rabbi Feinstein,[38] two years according to Rabbi Karelitz, and long enough to establish the medical necessity for AIH, in the opinion of Rabbi Waldenberg.

Procurement of semen for artificial insemination. Since most rabbinic opinion sanctions AIH under circumstances where pregnancy can be achieved in no other way, the question arises as to how to obtain the semen for the insemination without transgressing the prohibition of improper emission of seed or emission of semen for naught. This was the sin of Er and Onan (Genesis 38:7–10). This subject alone is of such broad dimensions as to require a separate essay, and the interested reader is referred to extensive discussions elsewhere.[39]

In brief, most rabbis (Frank, Feinstein, Waldenberg, Schwadron, Wolkin, Shapiro, Auerbach, Mintzberg, Baumohl) state that procurement of semen by acceptable means from the husband for insemination into his wife is permissible and does not constitute emission of seed for naught, since the semen will be used to fulfill the commandment of procreation. Some, like Rabbis Tannenbaum, Uziel, Hedaya, and Breisch, disagree, but they are in the minority. Two methods of obtaining the sperm are mentioned in the Talmud, where we find a discussion concerning a priest who is wounded in his testicles *(petzuah dakkah)* or whose membrum is cut off *(kerut shafchah):*

> Rabbi Judah stated in the name of Samuel: If it [the membrum] had a small perforation which was closed up, the man is deemed to be unfit if the wound reopens when semen is emitted, but if it does not reopen the man is regarded as fit. . . . Raba, the son of Rabbah, sent to Rabbi Joseph: Will our Master instruct us how to proceed [to test whether the semen will reopen the closed perforation]. The other replied: Warm barley bread is procured and placed upon the man's anus. Thereby the flow of semen sets in, and the effect can be observed. . . . Said Abaye, colored [women's] garments are dangled before him [exciting his passions thus causing semen emission].[40]

Both of these two methods, as well as others, are perfectly acceptable, according to Rabbi Feinstein.[41] In addition, it is permissible to think of a woman in order to excite the emotions and to cause semen emission for the purpose of artificial insemination into one's wife. The least objectionable method is the procurement of sperm from *coitus interruptus*, or, if this is unsatisfactory for any reason, a condom may be applied on the male membrum prior to coitus. These latter two procedures involve the natural sex act and are, therefore, most acceptable to Jewish law. Masturbation to obtain sperm is strongly condemned by Rabbi Feinstein, based upon the following talmudic passage: "Rabbi Eleazer stated: Who are referred to in the scriptural text *Your hands are full of blood* [Isaiah 1:15]? Those that commit masturbation with their hands. It was taught at the school of Rabbi Ishmael: *Thou shalt not commit adultery* [Exodus 20:13] implies that thou shalt not practice masturbation either with hand or with foot."[42]

To have sexual intercourse in the physician's office and for the physician to retrieve the sperm from the vagina of the woman to combine several ejaculates for subsequent insemination is considered licentious and improper, according to Rabbi Feinstein, although Rabbi Waldenberg allows this practice.[43] Rabbi Waldenberg also permits masturbation to obtain semen if all the other methods cannot be employed. He states that, if possible, the physician should perform the masturbation, but if that is not feasible, the husband can do it. Rabbi Waldenberg further states that one is permitted to extract semen directly from the testicle.

Two recent reviews of the subject of artificial insemination in Jewish law have been published, one of which, by M. Stern, is a twenty-six-chapter, profusely annotated and exhaustive review with 186 bibliographic citations.[44]

Conclusions

Artificial insemination using the semen of a donor other than the husband is considered by most rabbinic opinion to be an abomination and strictly prohibited for a variety of reasons, including the possibility of incest, lack of genealogy, and the problems of inheritance. Some authorities regard AID as adultery, requiring the husband to divorce his wife and her forfeiture of the *ketubah*, and even the physician and the donor are guilty when involved in this act akin to adultery. Some rabbinic opinion, however, states that without a sexual act involved, the woman is not guilty of adultery and is not prohibited to cohabit with her husband.

Regarding the status of the child, rabbinic opinion is divided. Most consider the offspring to be legitimate, as was Ben Sira, the product of conception *sine concubito;* a small minority of rabbis consider the child illegitimate; and at least two authorities take a middle view and label the child a *sofek mamzer.* Considerable rabbinic opinion regards the child (legitimate or illegitimate) to be the son of the donor in all respects (i.e., inheritance, support, custody, incest, levirate marriage, and the like). Some regard the child to be the donor's son only in some respects but not others. Some rabbis state that although the child is considered the donor's son in all respects, the donor has not fulfilled the commandment of procreation. A minority of rabbinic authorities asserts that the child is not considered the donor's son at all.

The woman, following AID or AIH, is considered to be the nursing or pregnant wife of another and, if her husband dies or divorces her, she cannot remarry another until after she has finished nursing the child. Several rabbis also invoke this rule to prohibit a man from cohabiting with his pregnant or nursing wife following AID.

There is near unanimity of opinion that the use of semen from the husband is permissible if no other method is possible for the wife to become pregnant. However, certain qualifications exist. There must have been a reasonable period of waiting since marriage (two, five, or ten years or until medical proof of the absolute necessity for AIH), and, according to many authorities, the insemination may not be performed during the wife's period of ritual impurity.

It is permitted by most rabbis to obtain sperm from the husband both for analysis and for insemination, but difference of opinion exists as to the method to be used in its procurement. Masturbation should be avoided if at all possible, and *coitus interruptus* or the use of a condom seem to be the preferred methods.

Since many important legal and moral considerations which cannot be enunciated in the presentation of general principles may weigh heavily upon the verdict in any given situation, it seems advisable to submit each individual case to rabbinic judgment, which, in turn, will be based upon expert medical advice and other prevailing circumstances.

Notes

1. D. P. Murphy and E. F. Torrano, "The Day of Conception: A Study of 48 Woman Having Two or More Conceptions by Donor Insemination," *Fertility and Sterility* 14 (1963): 410–415.

2. Chagigah 14b.

3. Rozanes, Commentary *Mishneh Lemelech* on Maimonides' *Mishneh Torah, Hilchot Ishut* 15:4.

4. Azulai, quoted by I. Jakobovits, in "Artificial Insemination, Birth Control and Abortion," *Harofé Haivri 2* (1953): 169–183 (Eng.) and 114–129 (Heb.); Eybeschutz, Commentary *Bnei Ahuvah* on Maimonides' Code, *Hilchot Ishut* 15:6; Ettlinger, Commentary *Aruch Lenair* on Yebamot 12b.

5. M. Schick (known as *Maharam Schick*), *Taryag Mitzvot*, no. 1; S. Schick, Responsa *Rashbam, Even Haezer*, no. 8.

6. Quoted by J. Sirkes, known as *Bach* or *Beth Chadash*, in his commentary on Jacob ben Asher's *Tur Shulchan Aruch, Yoreh Deah* 195. Also quoted by David ben Samuel Halevy, known as *Taz* or *Turei Zahav*, in his commentary on Joseph Karo's *Shulchan Aruch, Yoreh Deah* 195:7.

7. I. D. Eisenstein, "Alpha Betha de ben Sira," in *Otzar Midrashim* (New York, 1928), p. 43.

8. J. Preuss, *Biblical and Talmudic Medicine*, trans. F. Rosner (New York: Hebrew Publishing Co., 1978), p. 464; H. Friedenwald, *The Jews and Medicine* (Baltimore: Johns Hopkins Press, 1944), vol. 1, p. 386; I. Jakobovits, *Jewish Medical Ethicis* (New York: Bloch, 1959), Appendix on artificial insemination, pp. 244–250.

9. Gans, Responsa *Tzemach David*, p. 14b.

10. Verga, Responsa *Shevet Yehudah*.

11. Leviticus 21:14.

12. Rozanes, Commentary *Mishneh Lemelech* on Maimonides' *Mishneh Torah, Hilchot Issurei Biyah* 17:13.

13. Leviticus 12:2.

14. Uziel, Responsa *Mishpatei Uziel. Even Haezer*, no. 19.

15. Feinstein, Responsa *Iggrot Moshe, Even Haezer*, no. 10.

16. Schwadron, Responsa *Maharsham*, p. 3, no. 268; Baumol, Responsa *Emek Halachah*, no. 68; Wolkin, Responsa *Zekan Aharon*, p. 2, no. 97.

17. Zirelsohn, Responsa *Marchei Lev*, no. 73.

18. Lurie, in *Haposek* (Tel Aviv). Cheshvan–Kislev (5710) 1949; Hedaya, in *Noam* (1948/5718): 130–137.

19. Waldenberg, Responsa *Tzitz Eliezer*, vol. 9, no. 51:4.

20. Breisch, Responsa *Chelkot Yakov*, no. 24.

21. Nathanson, Responsa *Shoel Umeshiv*, 2d ed., p. 3, no. 133; Kirshbaum, Responsa *Menachem Meshiv*, p. 2, no. 26; Pladi, Responsa *Yad Ramah*, quoted by D. B. Kranzer, in *Noam* 1 (1958): 111–123; Neemrok, in *Noam* (1958/5718): 143–144; Auerbach, in ibid., pp. 145–166.

22. Genesis 17:7.
23. *Rashi's* commentary on Yevamot 42a.
24. Leviticus 18:20.
24. Commentary *Chelkat Mechokek* on Joseph Karo's *Shulchan Aruch, Even Haezer* 1:6.
25. Commentary *Beth Shmuel* on Karo's *Shulchan Aruch, Even Haezer* 1:6.
26. Ben Samuel, Responsa *Beit Yakov*, no. 122; Mintzberg, in *Noam* 1 (1958/5718): 129; Duran, Responsa *Tashbatz*, p. 3, no. 263; Ettlinger, Commentary *Aruch Lenair* on Yevamot 10a.
27. Emden, Responsa *She'elat Yavetz*, p. 2, no. 96.
28. M. A. L. Shapiro, in *Noam* 1 (1958/5718): 138–142.
29. Yevamot 36b and 42a.
30. *Tosafot* (various French and German authors of the twelfth and thirteenth century), Commentary on Sotah 42b, s.v. *me'ah pappi;* Jerusalem Talmud, Yevamot 4:2.
31. Commentary of *Rashi* on Sotah 42b, s.v. *bar me'ah pappi.*
32. Maimonides, *Mishneh Torah, Hilchot Gerushin* 11:25.
33. Ben Asher, *Tur Shulchan Aruch, Even Haezer* 13:11; Karo, *Shulchan Aruch, Even Haezer* 13:11.
34. Tanenbaum, Responsa *Divrei Malkiel*, p. 4, nos. 107–108.
35. Azulay, Commentary *Birkei Yoseph, Even Haezer* 1 and 13.
36. Feinstein, Responsa *Iggrot Moshe, Even Haezer*, p. 2, no. 18; A. Wolkin Responsa *Zekan Aharon, Even Haezer*, p. 2, no. 97; Frank, Commentary *Har Zvi, Tur Even Haezer*, no. 1; Yosef, Responsa *Yabeeya Omer*, p. 2, no. 1.
37. Weiss, Responsa *Minchat Yitzchak*, p. 1, no. 50 and p. 3, no. 47.
38. Feinstein, Responsa *Iggrot Moshe, Even Haezer*, p. 2, no. 16.
39. D. M. Feldman, *Birth Control in Jewish Law*, (New York: New York University Press, 1968), pp. 109–169; L. M. Epstein, *Sex Laws and Customs in Judaism* (New York: Ktav, 1967), pp. 144–147; S. J. Zevin in *Talmudic Encyclopedia* (Jerusalem, 1965), vol. 11, pp. 129–141.
40. Yevamot 76a.
41. Feinstein, Responsa *Iggrot Moshe, Even Haezer*, no. 70.
42. Niddah 13b.
43. Waldenberg, Responsa *Tzitz Eliezer*, vol. 3, no. 27 and vol. 9, no. 51.
44. M. Stern, "Artificial Insemination," in *Harefuah Le'or HaHalachah* (Jerusalem. 1980), vol. 1, p. 2, pp. 1–102; A. Steinberg, "Artificial Insemination in Jewish law," *Assia* (1976): 128–141.

9

In Vitro Fertilization, Surrogate Motherhood, and Sex Organ Transplants

General and Medical Aspects

The efforts of Drs. Patrick C. Steptoe and Robert G. Edwards in England culminated in the birth of Louise Brown on July 25, 1978 as a result of *in vitro* fertilization and reimplantation of the human embryo into the mother's womb.[1] The same investigators later reported the birth of a boy by this technique.[2] Since then, several hundred babies have been born by this methodology. More recently, fertilized ovum removal from the womb of one woman and its implantation into a recipient mother has been accomplished with the birth of healthy infants.

This chapter examines the legal, moral, ethical, and religious issues involved in *in vitro* fertilization and reimplantation of the human zygote either into the biologic mother's womb or into a surrogate or host mother's womb. Other related issues will also be mentioned where appropriate. For example, basic principles related to the paternity or maternity of the offspring of *in vitro* fertilization and reimplantation are derived from experience and knowledge about artificial insemination. The latter subject in turn relates to genetic screening and prenatal diagnosis. If amniocentesis reveals the presence of twins, one of whom is normal, the other being afflicted with a serious genetic defect, a serious medical and moral dilemma occurs. It is now possible to selectively terminate or abort the abnormal fetus by intracardiac puncture and exsanguination and to deliver the normal fetus at term,[3] an accomplishment highly publicized in the lay press in view of the danger to the normal fetus.[4] Although it is medically feasible, is this procedure ethically and morally justified?

The transmission of serious genetic defects by artificial insemination using donor sperm from individuals not screened for genetic diseases is also being recognized with increasing frequency.[5] In a recent review of current practice of artificial insemination by donor in the United States, the authors concluded that the screening of sperm donors for genetic diseases is inadequate and that a list of genetic traits needs to be established that can be used routinely for screening donors.[6] This procedure will ensure that children born through artificial insemination have a minimum of genetic defects. What are the ethical, moral, and legal considerations in the establishment and implementation of such procedures?

It is now possible, even if a single unborn fetus is severely abnormal, to perform delicate intrauterine surgery to correct the fetal defect.[7] The ethical dilemmas of this issue were discussed by Fletcher in an editorial,[8] and need to be further explored.

Are there alternatives to *in vitro* fertilization? In a monkey, it is possible to remove an egg from the ovary and to reinsert it low in the Fallopian tube below the point of blockage with subsequent fertilization *in vivo*.[9] Another technique is to bypass the Fallopian tube altogether and to place the ovum directly within the uterine lumen, anticipating that fertilization, cleavage of the embryo, and nidation might all be accomplished within the uterus. A third technique is to insert an egg-embryo chamber in the abdomen into which the fertilized egg is placed, to be transferred at an appropriate time to the uterus. These procedures are still experimental but may, in the future, provide the woman suffering from a "hopeless" tubal condition with several effective therapeutic courses from which to select that may enhance her prospects of successful pregnancy.

Another related issue is the subject of sex organ transplants. Fallopian tube transplantation followed by successful pregnancy has been observed on several occasions in animals and humans, thus providing another alternative to *in vitro* fertilization for Fallopian tube disease.[10] Ovarian transplantation has also been accomplished in both animals and in the human female.[11] Testicular transplantation of an intraabdominal testicle into the scrotum of the same person is technically feasible.[12] Testicular transplantation from one identical twin born with two normal testes to the other twin born with no testicles, with subsequent siring of a child by the previously sterile recipient twin, has also been achieved.[13]

If the ovary of a fertile woman is transplanted into the body of a previously barren woman to enable her to become pregnant and bear children, to whom do the children legally belong, the donor or the recipient of the ovary? What is the filial relationship of a child born following a testicular transplant? These and other moral and ethical questions are tangential but related to the question of the parenthood of a fertilized egg or fetus implanted in a host mother.

Legal Issues and Public Policy

Numerous legal issues have been raised by surrogate mother arrangements. In the typical case, a woman agrees to be artificially inseminated with the sperm from a man whose wife cannot conceive. The surrogate mother also agrees to relinquish her parental rights and turn over the baby to its biological father and his wife, who may then become its adoptive parents. One of the main legal controversies is whether or not the surrogate mother can be paid for these services.

In an article entitled "Contracts to Bear a Child: Compassion or Commercialism?" some of the following legal questions are raised:[14] If a surrogate mother receives a fee, is she being compensated for inconvenience and out-of-pocket expenses, or is she being paid for her baby? Should the surrogate be married or single; have other children or have no children? Should the adoptive parents (including the biological father) meet the surrogate? Should the child know about the surrogate arrangement when he or she grows up? Is monetary compensation the real issue? What kind of counseling should be done with all parties, and what records should be kept? And isn't this a strange thing to be doing in a country that records more than a million and a half abortions a year? Why not attempt to get women who are already pregnant to give birth instead of inducing those who are not pregnant to go through the "experience"?

Is it proper for surrogates to have children to be turned over to single people or homosexual couples? Does the impregnation of the surrogate mother with a married man's sperm amount to adultery? Does the impregnation of a woman with her brother-in-law's sperm constitute a type of incest? What if the surrogate mother decides to have an abortion or to keep the baby? What if the adoptive parents die or get divorced before the birth, or decide they do not want the baby after all? What if the child is born defective? These questions, and many others, merit serious consideration. So far, legal debate has focused primarily on the issue of whether or not surrogate parenting is to be considered baby selling.

Some legal issues related to human *in vitro* fertilization were recently highlighted by Evans and Dixler.[15] The four principal areas of legal concerns are the rights, if any, of the fertilized human egg before implantation (there is a rich body of law on the rights of the unborn but no law on the rights of the test tube embryo); the rights of the would-be parents; the rights and liabilities of the physician and hospital; and the public interest expressed through governmental regulation of the procedure. Because of the legal complexities involved with the *in vitro* fertilization procedure, and because of the lack of legal precedent to guide the parties, the above authors suggest that a written contract be drawn up and make specific proposals about the format and content of such a contract.

Moral and Ethical Issues

Long before the birth of Louise Brown in 1978 by *in vitro* fertilization, the ethical and moral issues involved in this procedure were discussed and debated. On the negative side, one author questions the propriety of perfecting the technologies of human reproduction by experiments on the newborn and the unconceived.[16] He further argues that because the new procedures for *in vitro* fertilization and laboratory culture of human embryos may carry a serious risk of damage to any child so generated, there appears to be no ethical way to proceed. One cannot ethically choose for a child the unknown hazards that he must face, and simultaneously choose to give him life in which to face them. Also strongly opposed to *in vitro* fertilization is a prominent theologian who asserts that this procedure "constitutes unethical medical experimentation on possible future human beings, and, therefore, it is subject to absolute moral prohibition."[17] He rejects rejoinders to all his arguments and concludes that "unless the ethics of the medical research profession is to be radically revised or abandoned we ought not to manipulate or risk the child-to-be." He abhors the extent to which human procreation has been replaced by the idea of "manufacturing" our progeny. He further urges more "animal work" before proceeding to human experimentation, considers *in vitro* fertilization to be pure medical research and not therapeutic in the usual sense, and charges that it is immoral to discard or "terminate the lives of the zygotes, the developing cluster of cells, the blastocysts, the embryos, or the fetuses it will be necessary to kill in the course of developing this procedure."

On the other hand, one of the physicians who was responsible for the birth of Louise Brown justifies his work by saying that in animals the preimplantation embryo is highly resistant to malformation, and that human volunteers are not only experimental subjects but have a chance of ultimately personally benefiting from the work while the methods and technology are being developed.[18] The reimplantation of a human embryo into the mother for the cure of infertility seems to need no moral justification if no other method can be used. Although the underlying infertility is not cured, the desire of (and biblical command to) the parents to have children is fulfilled. The situation is perhaps analogous to a diabetic whose clinical signs and symptoms are treated by insulin but whose underlying disorder is not cured thereby. Edwards is more cautious, however, in his moral approach to the case of surrogate mothers, since there might develop conflicting claims on the child by the embryo donor and the uterine mother, and divided loyalty of the child itself. Further, the surrogate mother might request an abortion or refuse to hand over the child, the donor might reject the child at birth, or the child might suffer psychologically on learning of the circumstances of its birth.

Does one tell the child born of a surrogate mother and/or following *in vitro* fertilization of the circumstances surrounding its birth? What does the surrogate mother tell her own children or friends and neighbors or colleagues at work about the "loss" of the baby if she surrenders it to the adoptive parents? Should she lie, saying the baby had died? What if the adoptive parents die or get divorced before the birth of the child, or decide they do not want the baby after all? What if the child is born defective?

The discussion about the morality and ethics of *in vitro* fertilization and surrogate motherhood relate to similar discussions in regard to abortion, contraception, artificial insemination, genetic engineering, cloning, and the like. These subjects are clearly beyond the scope of this essay. I will also not review the discussions defining the moment when human life begins, the Divine nature of procreation and the marital relationship, the possible "debiologization" of family life,[19] and related issues.

Suffice it to say that *in vitro* fertilization is strongly opposed on moral and ethical grounds by some writers,[20] and just as strongly justified by others, who argue that the procedure "does not pose any moral problems."[21] To assist in resolving the issues following several years of debate in scholarly and professional journals, a 1975 ban on government funding of human research in this area, and the work of the National Commission for the Protection of Human Subjects on fetal research, the Secretary of the United States Department of Health, Education and Welfare established an Ethics Advisory Board. The board rendered its report on March 16, 1979 and concluded that, with certain constraints, research on *in vitro* fertilization and embryo transfer is ethically acceptable. The board agreed "that the human embryo is entitled to profound respect; but this respect does not necessarily encompass the full legal and moral rights attributed to persons." The board expressed concern about the still unanswered questions of safety for both mother and offspring of *in vitro* fertilization and embryo transfer, and about the health and legal status of the children born following such a procedure.[22]

To show respect for life when *in vitro* fertilization is coupled with embryo transfer because an infertile couple is being helped to have a child, the Ethics Advisory Board recommended that the government support research provided that:

A. If the research involves human *in vitro* fertilization without embryo transfer, the following conditions are satisfied:
   1. the research complies with all appropriate provisions of the regulations governing research with human subjects;
   2. the research is designed primarily to establish the safety and efficacy of embryo transfer and to obtain important scientific information toward that end not reasonably attainable by other means;
   3. human gametes used in such research will be obtained exclusively from persons who have been informed of the nature and purpose of the research in which such materials will be used and have specifically consented to such use;
   4. no embryos will be sustained *in vitro* beyond the stage normally associated with the completion of implantation (14 days after fertilization); and
   5. all interested parties and the general public will be advised if evidence begins to show that the procedure entails risk of abnormal offspring higher than those associated with natural human reproduction.

B. In addition, if the research involves embryo transfer following human *in vitro* fertilization, embryo transfer will be attempted only with gametes obtained from lawfully married couples.

A critic of the board's report asks whether it is appropriate for such a board to be so structured that more than half of the members represent the medical and research community. The critic questioned whether a board constituted largely of researchers and oriented to their ethical concerns can be relied upon to say no to research, or whether they may be overwhelmingly disposed to judge research as "ethically defensible."[23] Responding to this criticism, one of the members of the board writes that it would have been inappropriate for the board to have made ethical recommendations and taken public policy stances by adopting any one of the following three positions: that the fertilized ovum is a person with all the claims and rights of persons; that the fertilized ovum is disposable material; or that the fertilized ovum is a living human being, deserving of awe and respect even if not meriting the fullest range of protection we accord persons.[24] To decree or stipulate that one of these positions is certainly the right one would have been impossible for the board; hence, the phrase "acceptable from an ethical standpoint" must be understood to mean "ethically defensible but still legitimately controverted."[25] However, that which is ethically defensible may not necessarily be morally right. "Active euthanasia, deception in research, amniocentesis for sex choice, bypassing informed consent, and possibly even infanticide are all issues where serious, plausible and favorable arguments have been made. Are they ethically acceptable because defensible?"[26] A stalemate on federally funded test tube baby research has developed,[27] while *in vitro* fertilization moves ahead clinically.

The 1981 Principles of Medical Ethics of the American Medical Association state that it is not unethical for a physician to perform *in vitro* fertilization and embryo transplantation within the confines of the professional physician-patient relation upon obtaining the patient's voluntary and informed consent.[28] Only physicians with special knowledge and competence in the use of such procedures should perform them. The patient's expectations of confidentiality should be preserved in all instances. The AMA statement continues by asserting that since *in vitro* fertilization and embryo transplantation is a new and experimental procedure, research studies are needed for the necessary medical knowledge and skills to be developed. Selecting and screening donors to control the transmission of infectious and genetic disease, to the extent current knowledge permits, should be required. To protect the interests of women wishing to be involved in such research projects, the following guidelines should apply:

A. Voluntary and informed consent, in writing, should be given by the patient.
B. Alternative treatment or methods of care should be carefully

evaluated and fully explained to the patient. If simpler and safer treatment is known, it should be pursued.

C. If possible, the risk to the embryo or fetus should be as minimal as is scientifically known to be possible.

These standards should also protect the interest of the fetus and potential newborn, to as great an extent as seems analytically possible.

The debates about the moral and ethical issues involved in *in vitro* fertilization, surrogate motherhood, and related subjects will probably continue for many years to come.

The Jewish View

It is a cardinal principle in Judaism that life is of infinite value and that each moment of life is equal to seventy years thereof. In Jewish law, all biblical and rabbinic commandments are set aside for the overriding consideration of saving a life. It is, therefore, permitted and even mandated to desecrate the Sabbath to save the life of someone who may only live for a short while and certainly for a patient who may recover from illness or traumatic injuries.

A second fundamental principle of Judaism concerns the sanctity of human life. Man was created in the image of God and, hence, human beings are holy and must be treated with dignity and respect, in life and after death. Our bodies are God-given, and we are commanded to care for our physical and mental well-being and to preserve and hallow our health and our lives. Only God gives and takes life.

Are we tampering with life itself when we perform *in vitro* fertilization? Are we interfering with the Divine plan for humanity? If God's will is for a man and/or a woman to be infertile, who are we to undertake test-tube fertilization and embryo reimplantation into the natural or genetic mother, or into a host or surrogate mother, to overcome the infertility problem?

Judaism teaches that nature was created by God for man to use to his advantage and benefit. Hence, animal experimentation is certainly permissible provided one minimizes the pain or discomfort to the animal. The production of hormones such as insulin from bacteria or in tissue culture or in animals by recombinant DNA technology for man's benefit also seems permissible. Gene therapy, such as the replacement of the missing or defective gene in Tay-Sachs disease or hemophilia, if and when it becomes medically possible, may also be sanctioned in Jewish law. But is man permitted to alter humanhood and/or humanity by *in vitro* fertilization, by transfer of the embryo from a woman inseminated with her husband's (or other) sperm into another woman's womb, or by artificial gestation in a test tube or glass womb, or by sex organ or gene transplants, or by genetic screening and/or counseling, and the like?

There exists a considerable body of rabbinic writings devoted to artificial insemination,[29] and many of the principles cited therein apply equally to *in vitro* fertilization. In a recent review, Stern cites Jewish sources which describe pregnancy *sine concubito*, including impregnation in a bathhouse, and discusses the following questions: the legal relationship of the offspring to the sperm donor; the possible fulfillment of the commandment of procreation by the sperm donor; the legality of procurement of sperm from the husband for artificial insemination and the preferred methods for its procurement; the insemination of the husband's sperm into his wife during or shortly after her menstrual cycle when she is *niddah* (ritually unclean); the possibility of the insemination itself rendering her ritually unclean by "opening the mouth of the womb"; the question of the woman becoming ritually unclean following birth after artificial insemination; whether such a male child may be circumcized on the Sabbath; whether such a child absolves the obligation of levirate marriage; whether or not a woman who is inseminated with donor sperm becomes prohibited to her husband; the legitimacy or bastardy of the offspring of artificial insemination using donor sperm; the case where sperm of the husband was mixed with donor sperm prior to insemination; whether or not a woman who claims she became pregnant in a bathhouse is believed; whether or not a husband can divorce his wife if she underwent artificial insemination without his knowledge; the obligation of the father to support his child born after artificial insemination; the status of the child if the sperm donor was a bastard; the case of insemination of semen from a priest into a profaned woman; whether levirate marriage can be consummated through artificial insemination; and the possible legality of using sperm from a gentile donor for artificial insemination into a Jewish woman.[30]

In brief, there is near unanimity of opinion that the use of semen from the husband is permissible if no other method is possible for the wife to become pregnant. However, certain qualifications exist. There must have been a reasonable period of waiting since marriage (two, five, or ten years or until medical proof of the absolute necessity for artificial insemination), and, according to many authorities, the insemination may not be performed during the wife's period of ritual impurity. Artificial insemination using the semen of a donor other than the husband is considered by most rabbinic opinion to be an abomination and strictly prohibited for a variety of reasons, including the possibility of incest (the child born of such insemination may later marry a sibling, unknowingly), lack of genealogy (the father's identity is unknown), and the problems of inheritance (does the child inherit the real father, the adopted father, or both). A few rabbis regard such insemination as adultery, requiring the husband to divorce his wife and her forfeiture of the marriage settlement *(ketubah)*. Most rabbinic opinion, however, states that without a sexual act involved, the woman is not guilty of adultery and is not prohibited to cohabit with her husband.

Regarding the status of the child, rabbinic opinion is divided. Most consider the offspring to be legitimate, as was Ben Sira, the product of conception *sine concubito;* a small minority of rabbis consider the child illegitimate, and at least two authorities take a middle view. Considerable rabbinic opinion regards the child (legitimate or illegitimate) to be the son of the donor in all respects (i.e., inheritance, support, custody, incest, levirate marriage, and the like). Some regard the child to be the donor's son only in some respects but not others. Some rabbis state that although the child is considered the donor's son in all respects, the donor has not fulfilled the commandment of procreation. A minority of rabbinic opinion asserts that the child is not considered the donor's son at all.

It is permitted by most rabbis to obtain sperm from the husband both for analysis and for insemination, but difference of opinion exists as to the method to be used in the procurement of it. Masturbation should be avoided if at all possible, and *coitus interruptus*, retrieval of sperm from the vagina, or the use of a condom seem to be the preferred methods.

In vitro fertilization, embryo transfer, host motherhood and sex organ transplants in Jewish law have been the subjects of several recent publications in Hebrew and in English.[31] In a situation in which the husband produces far too few sperm with each ejaculate to impregnate his wife or where a woman is unable to move the egg from the ovary into the uterus because of blocked Fallopian tubes, the former Israeli Chief Rabbi Ovadiah Yosef gave his qualified approval to the *in vitro* fertilization of the woman's egg with the husband's sperm and the reimplantation of the fertilized zygote or tiny embryo into the same woman's womb.[32] Another former Chief Rabbi, Shlomo Goren, asserted that conception in this manner is morally repugnant but legally unobjectionable. This situation represents a type of barrenness akin to physical illness and, therefore, justifies acts which entail a small amount of risk, such as the procurement of eggs from the mother's ovary by laparoscopy, a minor surgical procedure.

There is certainly no question of adultery involved, since the sperm used is that of the husband. Sperm and egg procurement for this procedure are permissible because the aim is to fulfill the biblical commandment of procreation. The offspring is legitimate and the parents thereby fulfill their obligation of having children. However, certain serious moral and Jewish legal problems relate to this type of test-tube baby.[33] If one uses sperm other than that of the husband, objections as discussed above under artificial insemination exist. Furthermore, if one obtains several eggs from the mother's ovary at one time and fertilizes all of them so as to select the best embryo for reimplantation, is one permitted to destroy the other fertilized eggs? Do they not constitute human seed and, therefore, should not be "cast away for naught"? Is one permitted to perform medical research on the unused fertilized eggs? What is the status of other fertilized ova in the test tube? Is the destruction of such fertilized ova tantamount to abortion? Is such a fertilized ovum regarded as "mere water" during the first forty days of its development?

In Judaism there is no concept of waste applied to the tens of millions of superfluous sperm which are lost following normal coitus. Perhaps excess fertilized eggs might be implanted into non-ovulating women. What, then, should be the approach if no woman is available for an additional implant and there has been more than one successful fertilization? If a fertilized ovum is "more than nothing," would Jewish law mandate *in vitro* procedures with only one ovum at a time? There may well be a Jewish legal and ethical distinction between a fertilized egg in a test tube and a fertilized egg in a uterus. The question of the possible independent existence of a zygote has legal import. Jewish law requires the desecration of the Sabbath to preserve the existence of an embryo in the mother's womb even less than forty days old. If there is no human fetal life outside the uterus, a superfluous fertilized ovum could be disposed of by any means, such as flushing down the drain. An alternative course of action would be to refrain from supplying nutrients to the ovum, thereby allowing it to perish. One can redefine the question in terms of whether or not an unfertilized egg may be deemed to be of ethical import as potential life. Since the vast majority of unfertilized sperm and eggs are never fertilized and do not constitute new life, only a fertilized ovum might be considered as potential life. If a fertilized ovum were equated with human life, Jewish law would even require the expenditure of substantial sums of money to transport a superfluous fertilized ovum great distances, if necessary, for implantation into a nonovulating woman.

The Committee on Medical Ethics of the Federation of Jewish Philanthropies of New York concluded that a fertilized egg not in the womb, but in an environment—the test tube—in which it can never attain viability, does not have humanhood and may be discarded or used for the advancement of scientific knowledge.[34] It should also be stressed that even in the absence of Jewish legal or moral objections to *in vitro* fertilization using the husband's sperm, no woman is required to submit to this procedure. The obligations of women, whether by reason of the scriptural exhortation to populate the universe or by virtue of the marital contract, are limited to bearing children by means of natural intercourse.[35]

If and when medical science develops more advanced techniques of test-tube gestation, it may be necessary to reexamine these moral and legal questions. Herschler addresses the issue of a fetus incubated for its full gestation in a totally artificial womb or incubator without using either the natural mother or a surrogate mother's uterus.[36] Is such a child human when it is "born"? Although this creature may have the hereditary characteristics of its biological parents, humanhood is usually assumed to occur following natural conception, pregnancy, and birth through a woman's womb. Does the interruption of this natural process even for a short period, such as for *in vitro* fertilization, negate the humanhood of such an infant? Is such an infant to be considered as a *golem* (artificially created "human" being) or as an angel, neither of whom are conceived and born from a woman's womb, and neither of whom are included in the human race? If so, destroying them might not be considered an act of murder. Would the destruction of a baby "born" in an artificial womb or incubator without ever having been in a human uterus be an act of murder?

Herschler cites numerous sources, including the famous talmudic passage which describes a *golem*, and concludes that the latter is not human but akin to a robot. On the other hand, a baby born after *in vitro* fertilization is derived from human seed, both egg and sperm, and matures and grows according to the laws of nature. Therefore, such a baby—even if totally gestated in an artificial womb—should be considered human with all the legal and moral responsibilities of a similar child born in the usual manner. Yet Herschler simultaneously concludes that destroying an infant that came into being outside a human uterus may not be legally considered an act of murder. Perhaps if someone had killed Adam, the first man in this world, he would not have been guilty of murder, because Adam was not born from a woman's womb but was created by Almighty God. The question, therefore, arises as to whether or not one is permitted to desecrate the Sabbath and other laws to save the life of such a zygote or fetus or baby born in an artificial incubator, just as one is so obligated in Jewish law for the usual fetus in its mother's womb.

Finally, in regard to *in vitro* fertilization, it may be possible to separate male-producing from female-producing sperm and thereby to predetermine the sex of one's baby, either by artificial insemination of male- or female-producing sperm or the use of the appropriate sperm to fertilize an egg in the test tube for reimplantation into the mother. Is such sex predetermination permissible in Jewish law? This subject is discussed in some detail elsewhere.[37] The freezing of human sperm and eggs for later use is another subject not yet adequately addressed by Jewish authorities.

The case of host motherhood in Jewish law concerns the implantation of a fertilized egg or tiny embryo into the womb of a woman other than the donor of the egg, perhaps because the true mother is unable to carry a fetus to term.[38] The host mother thus serves as a surrogate and "incubates" the fetus for the true mother. The fetus can either be transplanted from one mother to another or the egg and sperm are united *in vitro* in a test tube and directly implanted into the host mother. Another recent development is called adoptive pregnancy, in which a woman is artificially inseminated and within a week after conception, the embryo is flushed from her womb and transferred to another woman who carries it to term and "becomes the mother." There is a serious question in Jewish law whether or not the biological mother is allowed to give up her child for transplantation into another "womb" and whether or not the host mother is allowed to accept it. What is the legal parenthood of the child? If a married woman becomes a host mother, would Jewish law require her to abstain from sexual relations with her husband for ninety days, in order to ensure that the child is not his, that is to say, that she did not miscarry the implanted fetus and become pregnant by her husband? The husband would certainly not have to divorce his wife for serving as a host mother, since no act of adultery was committed.

Regarding the permissibility of host motherhood in Judaism, the Federation's Committee on Medical Ethics states that such procedures are only permissible in the absence of an alternative and may not be resorted to by fertile parents who prefer the services of a host mother.[39] While the use of surrogate mothers for the convenience of couples able to have children cannot be condoned, an infertile couple may have recourse to a surrogate mother in the absence of alternatives "to save a marriage or bring happiness to the depressed." There should, of course, be absolute assurance that the surrogate is participating without coercion and with fully informed consent, and that the arrangement is protected by all necessary legal and social safeguards.

According to Britain's Chief Rabbi Immanuel Jakobovits, to abort a mother's naturally fertilized egg and to reimplant it in a host mother for reasons of "convenience for women who seek the gift of a child without the encumbrance and disfigurement of pregnancy is offensive to moral susceptibilities." Furthermore, says Jakobovits, "to use another person as an 'incubator' and then take from her the child she carried and delivered for a fee is a revolting degradation of maternity and an affront to human dignity."[40]

In order to apply the laws pertaining to the firstborn, it is important to know whether the biological or the host mother is regarded as having given birth to the infant. If fetal transfer to a host mother is performed after forty days postconception, Rosenfeld considers the child to be the legal offspring of its biological parents, since the child became "completed" while still in the biological mother's body, and she is regarded as having given birth to it.[41] Jewish law may view differently the situation of fetal transfer prior to forty days after conception or *in vitro* fertilization followed by host motherhood.

Hershler states that the laws of genealogy are laws of the Torah and are not based on the laws of heredity or genetics.[42] In Jewish law, a child is considered to be genealogically descended from its father. If the father is a priest or a Levite, so is the son. In genetics and heredity, continues Hershler, father and mother play equal roles, as it is written: *male and female did He create them.*[43] The Talmud states:

> There are three partners in man: the Holy One, blessed be He, his father, and his mother. His father supplies the semen of the white substance out of which are formed the child's bones, sinews, nails, the brain in his head, and the white in his eye. His mother supplies the semen of the red substance out of

> which are formed his skin, flesh, hair, blood, and the black of his eye. And the Holy One, blessed be He, gives him the spirit and the breath, beauty of features, eyesight, the power of hearing and the ability to speak and walk, understanding, and discernment.[44]

Hershler also postulates that a baby born from a totally artificial womb may have no genealogical relationship to the biologic father. On the other hand, it may be logical to assume that the genealogical relationship is established immediately at the time of ejaculation during normal intercourse or at the time of *in vitro* fertilization, even long before the development of an embryo or fetus. The sperm itself establishes the filial relationship. Hershler cites several rabbinic sources to support the above views.

Finally, based on the biblical story of the birth of Dinah to Leah and the talmudic discussion thereon,[45] Hershler concludes that the maternity of the child is determined by the mother who nurtures and gives birth to the baby, not necessarily the biologic mother. Bleich expands on this subject by pointing out that the Talmud declares that Dinah was born a female as a result of Leah's prayers during her pregnancy.[46] Knowing that Jacob would become the father of a total of twelve sons, and not wishing her sister Rachel to bear their husband fewer sons than the maidservants Bilhah and Zilpah, Leah prayed that her already conceived fetus would be born a female. It is clear from the parallel narrative in the Palestinian Talmud,[47] continues Bleich, that the phenomenon described by the sages involved an *in utero* sex change. However, one biblical commentator states that what transpired was not a sex change in Leah's fetus but a physical exchange of the fetus from the womb of Leah to the womb of Rachel, and vice versa, i.e., an embryo transfer.[48] Dinah was thus conceived by Rachel but transferred to the womb of Leah, while Joseph was conceived by Leah and transferred to the womb of Rachel. Bleich further points out that a talmudic commentary[49] asserts that this double embryo transfer is also the correct interpretation of the talmudic narrative.[50] Finally, Bleich cites an alternative rabbinic opinion which concludes that maternal relationship is established by conception rather than birth.

Bleich had earlier addressed the issue of maternal identity by citing a rabbinic responsum by Rabbi Y. A. Kamelher which discusses a case in which the ovary of a fertile woman was transplanted into the body of a previously barren woman to enable her to become pregnant and bear children.[51] The same type of case was also discussed in two other rabbinic responsa cited by Bleich. Adultery is certainly not involved on the part of the recipient women even if the donor of the ovary was a married woman. The recipient of the ovarian transplant would probably be considered the legal mother of any child subsequently conceived and born because a transplanted organ is ordinarily deemed to become an integral part of the body of the recipient.

Another view cited by Bleich is that the ovary alone is an inert organ and incapable of reproduction were it not for the physiological contributions of the recipient. Furthermore, in the case of fetal transplantation, the host mother nurtures the embryo and sustains gestation and, perhaps, should be considered the legal mother of the offspring. According to other authorities, the donor mother alone may be viewed as the mother in the eyes of Jewish law, since the prohibition against feticide is applicable from the moment of conception. These authorities deem the fetus to be a human being with identity and parentage from the earliest stages of gestation. One can also raise the possibility of two maternal relationships existing simultaneously, the child thus having two mothers, the donor or biological mother and the host mother.

Jewish sources do not discuss testicular transplants, but similar principles would probably apply. The question of paternity in the case of a testicular transplant and maternity in the case of an ovarian transplant is related to the question discussed above of the parenthood of a fertilized egg or fetus implanted in a host mother. There may be a distinction between the transplantation of a sex organ and the transplantation of any other organ. The rule that a transplanted organ becomes an integral part of the body of the recipient may not apply to the implantation of a zygote or embryo into a host mother's womb or to the transplantation of ovary or testicle. Sperm and egg retain the full genetic identity of their donors. The process of fertilization whether *in vivo* or *in vitro* does not alter the genetic paternity or maternity of the eventual fetus. An "incubator mother" may not have maternal status. If it were possible for a full nine-month gestation to occur in an artificial incubator, the artificial incubator would certainly not be considered to be the mother of the infant.

Since sperm is produced within the testicle, after the first ejaculation in a case of testicular transplant, the sperm are produced by the recipient rather than by the donor. Similarly, following an ovarian transplant, the nourishment and maturation of eggs within the ovary depend upon the recipient and not the donor. There may, however, be a difference between a testicular transplant, where the sperm are to be produced in the future, and an ovarian transplant, where the ovary already contains the primordial egg cells at the time of the transplant. A transplanted ovary is an organ which functions within the existing physiology of the recipient, whereas a transplanted testicle is more like germ-plasm which constitutes a reservoir of genetic material. However, one should note that a gamete maintains its own individuality and retains the genetic code of the donor without reflecting the genetic code of the recipient. Because of genetic constancy, the transplanted ovary or testes are not free of the donor. For example, if the donor is a carrier of a detrimental trait, such as hemophilia or Tay-Sachs disease, the trait might appear in the offspring.

Is there a difference in Jewish law between a testicular transplant from a random donor and one from an identical twin brother of the recipient, in which case the genetic material of the donor is identical to that of the recipient? The source of the donor also raises a specific Jewish legal issue; since castration is biblically prohibited except for the preservation of human life, must one resort nearly exclusively to the use of cadaver ovaries and testicles for transplantation?

The medical problems of removing the ovum, modifying some of its genes by microsurgical techniques, and replacing the viable ovum in the mother have not yet been surmounted. However, assuming such surgery can be successfully performed, Rosenfeld contends that gene surgery might be permissible in Jewish law because genes are submicroscopic particles and no process invisible to the naked eye could be forbidden in Jewish law.[52] Laws of forbidden foods do not apply to microorganisms. The priest only declares ritually unclean that which his eyes can see. On the other hand, a newborn infant with ambiguous genitalia would probably need a chromosome analysis (microscopic examination) to establish genetic sex.

Another argument for the permissibility of gene surgery is the fact that the ovum (or sperm) is not a person, since conception has not yet taken place. Thus, gene manipulation would not be considered as tampering with an existing human being but only with a potential one. Some authorities, however, would argue that the destruction of even a potential human being (either the unborn fetus or the unfertilized human seed) is prohibited in Jewish law.[53]

Rosenfeld also argues that any surgery performed on a live human being must certainly be permitted on an ovum (or sperm) before conception. For example, if a surgical cure for hemophilia or Tay-

Sachs disease were possible, it would surely be permissible; hence, it would certainly be permissible to cure hemophilia or Tay-Sachs disease by gene surgery.

If it were possible to transplant one or more genes of one person into the ovum or sperm of another, the following Jewish legal questions would arise: Are gene transplants considered to be a type of perverted sex act between the gene donor and the recipient? Would such transplants be forbidden, in particular, if donor and recipient were close relatives? Would a child conceived from such a manipulated ovum or sperm be regarded as related to the gene donor? Can one draw parallels from the rabbinic responsa dealing with ovarian transplants and conclude that since no sex act is involved in a gene transplant, the recipient is not forbidden to marry the donor's relatives, and the child conceived and born following a gene transplant is not related to the gene donor? As already mentioned, in most organ transplants (kidney, cornea, heart, ovary, "gene") the organ becomes an integral part of the recipient.[54] The only exception may be the brain, since there is evidence to support the position that the legal identity of a person follows the brain.[55]

Notes

1. P. C. Steptoe, and R. G. Edwards, "Birth After the Reimplantation of a Human Embryo," *Lancet* 2 (1978): 366.

2. R. Edwards and P. Steptoe, *A Matter of Life* (London: Hutchinson, 1980).

3. T. D. Kerenyi and U. Chitkara, "Selective Birth in Twin Pregnancy with Discordancy for Down's Syndrome," *New England Journal of Medicine* 304 (1981): 1525–1527.

4. H. M. Schmeck, Jr., "Twin Found Defective in Womb Reported Destroyed in Operation," *New York Times*, June 18, 1981, pp. 1 and 19; E. Edelson, "Rare Abortion Saves a Twin," *New York Daily News*, June 18, 1981, p. 4.

5. W. G. Johnson, R. C. Schwartz and A. M. Chutorian, "Artificial Insemination by Donors: The Need for Genetic Screening, Late-Infantile G_{M2}—Gangliosidosis Resulting from This Technique," *New England Journal of Medicine* 304 (1981): 755–757; D. N. Shapiro and R. J. Hutchinson, "Familial Histiocytosis in Offspring of Two Pregnancies After Artificial Insemination," ibid., pp. 757–759.

6. M. Curie-Cohen, L. Luttrell and S. Shapiro, "Current Practice of Artificial Insemination by Donor in the United States," *New England Journal of Medicine* 300 (1979): 585–590.

7. M. R. Harrison, M. S. Golbus, and R. A. Filly, "Management of the Fetus with a Correctable Congenital Defect," *Journal of the American Medical Association* 246 (1981): 775–777.

8. J. C. Fletcher, "The Fetus as Patient: Ethical Issues," *Journal of the American Medical Association* 246 (1981): 772-774.

9. G. D. Hodgen, "In Vitro Fertilization and Alternatives," *Journal of the American Medical Association* 246 (1981): 590–597.

10. B. M. Cohen, "Fallopian Tube Transplantation and Its Future," *Clinical Obstetrics and Gynecology* 23 (1980): 1275–1292.

11. S. H. Sturgis and H. Castellanos, "Ovarian Homografts in Organic Filter Chambers," *Annals of Surgery* 156 (1962): 367–376; R. Blanco, "Ovarian Transplantation in the Human Female" (Paper presented before the Eighth Congress of Fertility and Sterility, Buenos Aires, 1974).

12. S. J. Silber "The Intra-Abdominal Testes: Microvascular Autotransplantation," *Journal of Urology* 125 (1981): 329–333.

13. S. J. Silber, "Transplantation of a Human Testis for Anorchia," *Fertility and Sterility* 30 (1978): 181–187.

14. G. J. Annas, "Contracts to Bear a Child: Compassion or Commercialism," *Hastings Center Report* 11 (1981): 23–24.

15. M. I. Evans and A. O. Dixler, "Human In Vitro Fertilization: Some Legal Issues," *Journal of the American Medical Association* 245 (1981): 2324–2327.

16. L. R. Kass "Babies by Means of *In Vitro* Fertilization: Unethical

Experiments on the Unborn?" *New England Journal of Medicine* 285 (1971): 1174–1179.

17. P. Ramsey, "Shall We 'Reproduce'? I. The Medical Ethics of *In Vitro* Fertilization. II. Rejoinders and Future Forecast," *Journal of the American Medical Association* 220 (1972): 1356–1360 and 1480–1485.

18. R. G. Edwards, "Fertilization of Human Eggs *In Vitro:* Morals, Ethics and the Law," *Quarterly Review of Biology* 49 (1974): 3–26.

19. R. McCormick, "Genetic Medicine: Notes on the Moral Literature," *Theological Studies* 32 (1972): 531–552.

20. Kass, op. cit., Ramsey, op. cit.

21. Edwards, op. cit.

22. M. O. Steinfels, "*In Vitro* Fertilization: Ethically Acceptable Research," *Hastings Center Report* 9 (1979): 5–8.

23. Ibid.

24. R. A. McCormick, "The EAB and *In Vitro* Fertilization," *Hastings Center Report* 9 (1979): 4.

25. M. O. Steinfels, "The EAB and *In Vitro* Fertilization," *Hastings Center Report* 9 (1979): 4 and 46.

26. Ibid.

27. S. Abramowitz, "A Stalemate on Test Tube Baby Research," *Hastings Center Report* 14 (1984): 5–9.

28. "Recent Opinions of the Judicial Council of the American Medical Association," *Journal of the American Medical Association* 251 (1984): 2078–2079.

29. F. Rosner, "Artificial Insemination in Jewish Law," *Judaism* 19 (1970): 452–464; I. Jakobovits, "Artificial Insemination," in *Jewish Medical Ethics* (New York: Bloch, 1975), pp. 244–250 and 261–266.

30. M. Stern, *Harefuah Le'Or Hahalachah* [Medicine in the light of Halachah], vol. 1 (Jerusalem: Institute for Research in Medicine and Halachah, 1980), pt. 1, Abortion, pt. 2, Artificial Insemination.

31. M. Hershler, "*Bayoth Hilchatiyoth Betinok Mavchanah*" [Jewish legal issues relating to test-tube babies], *Halachah Urefuah 1* (1980): 307–320; M. Drori, "*Hahanadassah Hagenetis: Iynn Rishoni Beheebatim Hamishpatiyim Vehahalachotiyim* [Genetic engineering: Preliminary discussion of its legal and halachic aspects], *Techumin* 1 ed. Wahrhaftig, Winter 5740 [1980]: 280–296; A. Steinberg, "*Tinok Mavchanah*" [Test-tube baby], *Assia* 6, no. 3 (1979): 11–16; J. D. Bleich, "Test Tube Babies," in *Jewish Bioethics*, ed. F. Rosner and J. D. Bleich (New York: Hebrew Publishing Co., 1979), pp. 80–85; idem, *Judaism and Healing: Halakhic Perspectives* (New York: Ktav Publishing House, 1981), pp. 85–95; idem, "Host Mothers," in *Contemporary Halakhic Problems* (New York: Ktav and Yeshiva University Press, 1977), pp. 106–108; D. M. Feldman and F. Rosner eds., *A Compendium on Medical Ethics: Jewish Moral, Ethical and Religious Principles in Medical Practice*, 6th ed. (New York: Federation of Jewish Philanthropies, 1984). pp. 51–52; A. Rosenfeld, "Generation, Gestation and Judaism," *Tradition* 12 (1971): 78–87.

32. Bleich, "Test Tube Babies" and "Host Mothers."

33. F. Rosner. In vitro Fertilization and Surrogate motherhood: the Jewish View. *Journal of Religion and Health* 22 (1983): 139–160.

34. Feldman and Rosner, *Compendium on Medical Ethics.*

35. Bleich, *Judaism and Healing*, p. 88; idem, "Host Mothers."

36. Hershler, "Bayoth Hilchatiyoth Betinok Mavchanah."

37. F. Rosner, "Sex Determination as Described in the Talmud," in *Medicine in the Bible and the Talmud* (New York: Ktav and Yeshiva University Press, 1977), pp. 173–178; idem, "The Biblical and Talmudic Secret for Choosing One's Baby's Sex," *Israel Journal of Medical Sciences* 15 (1979): 894–898.

38. Hershler, "Bayoth Hilchatiyoth Betinok Mavchanah"; Drori, "Hahanadassah Hagenetis"; Steinberg, "Tinok Mavchanah"; Bleich, "Test Tube Babies," *Judaism and Healing*, pp. 92–95, and "Host Mothers"; Feldman and Rosner, *Compendium on Medical Ethics*, pp. 51–52; Rosenfeld, "Generation, Gestation and Judaism."

39. Feldman and Rosner, *Compendium on Medical Ethics.*

40. Jakobovits, "Artifical Insemination," pp. 261–266.

41. Rosenfeld, "Generation, Gestation and Judaism," pp. 78–87.

42. Hershler, "Bayoth Hilchatiyoth Betinok Mavchanah," pp. 307–320.

43. Genesis 5:2.

44. Niddah 31a.

45. Genesis 30:21; Berachot 60a.

46. J. D. Bleich, "Maternal Identity," *Tradition* 19 (1981): 359–360.

47. Berachot 9:3.

48. *Targum Yonatan* on Genesis 30:21.

49. Commentary of Rabbi Samuel Edels, known as *Maharsha*, on Niddah 31a.

50. Berachot 60a.

51. Bleich, *Judaism and Healing*, p. 93; "Host Mothers."

52. A. Rosenfeld, "Judaism and Gene Design," *Tradition* 13 (1972): 71–80.

53. F. Rosner, "The Jewish Attitude Toward Abortion," *Tradition* 10 (1968): 48–71.

54. F. Rosner, "Organ Transplantation in Jewish Law," In *Jewish Bioethics* (New York: Hebrew Publishing Co., 1979), pp. 358–374.

55. A. Rosenfeld, "The Heart, the Head and the Halakhah," *New York State Journal of Medicine* 70 (1970): 2615–2618.

10

Sex Preselection and Predetermination

There are several methods of sex preselection. One of the most reliable is to determine the sex of an unborn fetus by chromosome analysis of cultured amniotic fluid cells. Since this procedure takes two to three weeks, recombinant DNA analysis of amniotic fluid and chorionic villus biopsy have been introduced as rapid screening tests for antenatal sex determination.[1] Noninvasive methods such as sonography can also help determine fetal sex *in utero*. If the fetus is not of the desired sex, it can be aborted. Judaism, however, unequivocally rejects the option of terminating a pregnancy simply because the fetus is not of the desired sex.[2] A more detailed discussion of the Jewish attitude toward abortion is presented elsewhere in this book (see chap. 12).

Another method of sex preselection involves procurement of sperm from the prospective father, the separation of androsperm (for males) from gynosperm (for females), and the artificial insemination of androsperm, if a male offspring is desired, into the prospective mother. This procedure results in a lower pregnancy rate than the insemination of the unseparated and less manipulated sperm but about 70 percent male progeny.[3] The Jewish legal and ethical issues pertaining to artificial insemination are also discussed in detail elsewhere in this book (see chap. 9).

A third method of sex preselection is the timing of intercourse. The proportion of male births is highest if intercourse occurs several days before ovulation.[4] In Jewish law, husband and wife are forbidden to cohabit during her menstrual period and for seven "clean" days thereafter (*niddah* period), effectively eliminating this method from consideration. Another study, however, has shown that more boys (65.5 percent) than girls are born to Jewish women who observe the Orthodox ritual of *niddah* and resume intercourse two days after ovulation.[5]

A fourth method of sex preselection is the manipulation of the acidity and alkalinity of the cervical and vaginal secretions. In human sperm, the larger, oval-shaped, female-producing sperm are said to be resistant to an acid environment, whereas the smaller, round-headed, but more numerous male-producing sperm succumb in an acid environment.[6] A variety of techniques are recommended to increase the alkalinity in the female lower genital tract if a male offspring is desired.

The secret of sex preselection and sex predetermination was already known in biblical and talmudic times,[7] thus fulfilling King Solomon's assertion that *there is nothing new under the sun.*[8] The key talmudic passage on this subject is as follows:[9]

> Rabbi Isaac, citing Rabbi Ammi, stated: If the woman emits her semen first she bears a male child; if the man emits his semen first she bears a female child; for it is said: *If a woman emits semen and bears a manchild.*[10] Our rabbis taught: At first it used to be said that if the woman emits her semen first she will bear a male, and if the man emits his semen first she will bear a female, but the sages did not explain the reason, until Rabbi Zadok came and explained it: *These are the sons of Leah, whom she bore unto Jacob in Paddan Aram with his daughter Dinah.*[11] Scripture thus ascribes the males to the females [i.e., sons of Leah] and the females to the males [i.e., his daughter Dinah].
>
> *And the sons of Ulam were mighty men of valor, archers, and had many sons, and sons' sons.*[12] Now is it within the power of man to increase the number of sons and sons' sons? But the fact is that because they contained themselves during intercourse, in order that their wives should emit their semen first, so that their children should be males, Scripture attributes to them the same merit as if they had themselves caused the increase of the number of their sons and sons' sons. This explains what Rabbi Kattina said: "I could make all my children to be males."

Although *many sons and sons' sons* could refer to offspring in general, both male and female, Rabbi Samuel Edels, known as

Maharsha, in his commentary on the above talmudic passage, explains that the phrase *men of valor and archers* indicates they were all males. The Talmud seems to be referring to orgasm and recommends that a woman reach orgasm first if a male offspring is desired. This is what Rabbi Kattina meant in his assertion, "I could make all my children males," indicating that with proper restraint to assure that his wife experienced orgasm prior to his own ejaculation, the desired result would be obtained.

The Talmud continues with the statement that "he who desires all his children to be males should cohabit twice in succession."[13] This advice to the husband to repeat the coital act in order to increase the chance of a male birth is explained by Rabbi Solomon ben Isaac, popularly known as *Rashi*, that during the second intercourse the woman will certainly "emit seed first." Apparently, if she did not reach orgasm first and did not conceive with the first ejaculation, she may be impregnated as a result of the second intercourse, during which she should be allowed to reach orgasm first. Perhaps *Rashi* is describing the postcoital refractory period in the man and assumes that the woman would certainly reach orgasm first during the second intercourse and therefore a male offspring would result.

Two discussions in the Talmud raise the question of what happens if both man and woman emit seed simultaneously.[14] Several possible answers are given: the offspring may be a hermaphrodite *(androginos)*, one whose sex is unknown *(tumtum)*, or twins, one male and one female.

Elsewhere, the Talmud describes a "village of males" (*kfar dikraya*), so called because women used to bear male children first, finally a girl, and then no more.[15]

Another talmudic passage states that if a man's wife is pregnant and he prays that God grant that his wife bear a male child, it is a vain prayer.[16] The Talmud then asks:

> Does such a prayer avail? Has not Rabbi Isaac, the son of Rabbi Ammi, said that if a man first emits seed, the child will be a girl; if the woman first emits seed, the child will be a boy? [which shows that it is fixed beforehand]. With what case are we dealing here? For instance, they both emitted seed at the same time.[17]

Apparently, since the sex of the fetus is already determined at the time of intercourse, a prayer to change the sex of the child is considered vain. The only exception seems to be the situation where both husband and wife "emitted seed" simultaneously, in which case the sex of the fetus remains indeterminate for forty days, during which time prayer may be efficacious to ensure a male offspring.

The Talmud also declares that "the world cannot exist without males or without females. Happy is he whose children are males, and woe unto him whose children are females."[18] One can only offer speculations about the meaning of this statement. It is possible that the agricultural society of talmudic times required considerable physical labor, and hence the strength of the male gender was a desirable goal. Another reason might be the pragmatic concern for the need to raise a dowry for one's daughters. The real reason is not important for the present essay.

Other advice to sire male offspring is offered by the Talmud, which asserts: "What should a person do so that his children will be males? Rabbi Eliezer says: He should distribute money among the poor. Rabbi Joshua says: He should gladden his wife prior to intercourse."[19]

A final talmudic passage concerns one of twelve questions that the Alexandrians addressed to Rabbi Joshua ben Chananiah:

> What should a man do that he may have male children? He replied: He should marry a wife that is worthy of him, and conduct himself in modesty at the time of marital intercourse. They said to him: Did not many act in this manner but it did not avail them? Rather, let him pray for mercy from Him to whom are the children, for it is said: *Lo, children are a heritage of the Lord, the fruit of the womb is a reward.*[20] [Seeing that one has in any case to pray for mercy], what then does he teach us? That one without the other does not suffice. What is exactly meant by "the fruit of the womb is a reward"? Rabbi Chama, son of Rabbi Chaninah, replied: As a reward for containing oneself [during intercourse] in the womb, in order that one's wife may emit the semen first, the Holy One, blessed be He, gives one the reward of the fruit of the womb.[21]

The often-repeated talmudic advice to have the woman "emit semen first" in order to have male offspring is usually assumed to refer to orgasm. Is it possible that it refers to ovulation? If so, then Shettles's hypothesis[22] may in fact explain the talmudic discussion in that ovulation represents a time when cervical secretions are alkaline, allowing the male-producing sperm to predominate. Does the phrase "if a woman emits seed" refer to female orgasm? We know that orgasm increases the flow of alkaline secretions, which would also enhance the activity of the male-producing sperm. It would seem obvious from a number of the previous citations that the meaning must be orgasm rather than ovulation, for otherwise it would not make sense to speak of the men restraining themselves during intercourse in order to allow their wives to "emit seed" first.

Let us turn to biblical commentaries for assistance in the interpretation of the key scriptural phrase, *if a woman emits semen [tazria] and bears a manchild,*[23] on which is based the talmudic pronouncement regarding sex determination. Rabbi Abraham Ibn Ezra asserts:

> Many say that if the woman emits her seed first she bears a male child. . . . the view of the Greek savants is that the woman has the seed and the male seed causes it to jell and the entire son comes from the blood of the woman. Actually, the explanation of the word *tazria* is "to give forth seed," because she is like earth.

The phrase "she is like earth" is explained by a later biblical commentator, known as *Sifsei Chachamim*, that "a woman is like earth, which sprouts that which one plants therein, and man was created from earth." Rabbi Meir ben Yechiel Michael, known as *Malbim*, echoes the same sentiment: "The fetus comes out from the site of semen implantation like the earth, which sprouts that which is planted."

Rabbi Moses ben Nachman, known as Nachmanides or *Ramban*, in his commentary on the pertinent passage in Leviticus, states:

> When the sages interpreted the phrase *if a woman conceives [tazria]* to mean that if a woman emits her seed first she bears a male child,[24] their intention was not to imply that the fetus is formed from the seed of the woman. For even though the woman has eggs [i.e., ovaries] like the eggs of a male [i.e., testicles], either she creates no seed in them at all or the seed jells and contributes nothing to the fetus. The sages said that "she conceives" refers to the blood of the uterus that gathers in the mother at the end of intercourse and unites with the male seed because, in their view, the fetus is formed from the blood of the female and the white [semen] of the man, and both are called seed. Similarly, they stated that man has three partners [in his creation]: the father supplies the white [semen] from which are formed sinews, bones, and the white of the eye; the mother provides the red [semen] from which are formed skin, flesh,

> blood, and hair and the black of the eye; and God gives the spirit and the breath, beauty of features, eyesight, the power of hearing, the ability to speak and to walk, understanding and discernment. And this is also the view of physicians of human creation. And, according to the Greek philosophers, the entire body of the fetus comes from the blood of the mother. The father only has the power known as *heyuli* in their language: that is, he gives form to the matter. . . . so too renders *Targum Onkelos*, she carries seed.

Nachmanides is saying several things. First, a fetus or embryo is initiated from uterine blood, which is called seed. Second, the ovaries either do not contain seed or contain seed that is useless. Contrary to Ibn Ezra and the ancient Greeks, who claim that the entire baby comes from the mother's blood, Nachmanides asserts that the baby is produced from the contributions of both the mother's uterine blood and the father's seed.

Rabbi Ovadiah Seforno interprets the phrase in Leviticus as follows:

> The sages have already stated that if a woman emits seed first she bears a male child, because in fact it is the seed of the woman. And it is the liquid that emanates from her at times during intercourse that plays no role at all in the formation of the male fetus; rather her uterine blood jells in the seed of the father. When some of her liquid seed enters her jelled blood, then liquid seed is in excess, and the offspring is a girl.

Seforno seems to be saying that ovarian seed is useless for the production of male offspring but does play a role in the formation of girls. In either case, the essential reproductive force is the woman's blood. Scientifically, one might interpret Seforno to be saying that female orgasm after male ejaculation causes the fetus to develop as a female. The secretions entering the already fertilized egg cause the fetus to become a female. Female orgasm prior to ejaculation has no effect and allows the fetus to develop as a male.

Rabbi Shlomo Ephraim ben Aharon, in his biblical commentary known as *K'li Yakar*, simply states that the explanation of the rabbinic dictum that if a man emits seed first, the offspring is a female, and vice versa, is that "this is a matter of nature."

A very novel approach is found in the commentary called *Da'at Zekenim Mi-Baale Ha-Tosefot*.

> There are seven openings in a woman, three on the right, three on the left, and one in the middle. If the semen enters on the right side, a male offspring is born; if on the left side, a female offspring is born; but if in the middle, a *tumtum* [baby of unknown sex] or *androginos* [hermaphrodite] is born. If she lies on her right side, the seed will enter the openings on the right and she will give birth to a boy, and if she lies on the left side, she will give birth to a girl.

The above opinion seems to be based on Hippocrates, who in his famous *Aphorisms* (sec. 5:48) said that a male fetus matures better on the right side and a female fetus on the left side. In an earlier section (5:38), Hippocrates said that if a woman is pregnant with twins and one of her breasts shrinks, one of her fetuses will be aborted. If the right breast shrinks, the male fetus is aborted; if the left breast shrinks, the female fetus is aborted. Moses Maimonides criticizes Hippocrates for his statement that a boy is born from the right ovary and a girl from the left.[25] Maimonides remarks: "A man should be either prophet or genius to know this."

Rabbi Baruch HaLevi Epstein, in his commentary entitled *Torah Temimah*, offers the following observation:

> It seems clear that the matter was known to the Sages because this is the way it is in nature, because all is reckoned after the first power. Therefore, if the man emits semen first, his strength is finished first and the creation is determined by the last power, which is her seed, and therefore she bears a female child. And so too the reverse. There is only an allusion or hint of this fact in this scriptural phrase . . . for this well-known occurrence in nature.

In a recent publication of the Institute for Jewish Policy Planning and Research of the Synagogue Council of America, Roberts writes about societal risks in sex preselection with emphasis upon Jewish perspectives.[26] He describes the preference for male babies in contemporary society and discusses sociological and psychological consequences and potential biological problems stemming from male preselection. These psychosociological aspects of this subject are beyond the scope of my essay, which is limited to the biblical and talmudic references to sex preselection and sex predetermination. The Talmud and other authoritative Jewish writings emphatically state that if a woman "emits seed first," she will bear a male child.

Perhaps this phrase is to be understood in an ethical or humanistic sense in that a husband who shows consideration for his wife by delaying his own orgasm until his wife has been gratified is thereby assured of male offspring. Although orgasm seems to be the most likely explanation of this phrase, we have yet to precisely understand its meaning in modern scientific terms.

Notes

1. Y. F. Lau, J. C. Huang, A. D. Dozy, and Y. W. Kan, "A Rapid Screening Test for Antenatal Sex Determination," *Lancet* 1 (1984): 14–16; J. R. Gosden, C. M. Gosden, S. Christie, J. M. Morsman, and C. H. Rodeck, "Rapid Fetal Sex Determination in First Trimester Prenatal Diagnosis by Dot Hybridisation of DNA Probes," ibid., pp. 540–541.

2. J. D. Bleich, "Abortion in Halakhic Literature," in *Contemporary Halakhic Problems.* (New York: Ktav and Yeshiva University Press, 1977), pp. 325–371; D. M. Feldman, *Marital Relations, Birth Control, and Abortion in Jewish Law* (New York: Schocken, 1975), pp. 251–294; I. Jakobovits, "Jewish Views on Abortion," in *Jewish Bioethics*, ed. F. Rosner and J. D. Bleich (New York: Hebrew Publishing Co., 1979), pp. 118–133.

3. S. J. Behrman, "Artificial Insemination and Public Policy," *New England Journal of Medicine* 300 (1979): 619–620.

4. R. Guerrero, "Association of the Type and Time of Insemination within the Menstrual Cycle with the Human Sex Ratio at Birth," *New England Journal of Medicine* 291 (1974): 1056–1059.

5. S. Harlap, "Gender of Infants Conceived on Different Days of the Menstrual Cycle," *New England Journal of Medicine* 300 (1979): 1445–1448.

6. L. B. Shettles, "The Great Preponderance of Human Males Conceived," *American Journal of Obstetrics and Gynecology* 89 (1964): 130–133.

7. F. Rosner, "The Biblical and Talmudic Secret for Choosing One's Baby's Sex," *Israel Journal of Medical Sciences* 15 (1979): 784–787.

8. Ecclesiastes 1:9.

9. Niddah 31a–31b.

10. Leviticus 12:2.

11. Genesis 46:15.

12. I Chronicles 8:40.

13. Niddah 31b.

14. Ibid. 25b and 28a.

15. Gittin 57a.

16. Berachot 54a.

17. Berachot 60a.

18. Kiddushin 82b.

19. Baba Batra 10b.

20. Psalms 124:3.

21. Niddah 70b–71a.

22. Behrman, op. cit.

23. Leviticus 12:2.

24. Niddah 31a.

25. F. Rosner, *Moses Maimonides' Commentary on the Aphorisms of Hippocrates* (Haifa: Maimonides Research Institute, 1986).

26. H. J. Roberts, "Societal Risks in Sex Preselection with Emphasis upon Jewish Perspectives," *Analysis*, 68 (December 1980), pp. 1–6.

11

Abortion

Major impetus for abortion reform in the United States followed two incidents that occurred in the early 1960s. In 1962, an Arizona housewife, Mrs. Sherri Finkbine of Phoenix, early in pregnancy, took a tranquilizing pill called thalidomide. This drug had produced approximately seven thousand deformed babies, usually born without arms or legs, in women who took this medication during the first few months of pregnancy. Mrs. Finkbine, denied an abortion in her own state of Arizona and in several other states, went to Sweden, where an abortion verified the fact that her baby would have been born with only stumps instead of arms and legs.

Two years later, in 1964, a major German measles epidemic in the United States resulted in the birth of many thousands of physically and mentally deformed babies as well as many other thousands of stillborn infants, over and above the expected number for a comparable period. Thus, the thalidomide and German measles tragedies, occurring in rapid succession, provided the stimulus for Colorado to become the first state to reform its abortion law, on April 25, 1967, followed by North Carolina and California in the same year. Georgia and Maryland followed suit in 1968. Five additional states in 1969 (New Mexico, Arkansas, Delaware, Oregon, Kansas) and five more in 1979 (New York, Hawaii, Virginia, South Carolina, and Alaska) reformed their abortion laws. These fifteen states allowed abortion for pregnancy resulting from rape or incest, or where the fetus may be born malformed physically, or deficient mentally, or where the mother's life or health are threatened. In 1973, the United States Supreme Court decision in *Roe v. Wade* rendered all abortion statutes in this country unconstitutional and effectively legalized abortion on demand.

Tremendous interest in this subject continues, as evidenced by the flood of books, articles, and editorials in the medical literature as well as writings in the lay press. In addition, there is an abundance of papers and books in the legal, theological, and social science literatures, enumeration of which is beyond the scope of this essay. One of the reasons for this flurry of interest in abortion is the changing moral and legal attitudes toward therapeutic abortion. Is there a new moral climate in our society that has caused all the above changes? Why has our moral code been altered? By whom? Does increased premarital sex lead to more unwanted pregnancies for which abortion is sought as a solution? Are there more contraceptive failures with increased numbers of unwanted pregnancies? Numerous reasons put forth by protagonists of abortion reform have in fact been applicable for several decades. For example, population control and women's rights are points of controversy that have been debated for many years.

Religious attitudes concerning abortion play a paramount role in shaping the thoughts, decrees, and actions of various groups. The present essay is an attempt to survey the biblical, talmudic, and rabbinic literatures, and, from these sources, to describe in detail the Jewish legal and moral attitude toward abortion. For comparative purposes, the Catholic and Protestant positions on abortion are briefly outlined.

Catholic View

The Catholic church's attitude toward therapeutic abortion is that any direct attack on the fetus is considered murder, even if it is carried out with the best intentions. Neither man nor the state has the authority to destroy the life of an innocent person, and both criminal and therapeutic abortion involve a direct and deliberate destruction of an innocent life. The emphasis is on the word "innocent." The unborn child, from conception onward, is considered a human being with all the rights of any other human person. Therefore, even if a direct abortion would preserve the mother's life or health, it is not morally permissible.

On October 29, 1951, Pope Pius XII delivered an address on morality in marriage in which he stated:

> Every human being, even the infant in the mother's womb, has the right to life immediately from God, not from the parents or from any human society or authority. Therefore, there is no

man, no human authority, no science, no medical, eugenic, social, economic or moral indication, that can show or give a valid juridical title for direct deliberate disposition concerning an innocent life. . . . Thus, for example, to save the life of the mother is a most noble end, but the direct killing of the child as a means to this end is not licit.[1]

Further reasons for Catholic opposition to abortion include the teaching that all unbaptized fetuses and infants are forever excluded from participation in God's divinity and in the Beatific Vision reserved for those who have been baptized. No one has the right to exclude an unborn infant from such participation.[2]

The penalty for performing an abortion is stated in Canon 2350 of the church's Code of Canon Law: "Persons who procure abortion, the mother not excepted, automatically incur excommunication." The same penalty is incurred by all those who assist in procuring the abortion.

From the standpoint of the Catholic church, there seem to be neither psychiatric nor medical indications for terminating a pregnancy.

Protestant Views

Baptists consider abortion to be primarily "a medical problem and that the theological implications can be trusted to our Omniscient Heavenly Father."[3] Similarly, the Methodist church considers abortion a scientific, medical matter on which only competent medical opinion has any value.

The attitude of the Lutheran church is very similar to that of the Catholics in that "the use of abortifacients and of medicines designed to produce sterility is condemned."[4] The American Lutheran Conference, however, at its biennial meeting in 1952, issued a statement part of which reads as follows: "Abortion must be regarded as the destruction of a living being, and, except as a medical measure to save the mother's life, will not be used by a Christian to avoid an unwanted birth."

The Presbyterian church believes the life of the mother should receive first consideration. Ministers and members are allowed to follow "enlightened conscience with regard to this matter."[5] The Episcopalians also permit individual clergymen to make the decision.

The Unitarian church states that "judgment regarding therapeutic abortions rests upon the principle of preserving and extending human life and that this decision must be the patient's and the physician's—not the Church's or any other institution's."[6]

Jewish Legal Attitude Toward Abortion

An unborn fetus in Jewish law is not considered a person (Heb. *nefesh*, lit. "soul") until it has been born. The fetus is regarded as a part of the mother's body and not a separate being until it begins to egress from the womb during parturition. In fact, until forty days after conception, the fertilized egg is considered as "mere fluid." These facts form the basis for the Jewish legal view on abortion. Biblical, talmudic, and rabbinic support for these statements will now be presented.

Intentional abortion is not mentioned directly in the Bible, but a case of accidental abortion is discussed in Exodus 21:22–23, where Scripture states:

> *When men fight and one of them pushes a pregnant woman and a miscarriage results, but no other misfortune ensues, the one responsible shall be fined as the woman's husband may exact from him, the payment to be based on judges' reckoning. But if other misfortune ensues, the penalty shall be life for life.*

The famous biblical commentator Solomon ben Isaac, known as *Rashi*, interprets *no other misfortune* to mean no fatal injury to the woman following her miscarriage. In that case, the attacker pays only financial compensation for having unintentionally caused the miscarriage, no differently than if he had accidentally injured the woman elsewhere on her body. Most other Jewish Bible commentators, including Moses Nachmanides (*Ramban*), Abraham Ibn Ezra, Meir Leib ben Yechiel Michael (*Malbim*), Baruch Halevi Epstein (*Torah Temimah*), Samson Raphael Hirsch, Joseph Hertz, and others, agree with *Rashi*'s interpretation. We can thus conclude that when the mother is otherwise unharmed following trauma to her abdomen during which the fetus is lost, the only rabbinic concern is to have the one responsible pay damages to the woman and her husband for the loss of the fetus. None of the rabbis raise the possibility of involuntary manslaughter being involved because the unborn fetus is not legally a person and, therefore, there is no question of murder involved when a fetus is aborted.

Based upon this biblical statement, Moses Maimonides asserts as follows: "If one assaults a woman, even unintentionally, and her child is born prematurely, he must pay the value of the child to the husband and the compensation for injury and pain to the woman."[7] Maimonides continues with statements regarding how these compensations are computed. A similar declaration is found in Joseph Karo's *Shulchan Aruch*.[8] No concern is expressed by either Maimonides or Karo regarding the status of the miscarried fetus. It is part of the mother and belongs jointly to her and her husband, and thus damages must be paid for its premature death. However, the one who was responsible is not culpable for murder, since the unborn fetus is not considered a person.

Murder in Jewish law is based upon Exodus 21:12, where it is written: *He that smiteth a man so that he dieth shall surely be put to death.* The word *man* is interpreted by the sages to mean a man but not a fetus.[9] Thus, the destruction of an unborn fetus is not considered murder.

Another pertinent scriptural passage is Leviticus 24:17, where it states: *And he that smiteth any person mortally shall surely be put to death.* However, an unborn fetus is not considered a person or *nefesh* and, therefore, its destruction does not incur the death penalty.

Turning to talmudic sources, the Mishnah asserts the following:[10] "If a woman is having difficulty in giving birth [and her life is in danger],[11] one cuts up the fetus within her womb and extracts it limb by limb, because her life takes precedence over that of the fetus. But if the greater part was already born, one may not touch it, for one may not set aside one person's life for that of another."

Rabbi Yom Tov Lippman Heller, known as *Tosafot Yom Tov*, in his commentary on this passage in the Mishnah, explains that the fetus is not considered a *nefesh* until it has egressed into the air of the world and, therefore, one is permitted to destroy it to save the mother's life. Similar reasoning is found in *Rashi*'s commentary on the talmudic discussion of this mishnaic passage, where *Rashi* states that as long as the child has not come out into the world, it is not called a living being, i.e., *nefesh*.[12] Once the head of the child has come out, the child may not be harmed because it is considered as fully born, and one life may not be taken to save another.[13]

The Mishnah elsewhere states: "If a pregnant woman is taken out to be executed, one does not wait for her to give birth; but if her pains of parturition have already begun [lit. she has already sat on the birth stool], one waits for her until she gives birth."[14] One does not delay the execution of the mother in order to save the life of the

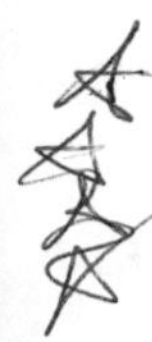

fetus because the fetus is not yet a person (Heb. *nefesh*), and judgments in Judaism must be promptly implemented. The Talmud also explains that the embryo is part of the mother's body and has no identity of its own, since it is dependent for its life upon the body of the woman.[15] However, as soon as it starts to move from the womb, it is considered an autonomous being (*nefesh*) and thus unaffected by the mother's state. This concept of the embryo being considered part of the mother and not a separate being recurs throughout the Talmud and rabbinic writings.[16] The Talmud continues: "Rab Judah said in the name of Samuel: If a [pregnant] woman is about to be executed, one strikes her against her womb so that the child may die first, to avoid her being disgraced."[17] *Rashi* explains that if the child escaped death and came forth after the mother's execution, it might cause bleeding and thus expose the executed mother to disgrace. Thus, we have evidence that an unborn fetus does not have the status of a living being, and destroying it to save the mother embarrassment is not prohibited if it is going to die anyway.

The talmudic commentary known as *Tosafot* states that "it is permissible to kill an unborn fetus."[18] Some rabbinic authorities accept these words of *Tosafot* verbatim,[19] whereas others are of the opinion that *Tosafot* is not to be interpreted literally.[20] Yet others believe that *Tosafot* is in error.[21]

Prior to forty days after conception, the Talmud considers a fertilized egg nothing more than "mere fluid,"[22] and one "need not take into consideration the possibility of a valid childbirth."[23] However, after forty days have elapsed, fashioning or formation of the fetus is deemed to have occurred. Laws of ritual uncleanliness must be observed for abortuses older than forty days.[24] This period of uncleanliness is similar to that prescribed following the birth of a child and is not the same as that for a menstruant woman. Furthermore, a woman who aborts after the fortieth day following conception is required to bring an offering just as if she had given birth to a live child.[25] These laws of ritual impurity and offerings apply even where the abortus "resembles cattle, a wild beast, or a bird" or a "shapeless piece of flesh." These rules imply that the unborn fetus, although not considered a living person (*nefesh*), still has some status. Nowhere in the Talmud, however, does it state that killing this fetus by premature artificial termination of pregnancy is considered murder.

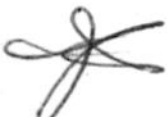

Based upon these talmudic sources as well as the scriptural

passages cited earlier, one may again ask why most rabbinic authorities prohibit abortion, except in certain situations, as a serious moral offense even though it is not considered legal murder. Distinguished Jewish physicians of ancient and more recent times also admonished against abortion. Denunciations of the practice of abortion are recorded in the medical oaths and prayers of Asaph Judaeus in the seventh century, Amatus Lusitanus in the sixteenth century, and Jacob Zahalon in the seventeenth century.[26] What are the objections to abortion in the opinion of these Jewish physicians in view of the fact that an unborn fetus does not have the status of a person (*nefesh*) in Jewish law? If abortion is not considered murder, on what legal basis is it prohibited?

Let us first establish the time that a fetus legally acquires the status equal to an adult human being. We have previously cited the main talmudic source upon which the Jewish legal attitude toward abortion is based.[27] The Talmud states in part that if the "greater part was already born, one may not touch it, for one may not set aside one person's life for that of another." Thus the act of birth changes the status of the fetus from a nonperson to a person (*nefesh*). Killing the newborn after this point is infanticide. Many talmudic sources and commentators on the Talmud substitute the word "head" for "greater part."[28] Others maintain the "greater part" verbatim.[29] Maimonides and Karo also consider the extrusion of the head to indicate birth.[30] They both further state that by rabbinic decree, even if only one limb of the fetus was extruded and then retracted, childbirth is considered to have occurred.[31]

Not only is the precise time of the birth of paramount importance in adjudicating whether aborting the fetus is permissible to save the mother's life, but the viability of the fetus must also be taken into account. The newborn child is not considered fully viable until it has survived thirty days following birth, as it is stated in the Talmud: "Rabban Simeon ben Gamliel said: Any human being who lives thirty days is not a *nephel* [abortus] because it is stated: *And those that are to be redeemed of them from a month old shalt thou redeem* [Num. 18:16], since prior to thirty days it is not certain that he will survive."[32] Further support for the necessity of a thirty-day postpartum viability period for adjudicating various Jewish legal matters pertaining to the newborn comes from Maimonides, who asserts: "Whether one kills an adult or a day-old child, a male or a female, he must be put to death if he kills deliberately . . . provided that the child is born after a full-term pregnancy. But, if it is born before the end of nine months, it is regarded as an abortion until it has lived for thirty days, and if one kills it during these thirty days, one is not put to death on its account."[33]

Thus, although the newborn infant reaches the status of a person or *nefesh*, which it didn't have prior to birth, it still does not enjoy all the legal rights of an adult until it has survived for thirty days post partum. The death penalty is not imposed if one kills such a child before it has established its viability, but killing it is certainly prohibited because "one may not set aside one person's life for that of another."[34]

The permissibility to kill the unborn fetus to save the mother's life rests upon the fact that such an embryo is not considered a person (*nefesh*) until it is born. Maimonides and Karo present a second reason for allowing abortion or embryotomy prior to birth where the mother's life is endangered, and that is the argument of "pursuit," whereby the fetus is "pursuing" the mother.[35] The argument of pursuit is based upon two passages in the Pentateuch.

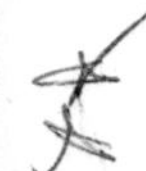

> Deuteronomy 25:22–12. *When men strive together one with another, and the wife of one draws near to save her husband from the hands of the one that smiteth him, and she puts her hand and taketh hold of his genitals, then you shall cut off her hand, your eye shalt have no pity.*
>
> Leviticus 19:16. *Thou shalt not stand idly by the blood of thy neighbor.*

In the former case, the woman is pursuing the man by maiming him, and she should be stopped. The latter case is interpreted by *Rashi* and most other commentators to mean that one should not stand idly by without attempting to rescue one's fellowman whose life is threatened by robbers, drowning, or wild beasts. Based upon these biblical passages, the Mishnah states: "These may be delivered at the cost of their lives: he that pursues after his fellowman to kill him . . ."[36] The Talmud follows with a lengthy discussion asserting that it is one's duty to disable or even take the life of the assailant to protect the life of one's fellowman.[37]

This discussion prompted Maimonides to state: "Consequently, the sages have ruled that if a pregnant woman is having difficulty in giving birth, the child inside her may be excised, either by drugs or manually [i.e., surgery], because it is regarded as pursuing her in order to kill her. But if its head has been born, it must not be touched, for one may not set aside one human life for that of another, and this happening is the course of nature [i.e., an act of God, that is, the mother is pursued by heaven, not the fetus]."[38] An identical statement is found in Karo's Code.[39]

Many rabbinic authorities pose the following question to Maimonides.[40] How can the argument of pursuit be invoked here, since if it were applicable, killing the fetus even after the head or greater part is born should be permissible? Rabbi Israel Lipschuetz, known as *Tiferet Israel*,[41] and others state that the argument of pursuit is totally inappropriate because the child's endangering of the mother's life is an act of God. The child does not intend to kill the mother. It is a case of heavenly pursuit. This concept of heavenly pursuit is discussed in the Talmud and mentioned by both Maimonides and Karo. Jakobovits amplifies the problem by stating that a contradictory ruling seems to be emerging.[42] On the one hand, we invoke the argument of pursuit to allow therapeutic abortion, and on the other hand, the validity of this argument is dismissed because nature and not the child pursues the mother.

The problem is resolved by many rabbis who state that the non-person status of the fetus prior to birth is not sufficient to warrant the embryo's destruction, since this would still constitute a serious moral offense, even if it is not a penal crime.[43] Thus one must invoke the additional argument of pursuit. After the baby's head has emerged, however, the fetus attains the status of a *nefesh*, even prior to proved thirty-day postpartum viability, and the "weak" argument of pursuit no longer justifies killing the child even if the mother's life is threatened, since it is a case of Heavenly pursuit. However, even after egress of the head, if both lives are threatened one may kill the fetus to save the mother.[44] The reason is that the mother's life is threatened, since it is a case of heavenly pursuit. viability of the fetus is in doubt until thirty days have elapsed following birth. This viewpoint is also espoused by Rabbis Moses Schick and David Hoffman.[45] Others dispute this ruling.[46]

We now return to the original question. If the unborn child is not considered a *nefesh*, why should its destruction not be allowed under all circumstances? Why is only a threat to the mother's life or health an acceptable reason for therapeutic abortion?

One answer is given by Rabbi Ya'ir Bacharach, who, contrary to the Mishnah in Tractate Arachin 1:4, states that one waits for a condemned pregnant woman to give birth because a potential human being can arise from each drop of human seed (sperm). Interference with pregnancy would constitute expulsion of semen for naught, an act akin to *coitus interruptus* and strictly prohibited in

Jewish law. This reason for prohibiting therapeutic abortion upon demand is also subscribed to by others.[47]

A second reason for not allowing abortion without specific indication is that the unborn fetus, although not a person, does have sufficient status, if it is aborted after forty days of conception, to require its mother to undergo the same ritual purification process as if she had given birth to a live child. The same process is also prescribed for a woman who has a spontaneous miscarriage. Thus, the fetus can be considered to be a "partial person."[48]

A third reason for prohibiting abortion on demand is that one is not permitted to wound oneself,[49] and a woman undergoing vaginal abortion by manipulative means is considered as intentionally wounding herself. At least two rabbinic authorities adhere to this viewpoint.[50]

A fourth reason for prohibiting abortion without maternal danger is that the operative intervention entails danger.[51] One is prohibited in Jewish law from intentionally placing oneself in danger, based upon Deuteronomy 4:15: *Take ye therefore good heed unto yourselves.*

Another reason for prohibiting therapeutic abortion in cases where no threat to the mother exists is offered by Rabbi Issur Yehuda Unterman, who states that one may desecrate the Sabbath to save the life or preserve the health of an unborn fetus in order that the child may observe many Sabbaths later.[52] As a result, destroying the fetus, although not legally murder, is nevertheless forbidden as an appurtenance to murder. Rabbi Bacharach, who permits abortion prior to forty days of pregnancy because the fetus has no status at all but is considered mere fluid, is taken to task by Rabbi Unterman, who states that even prior to forty days there is an appurtenance to murder.

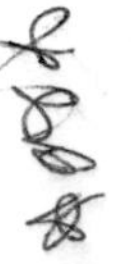

Another argument of Rabbi Unterman is that a fetus, even less than forty days after conception, is considered a potential (lit. questionable) human being which, by nature alone, without interference, will become an actual human being. Thus a potential person *(sofek nefesh)* has enough status to prohibit its own destruction.

A final argument of Rabbi Unterman comes from the interpretation of Rabbi Ishmael of the scriptural verse: *Whoso sheddeth man's blood, by man shall his blood be shed, for in the image of God did He make man*,[53] which can be translated "whoso sheddeth the blood of man in man, his blood shall be shed." The "man in man" is interpreted to mean a fetus.[54] This Noachidic prohibition of killing a fetus applies also to Israelites, even though the Jewish legal consequences might differ.

The final reason and perhaps most important for prohibiting abortion on demand in Jewish law is suggested by Rabbi Immanuel Jakobovits and Rabbi Moshe Yonah Zweig among others.[55] They point to the Mishnah in Oholoth 7:6 which permits abortion prior to birth of the child only when the mother's life is endangered. The implication is that when the mother's life is not at stake, it would be prohibited to kill the unborn fetus.

Handicapped Babies and Defective Newborns

Treatment or nontreatment of a newborn with major medical or mental defects is the subject of considerable controversy. Numerous "Baby Doe" cases have been widely publicized in recent years, and the medical and lay literatures are replete with articles on the subject.

The Talmud quotes the following unusual birth: "In the case of a birth given to a creature which possesses a double back or a double spine, Rab said: If it was a woman [who miscarried], it is not regarded as an offspring,[56] that is, the laws concerning a birth are not observed. However, once this creature has been born, it has the status of a person, and killing it is considered infanticide, which is prohibited in Jewish law.

Rabbi Judah the Pious, author of the thirteenth-century work *Sefer Chasidim*, describes the case of a child born with grotesque teeth and a tail.[57] It was feared that people might consider the infant to be a fish and eat it. Rabbi Judah was asked whether it was permissible to kill it. His reply was that one should remove the teeth and the tail in spite of the risks and raise the child as an otherwise normal human being. This ruling clearly prohibits the killing of handicapped babies.

Another ruling relating to a malformed child is that of nineteenth-century Rabbi Eleazar Fleckeles, who states that once a child is born it is a human being in all respects and may not be destroyed.[58] Starving it to death, as was suggested by the questioner, is considered infanticide and prohibited.

The problem of babies born without one or more limbs, technically known as phocomelia, to women who ingested the drug thalidomide early in pregnancy is discussed by Belgian Rabbi Zweig,[59] who condemns the killing of the thalidomide-deformed baby which resulted in the famous Liège trial involving parents, relatives, and physician charged with murder.[60] Rabbi Zweig's lengthy dissertation, however, deals primarily with abortion (i.e., antenatal) and not infanticide (i.e., postnatal).

Although the subject of genetic screening and Tay-Sachs disease is discussed elsewhere in this book (see chap. 13), it seems pertinent to point out that Rabbi Eliezer Waldenberg allows abortion up to the seventh month of pregnancy if amniocentesis reveals that the mother is carrying a Tay-Sachs fetus.[61] His reason is the "great need" of the enormous mental anguish of the mother in knowing the fatal outcome that awaits her diseased child. On the other hand, Rabbi Moshe Feinstein states that every case must be individualized and that "routine" abortion for Tay-Sachs disease is not permissible.[62] In fact, the amniocentesis itself, if performed for no valid medical indication, may be prohibited because of the small but significant risk that this procedure entails. Rabbi Yitzchak Silberstein suggests that a couple both of whom are carriers of a genetic chromosomal defect and/or where one can anticipate the birth of a defective child, should be advised not to marry.[63] If they marry, they should be divorced unless divorce is very difficult and undesirable for them, in which case they should still have children and hope for the best. If they already have two children, they are not obligated to have more, concludes Silberstein.

Rabbi Jakobovits summarizes succinctly the Jewish view of the treatment of handicapped newborns as follows: A physically or mentally abnormal child has the same claim to life as a normal child because it is considered a person *(nefesh)*. Furthermore, while only the killing of a born and viable child constitutes murder in Jewish law, the destruction of the fetus, too, is a moral offense and cannot be justified except out of consideration for the mother's life or health. Consequently, the fear that a child may or will be deformed is not in itself a legitimate indication for its abortion, particularly since there is usually a chance that the child might turn out to be quite normal. Killing a handicapped adult is similarly prohibited.[64]

Once a malformed child has been born, one cannot use the argument of euthanasia or mercy killing to sanction its destruction. This act is positively prohibited in Jewish law as nothing less than murder (infanticide). The Jewish attitude toward euthanasia in general is discussed elsewhere in this book (see chap. 15).

Summary of Rabbinic Opinion on Abortion

Prior to forty days after conception, the fertilized egg is considered by some rabbinic authorities as mere fluid. Such an early zygote has no status at all, is not a person or *nefesh*, is regarded as part of the mother's flesh, and aborting it is not considered legal murder. According to this minority view, the slightest reason might be sufficient to allow abortion at this early stage.[65] Such a reason might be the fear that a deformed child may be born, due to exposure of the mother early in pregnancy to German measles or a teratogenic drug such as thalidomide or possibly even for socioeconomic reasons or family planning. A small minority of rabbis also allow abortion for reasons such as incest and rape.[66] Justification for this position rests on the grounds of concern for the mother, i.e., that such a birth would adversely affect her mental or physical health by causing her anguish, shame, or embarrassment.

Such permissive rulings are vigorously denounced by most rabbinic authorities who prohibit therapeutic abortion in cases such as exposure of the mother early in pregnancy to German measles[67] or to thalidomide.[68] Most rabbis permit and even mandate abortion where the health or life of the mother is threatened. Some authorities are stringent and require the mother's life to be in danger,[69] however remote that danger, whereas others permit abortion for a serious threat to the mother's health.[70] Such dangers to maternal health may include deafness,[71] cancer,[72] pain,[73] or psychiatric illness.[74] Psychiatric indication for abortion must be certified by competent medical opinion or by previous experiences of mental illness in the mother, such as a postpartum nervous breakdown.

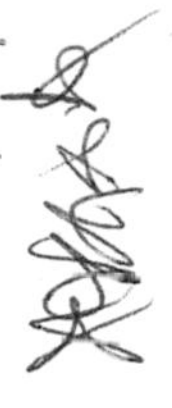

If the mother becomes pregnant while nursing a child and the pregnancy changes her milk, so that the suckling's life is endangered, abortion is permitted.[75] Once the baby is in the process of being born, it becomes a person for Jewish legal purposes and may not be harmed. The only exception is if *both* the baby's and the mother's lives are threatened. Then one may sacrifice the birthing child to save the mother because her life is a certainty without the fetal threat,[76] whereas the infant has not proved its viability until thirty days postpartum have elapsed. After thirty days of life, every human being, whether physically deformed, mentally deficient, or otherwise handicapped, is considered to be equal to every other human being and may not be harmed in any way.

For further discussion of the Jewish attitude toward abortion, the interested reader is referred to several recent reviews both in English and in Hebrew,[77] including one exhaustive review profusely annotated with 188 bibliographical citations.[78]

Since many important legal and moral considerations which cannot be spelled out in the presentation of general principles may weigh upon the verdict in any given case, it seems advisable to submit every individual case to rabbinic judgment in the light of the prevailing medical and other circumstances.

Jewish Moral Considerations on Abortion

The previous discussion has presented the Jewish legal principles relating to abortion. The destruction of the unborn fetus, although legally not considered murder, can be considered to constitute "moral murder." The unborn baby has a heartbeat, a brain, arms, legs, and nearly everything with which a healthy newborn baby is endowed. Thus, killing the unborn fetus, according to Rabbi Unterman, is an "appurtenance of murder" and strictly prohibited, although, because of a legal technicality, such an act is not considered murder for which the death penalty is imposed.

The major biblical citation dealing with abortion, Exodus 21:22–23, concerns accidental abortion, not intentional or induced abortion, a deed initiated at the outset *(lechatchilah)*. Therefore, one can argue that premeditated interruption of pregnancy is not allowed except to save the life or preserve the health (mental or physical) of the mother. Though some maintain that in Jewish law the death penalty may not be imposed upon the mother or the person performing the abortion, the rabbinic concept of a nonpenalized but prohibited act *(patur aval assur)* may prevail.

The concept of time seems all-important. If one destroys a baby five minutes *after* birth, it is considered murder in American and Jewish law; yet if one destroys the fetus five minutes *before* it is born, such an act is not murder. Why not? What is the difference? Certainly it is moral murder, although not legal murder. The same principle applies if one destroys a baby five hours, five days, or five months before and after birth. To some people, abortion is acceptable if done prior to the time the fetus might be expected to live. How then is life defined? Must there be a heartbeat? Limbs? Is not the fertilized zygote already alive? Does life mean that which is able to duplicate itself in the biological sense? Does life refer to the stage of fetal development when physical movement is first detected? Or is life the "breath of life" instilled in a newborn infant immediately after the birth process?

The next moral issue is the question of potentiality. The unborn fetus, if left alone, may turn out to be a genius. Or he may just be a person of normal intelligence. Of, if physically deformed, he may still make a positive contribution to society. In the secular world, should we not cite the contributions made by such handicapped or deformed human beings as Helen Keller, Ludwig van Beethoven, and Henri de Toulouse-Lautrec? Or in our religious experience, should we not marvel at the learned and soul-rending contributions made by the blind talmudic scholars Rav Sheshes and Rav Yosef, the unsightly Rabbi Yehoshua ben Chananyah, and the limbless Rabbi Amnon of Mayence, author of the renowned *Unethaneh Tokef* prayer recited on the High Holy Days? The potential of an unborn infant is unknown. However, as Rabbi Unterman points out, the potential human being, i.e., the unborn fetus, if left alone, will develop into an actual human being. Hence, this potential person *(sofek nefesh)* has enough status to prohibit its destruction. Jewish law also allows, and in fact requires, that one desecrate the Sabbath to save the life or health of the unborn fetus in order that the fetus may observe many Sabbaths later, after it is born.

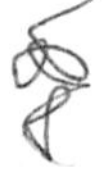

The Talmud compares the unborn fetus to an extra appendage of the mother *(ubar yerech imo hu)*, destruction or damage to which requires that financal remuneration be paid to the mother for pain, shame, anguish, medical bills, inability to work, and the like. However, how can one compare the unborn fetus to a finger of the mother? If one destroys a finger, the woman has lost a finger, which would never have become anything other than a finger. The unborn fetus, if left alone, would have developed into a full and complete human being.

Philosophical-moral arguments against abortion are also very potent. If a woman becomes pregnant, almost certainly Almighty God so willed it. How dare we interfere? Even if the child might be born physically deformed, this too is the will of God. One is reminded of the encounter between King Hezekiah and the Prophet Isaiah as described in the Talmud.

> The Holy One, Blessed be He, brought sufferings upon Hezekiah and then said to Isaiah: Go visit the sick, for it is written: *In those days Hezekiah was sick unto death, and Isaiah the prophet, son of Amoz, came to him and said unto him, Thus saith the Lord, set your house in order, for you shall die and not live, etc.* [Isaiah 38:1]. What is the meaning of *you shall die and not live?* You shall die in this world and not live in the world-to-come. [Hezekiah] said to [Isaiah]: Why so bad? [Isaiah] replied: Because you did not try to have children. [Hezekiah] said: The reason was because I saw by the holy spirit that the children issuing from me would not be virtuous. [Isaiah] said to [Hezekiah]: What have you to do with the secrets of the All-

Merciful? You should have done what you were commanded and let the Holy One, blessed be He, do that which pleases Him. [Although this defiance of God's will by Hezekiah was punished, the outcome of the story is a happy one: Hezekiah was healed and lived another fifteen years.][79]

King Hezekiah apparently knew that his children would be morally corrupt, so he put aside the "first" commandment of the Torah, *be fruitful and multiply*,[80] and did not take a wife. Isaiah charges him with lack of faith. In a similar vein, is not one's faith in the Almighty being challenged by the mother who requests abortion because she can see no way of solving her social or economic difficulty?

A further philosophical argument against abortion contends that throughout the ages, millions of Jews have perished at the hands of their enemies. Are we today to kill even more by performing indiscriminate abortion? Certainly not!

Let us turn to the possible consequences of legalized abortion. Will legal infanticide follow? Legal genocide? Legal extermination of social misfits, as Hitler proposed? Legal euthanasia? Where does the trend end? What about the psychological consequences to the mother? After the abortion, she cannot change her mind. The deed is done. Who decides whether an abortion is to be performed? Why only the mother? How about the father? Has he nothing to say? Why not? Why should not the boyfriend be consulted if an unwed pregnant girl seeks an abortion? How about the siblings of the unborn fetus? Should they have a say in this matter? Furthermore, who speaks for the fetus? We have a Society for the Prevention of Cruelty to Animals, a Society for the Prevention of Cruelty to Children, yet there is no Society for the Prevention of Cruelty to Fetuses. Theoretically, if we could communicate with the fetus and ask it whether it would choose life if it knew that it would be born without arms or legs, the answer would doubtless be a resounding yes. If the fetus were told he would be the twelfth child in a very poor family living in a very small apartment, it would still probably choose life. So who speaks for the fetus in the decision-making process concerning an abortion? Why is the mother the major, if not the only, determining factor? Why should we, society, not speak for the fetus? In divorce proceedings, the courts decide the disposition of the involved children, if any. Why should not the courts have a say about the continued life of the fetus?

Women, as human beings, were created in the image of God, and thus a woman is not the sole owner of her body and soul, to treat it as she pleases. A woman does not have the right to take her own life, i.e., to commit suicide. She is entrusted with her body and may use but not abuse it. She is commanded to care for her body and soul and do all that is necessary to protect and preserve both.

For an unwed girl who is pregnant, the dilemma is severe indeed. Which is better, to have the baby and give it away, or to destroy it before it is born? How would she feel in giving up her child for adoption to a foster mother? How would she feel in aborting the pregnancy? The argument that this unfortunate girl should not have become pregnant is no consolation to her in her present predicament. Should this mother-to-be be permitted to extinguish the life of what will probably be a healthy human being in order to avert her personal shame or a socially unpleasant situation?

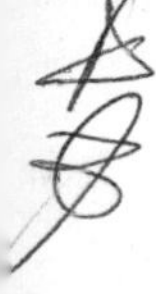

What are the moral issues involved in the various social reasons proposed for liberalizing abortion? Practically everyone loyal to Jewish law would subscribe to the proposition that to sacrifice a potential life to save an actual living person is permissible, if there is danger to the latter. But even if abortion in thalidomide and German measles cases were allowed, should abortion for social reasons, or abortion on demand, be permitted? In such a situation (i.e., poverty, inadequate housing, accidental pregnancy, etc.), one is sacrificing a potential life solely for the convenience or happiness of an adult, either mother or father, or both.

If one is told to kill somebody or be killed oneself, one is not allowed to kill, because one may not set aside one person's life for that of another. True, the unborn fetus is only a potential life, but why should the mother be able to spill her unborn baby's blood? Why is her convenience more valuable than a potential life?

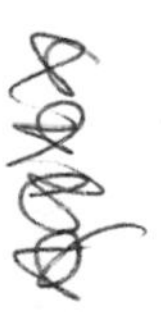

If a woman seeks an abortion for social reasons, might not the social conditions change? Perhaps the family's financial situation will improve. Perhaps larger living quarters will be provided to the family. Is not the abortion for social reasons a denial of one's faith in God and His ability to provide sustenance?

There are other reasons, moral and otherwise, which speak against legalized abortion. When a married woman or an unwed girl has an abortion, what guarantee does she have that she can ever become pregnant again? Is she so certain that the Divine mystery of conception will be hers again? Should she not pause and ask herself, "Will I ever regret denying myself this ultimate of feminine fulfillment, if I should never conceive again?"

Might it not happen that an abortion is contraindicated for

medical or psychiatric reasons? If a physician can reject a woman for abortion because of such a contraindication, why should the abortion request not be rejected by the physician or society because of a moral contraindication? If induced abortion becomes commonplace, will there not be an undermining or subversion of the ethics of medical practice? Will there be a shift from the "healer" physician to the "exterminator" physician?

Another moral issue is the sale or use of aborted fetuses for medical research. Who should have the say regarding the disposal of the fetus? The woman? The father? The gynecologist? The pathologist? Society? Who? Jewish morality and law require burial not only for a dead body but for removed human organs (e.g., as a result of an operation or an accidental amputation) as well. Our sages refer to the human body and its parts as "vessels which contain the human soul." How coarse, therefore, are those who would deal with, and profit from, the sale of the fetus, this potential "soul container."

Concluding Note

The Jewish legal and moral aspects of abortion have been presented in great detail in this essay. More questions are posed than answers given. I would like to leave the reader with the ancient pronouncement: "He who saves one life of the people of Israel is as if he had saved an entire world."[81] A single life, in Jewish teaching, is equivalent to a whole world. Furthermore, the fact that abortion on demand is legal in the United States and elsewhere does not mean that it is right. Legal permissibility is not synonymous with moral license.

Notes

1. C. Y. McFadden, *Medical Ethics*, 5th ed. (Philadelphia: F. A. Davis Co., 1961), pp. 140–141.
2. E. F. Healy, *Medical Ethics* (Chicago: Loyola University Press, 1956), pp. 357–358; J. Marshall, *The Ethics of Medical Practice* (London: Darton, Longman & Todd, 1960), pp. 152–153.
3. F. J. Curran, "Religious Implications," in *Therapeutic Abortion: Medical, Psychiatric, Legal, Anthropological and Religious Considerations*, ed. H. Rosen (New York: Julian Press, 1954), pp. 153–174.
4. Ibid.
5. Ibid.
6. Ibid.
7. Maimonides, *Mishneh Torah, Hilchot Chovel Umazik* 4:1.
8. Karo, *Shulchan Aruch, Choshen Mishpat* 423:1.
9. Sanhedrin 84b.
10. Oholot 7:6.
11. I. Lipschuetz, Commentary *Tiferet Yisroel* on *Oholot* 7:6.
12. Sanhedrin 72b.
13. Terumot 8:12.
14. Arachin 1:4.
15. Arachin 7a.
16. Talmud: Chullin 58a, Gittin 23b, Nazir 51a, Baba Kamma 88b, Temurah 31a, and elsewhere. Rabbinic writings: J. Trani, Responsa *Maharit*, pt. 1, nos. 97 and 99; Y. Bacharach, Responsa *Chavat Ya'ir*, no. 31; E. Landau, Responsa *Noda Biyehuda, Choshen Mishpat*, no. 59; Nachmanides, Novellae on Niddah 44b; J. Teomim, Commentary *Peri Megadim* on *Shulchan Aruch, Orach Chayim* 328:7:1; M. HaMeiri, Commentary *Beth Habechirah* on Sanhedrin 72b; Shneur Zalman of Lublin, Responsa *Torat Chesed, Even Haezer*, no. 42:32; Y. Emden, Responsa *She'elat Yavetz*, pt. 1, no. 43; S. Drimmer, Responsa *Bet Shlomo, Choshen Mishpat*, no. 132; E. Y. Waldenberg, Responsa *Tzitz Eliezer*, vol. 9, no. 5:3; and numerous others.
17. Arachin 7a.
18. Niddah 44b.
19. Waldenberg, Responsa *Tzitz Eliezer*, vol. 9, no. 51:3; and Bacharach, Responsa *Chavat Ya'ir*, no. 31.
20. I. Y. Unterman, in *Noam* 6 (1963): 1–11; and Emden, Responsa *She'elat Yavetz*, pt. 1, no. 43.
21. I. Schmelkes, Responsa *Bet Yitzchak, Yoreh Deah*, pt. 2, no. 162.
22. Yevamot 69b, Niddah 30b, and Keritot 1:3.
23. Niddah 3:7.
24. Niddah 3:2–6.
25. Keritot 1:3–6.
26. F. Rosner and S. Muntner, "The Oath of Asaph," *Annals of Internal*

Medicine 63 (1965): 317–320; H. Friedenwald, H. "The Oath of Amatus," in *The Jews and Medicine* (Baltimore: Johns Hopkins Press, 1944), pp. 368–370; H. Savitz, "Jacob Zahalon and His book *The Treasure of Life*," *New England Journal of Medicine* 213 (1935): 167–176; I. Simon, "La Prière des Medécins *Tephilat Harofim* de Jacob Zahalon, Médecin et Rabbin en Italie (1630–1693)," *Revue d'Histoire de la Medécine Hebraique* 8 (1955): 38–51; H. Friedenwald, "The Physician's Prayer of Jacob Zahalon of Rome," in *The Jews and Medicine* (Baltimore: Johns Hopkins Press, 1944), pp. 273–279.

27. Oholot 7:6.

28. Talmud: Sanhedrin 72b, Niddah 3:5 and 29a, and *Tosefta* (additional Talmud) Yevamot 9:9. Commentaries of Ovadiah of Bertinoro, known as *Bertinoro*, Asher ben Yechiel, known as *Rosh*, and Isaiah Berlin, known as *Rishon Letzion*, on Oholot 7:6; commentaries of *Rashi* on Sanhedrin 72b and *Tosafot* on Sanhedrin 59a.

29. Jerusalem (Palestinian) Talmud, Shabbat 14:4 and Avodah Zarah 2:2.

30. Maimonides, *Mishneh Torah, Hilchot Issurey Biyah* 10:3; Karo, *Shulchan Aruch, Choshen Mishpat* 425:2.

31. Maimonides, loc. cit., and Karo, *Shulchan Aruch, Yoreh Deah* 194:10.

32. Shabbat 135b.

33. Maimonides, *Mishneh Torah, Hilchot Rotze'ach* 2:6.

34. Oholot 7:3.

35. Maimonides, *Mishneh Torah, Hilchot Rotze'ach* 1:9; Karo, *Shulchan Aruch, Choshen Mishpat* 425:2.

36. Sanhedrin 8:7.

37. Sanhedrin 72b–73a.

38. Maimonides, *Hilchot Rotze'ach* 1:9.

39. Karo, *Choshen Mishpat* 425:1.

40. M. Y. A. Zweig, in *Noam* 7 (1964): 36–56; A. Eger, *Tosafot R. Akiva Eger* on Oholot 7:6; E. Landau, Responsa *Noda Biyehudah, Choshen Mishpat*, pt. 2, no. 59; Waldenberg, Responsa *Tzitz Eliezer*, vol. 9, no. 51:3; Bacharach, Responsa *Chavat Ya'ir*, no. 31.

41. I. Lipschuetz, Commentary *Tiferet Yisrael* on Oholot 7:6.

42. I. Jakobovits, *Jewish Medical Ethics* (New York: Bloch, 1975), pp. 170–191.

43. Waldenberg, loc. cit.; Bacharach, loc. cit.; Unterman, loc. cit.; Emden, loc. cit.; Zweig, loc. cit.; Eger, loc. cit.; Landau, loc. cit.; Lipschuetz, loc. cit.

44. Eger, loc. cit.; Lipschuetz, loc. cit.; and others.

45. Schick, Responsa *Maharam Schick, Yoreh Deah*, no. 155; Hoffman, Responsa *Melamed Leho'il, Yoreh Deah*, no. 69.

46. Ch. Sofer, Responsa *Machanei Chayim, Choshen Mishpat*, no. 50; M. A. Eisenstadt, Responsa *Panim Me' irot*, pt. 3, no. 8.

47. B. T. Frankel, Responsa *Ateret Chachamim*, *Even Haezer*, no. 1; Emden, Responsa *She'elatz Yavetz*, pt. 1, no. 43.
48. J. Rosen, Responsa *Tzofnat Pane'ach*, pt. 1, no. 49.
49. Baba Kamma 91b; Maimonides, *Mishneh Torah*, *Hilchot Chovel Umazik* 5:1.
50. J. Trani, Responsa *Maharit*, pt. 1, no. 99; Zweig, in *Noam* 7 (1964): 36–56.
51. S. Drimmer. Responsa *Bet Shlomo*, *Choshen Mishpat*, no. 132.
52. Nachmanides, Commentary *Ramban* on Niddah 44b. See also M. Hershler, in *Halachah Urefuah* 2 (1981): 57–64.
53. Genesis 9:6.
54. Sanhedrin 57b.
55. I. Jakobovits, "Jewish Views on Abortion," in *Abortion and the Law*, ed. D. T. Smith (Cleveland: Western Reserve University Press, 1967), pp. 124–143; Zweig, in *Noam* 7 (1964): 36–56.
56. Bechorot 43b.
57. Judah ben Samuel the Pious, *Sefer Chasidim*, no. 186.
58. Fleckeles, Responsa *Teshuva Me'Ahavah*, pt. 1, no. 53.
59. Zweig, loc. cit.
60. L. Colebrook, "The Liège Trial and the Problem of Voluntary Euthanasia," *Lancet* 2 (1962): 1225.
61. Waldenberg, Responsa *Tzitz Eliezer*, vol. 13, no. 102; also in *Assia* 2 (1981): 93–98.
62. M. Feinstein, in *Halachah Urefuah* 1 (1980): 304–306.
63. Y. Silberstein, in *Halachah Urefuah* 2 (1981): 106–113.
64. I. Jakobovits, in *The Jewish Review* (London), Nov. 14, 1962.
65. Schneur Zalman of Lublin, Responsa *Torat Chesed*, *Even Haezer*, no. 42:32.
66. Emden, Responsa *She'elatz Yavetz*, pt. 1, no. 43.
67. I. Y. Unterman, in *Noam* 6 (1963): 1–11.
68. I. Jakobovits, *Journal of a Rabbi* (New York: Living Books, 1966), pp. 262–266.
69. A. Lifschutz, Responsa *Aryeh Debei Ilay*, *Yoreh Deah*, no. 19; E. Deutsch, Responsa *Pri Hasadeh*, pt. 4, no. 50; S. Drimmer, Responsa *Bet Shlomo*, *Choshen Mishpat*, no. 132; D. Meislich, Responsa *Binyan David*, no. 47; M. Winkler, Responsa *Levushei Mordechai*, *Choshen Mishpat*, no. 39; I. Schorr, Responsa *Ko'ach Schor*, no. 21; A. J. Horowitz, Responsa *Tzur Yakov*, no. 141; Y. Teitelbaum, Responsa *Avnei Tzedek*, *Choshen Mishpat*, no. 19.
70. Yosef Chayim ben Eliyahu, Responsa *Rav Pa'alim*, *Even Haezer*, no. 4.
71. B. Z. Uziel, Responsa *Mishpetei Uziel*, *Choshen Mishpat*, pt. 3, no. 46.
72. G. Fiedler, Responsa *She'elatz Yeshurun*, pt. 1, no. 39.
73. I. M. Mizrachi, Responsa *Pri Ha'aretz*, *Yoreh Deah*, no. 21.

74. N. Z. Friedman, Responsa *Netzer Mata'ai*, pt. 1, no. 8.

75. Ch. Pallagi, Responsa *Chayim Veshalom*, pt. 1, no. 40; Y. Ayyas, Responsa *Bet Yehudah, Even Haezer*, no. 14; I. Oelbaum, Responsa *She'elat Yitzchak*, no. 69; Waldenberg, *Responsa Tzitz Eliezer*, vol. 9, no. 51:3.

76. Lipschuetz, Commentary *Tiferet Yisroel* on Oholot 7:6; A. Eger, Commentary *Tosefot Rabbi Akiba Eger* on Oholot 7:6.

77. D. M. Feldman, *Marital Relations, Birth Control and Abortion in Jewish Law* (New York: Schocken, 1975), pp. 251–294; J. D. Bleich, "Abortion in Halakhic Literature," in *Contemporary Halakhic Problems* (New York: Ktav and Yeshiva University Press, 1977), pp. 325–371; I. Jakobovits, "Jewish Views on Abortion," in *Jewish Bioethics*, ed. F. Rosner and J. D. Bleich (New York: Hebrew Publishing Co., 1979), pp. 118–133; M. Stern, "Abortion," in *Harefuah Le'or HaHalachah* (Jerusalem, 1980), vol. 1, pt. 1, pp. 1-147; O. Yosef, "Interruption of Pregnancy According to Halachah," *Assia* 1 (1976): 78–94; S. Y. Cohen, "Abortion According to Halachah," *Halachah Urefuah* 3 (1983): 86–90; A. Steinberg, "Abortion According to Halachah," *Assia* 1 (1976): 107–124.

78. Stern, "Abortion."

79. Berachot 10a.

80. Genesis 1:28, 9:1 and 7, 35:11.

81. Sanhedrin 4:5.

12

Pregnancy Reduction

Introduction

About 10 percent of all infertile women in whom ovulation is induced by hormonal manipulation become pregnant with multiple fetuses.[1] In vitro fertilization with insemination and implantation of multiple embryos may also result in multiple gestation.[2] The mother of multiple fetuses is subject to very high rates of pregnancy complications. Mothers of triplets have a 20 percent rate of pre-eclampsia and a 35 percent risk of serious postpartum hemorrhage.[3] Complication rates for mothers of four or more fetuses are likely to be even higher.[4] Venous stasis due to uterine distention coupled with long periods of confinement to bed with inactivity make patients with multiple gestation prime candidates for varicose veins, phlebothrombosis (clots in the veins), thrombophlebitis (inflammation of the veins), and embolic phenomena of a serious and even life-threatening nature.

There is also a very high fetal morbidity and mortality which is directly proportional to the number of fetuses in the uterus, primarily because of an increased predisposition to premature delivery. Sixteen percent of triplets, 21 percent of quadruplets and quintuplets, and 41 percent of sextuplets, respectively, do not survive the perinatal period.[5] There is also a very high incidence of infant morbidity and mortality in babies born from multiple gestation.[6]

To reduce or perhaps eliminate these maternal and fetal complications associated with multiple gestation pregnancies, one option is to selectively abort one or more fetuses so that the others remaining have a better chance of surviving normally. Berkowitz et al.

performed selective pregnancy reduction in eleven patients.[7] Two of the patients had each conceived six fetuses, one had five, five had four, and four were carrying triplets. The number of fetuses was reduced to two in eleven pregnancies, and to three in one pregnancy. Seven of the patients had healthy twins, one had a healthy single infant, and four had no liveborn infants. Other cases of selective termination in quintuple pregnancy with successful birth of two babies have been reported.[8]

Women who desperately want their pregnancies to go to term with the birth of one or more healthy infants have few options. To abort all the fetuses because of the danger to the mother of carrying a large number of fetuses defeats the purpose of the pregnancy. Furthermore, the chances of salvaging healthy infants in patients with five or more fetuses without a reduction procedure are poor. Therefore, those who believe that abortion may be appropriate under special circumstances must wrestle with the concept of sacrificing some fetuses so that others can survive.[9]

A related issue is the selective abortion of one or more fetuses that have a serious genetic defect, allowing the unimpeded birth of the other healthy fetuses. Redwine and Hays review twelve cases of twins, including four of their own, in which one twin with either Hurler's syndrome, Down's syndrome, microencephaly, Tay-Sachs disease, spina bifida, hemophilia A or thalassemia major was selectively aborted to allow the birth of the normal co-twin.[10] Eight healthy surviving twins in the first eleven cases gave a success rate of 70 percent.

Another issue is the management of multiple pregnancies complicated by the spontaneous or natural death of one or two fetuses.[11] Danger to the mother from consumption coagulopathy due to a retained dead fetus is a well-recognized medical fact in single and multiple pregnancies requiring intervention to promptly evacuate the dead fetus.[12] Disseminated intravascular coagulopathy causing brain damage in surviving twins after spontaneous intrauterine death of a co-twin is very rare.[13]

The Questions

Does Judaism sanction pregnancy reduction in multiple gestation under any circumstances? Is the abortion of one or more fetuses with a serious genetic or other disease or defect permissible to allow the other, normal fetus or fetuses to be born healthy? Is the selective reduction to two or three normal fetuses from quadruplets, quintuplets, sextuplets, or more, permissible to allow the others to be born healthy? Since the chances of salvaging healthy infants in women with five or more fetuses are extremely poor, can all the fetuses be aborted? Is it permissible to selectively abort a fetus that is endangering the life of the mother and perhaps the lives or health of the other fetuses as well? Is there a difference in Jewish law whether the multiple pregnancy was induced by hormonal stimulation of ovulation or whether multiple ova were inseminated and became implanted following *in vitro* fertilization?

Since these questions are intimately related to the issue of the abortion of even a single fetus, it is first necessary to understand the Jewish view of abortion. Hence, the reader is referred to the previous chapter.

Pregnancy Reduction in Jewish Law

It is axiomatic in Judaism that one may not sacrifice one human life to save another human life or even to save many human lives. Does this principle also apply to the unborn fetus, which is only a potential person and not yet a "human life"? Since all six embryos in a sextuplet pregnancy may not survive if all are left undisturbed, is it permissible to sacrifice three of the embryos by pregnancy reduction in order to allow the other three to live? It is quite possible, although not certain, that the principle of not sacrificing a life to save another life might not extend to the unborn fetus, thereby permitting the destruction of one or more healthy fetuses in order to allow the others to live. The alternative view is that it may be better to let all the fetuses die rather than kill one or more of them.

The latter approach is depicted in the Talmud in a situation in which heathens said to a group of Jewish women: "Surrender one of you to us so that we may defile her, or else we will defile you all."[14] The Talmud rules they should all suffer defilement rather than surrender a single woman to the heathens.

Maimonides extends this principle as follows:

> If heathens said to Israelites: "Surrender one of you to us so that we may put him to death; otherwise we will put you all to death," they should all suffer death rather than surrender a single Israelite to them. But if the heathens specified an individual, saying: "Surrender that particular person to us, or else we will put all to death," they may give him up, provided that he

> was guilty of a capital crime, like Sheba son of Bichri [who rebelled against King David. See II Samuel 20:21–22].[15]

The only exception to the principle that one may not sacrifice one life to save the life of another is the situation of "pursuit" (see previous chapter on abortion), where the pursuer who is threatening the life of his fellow man must be stopped even at the cost of the pursuer's life. Is it possible to argue that three of the six fetuses in a multiple gestation are endangering the life of the other three fetuses and may, therefore, be destroyed to save the lives of the latter three? Clearly, as discussed above, this is a situation of "heavenly pursuit," or an act of God. Secondly, even if one here invokes the argument of pursuit, it is unclear which fetuses are endangering which of the other fetuses. Therefore, it might be inappropriate in Jewish law to permit pregnancy reduction of healthy fetuses for this reason.

On the other hand, in the famous case of Siamese twins joined at the chest and sharing a single six-chambered heart that could not be divided so that both could live, the rabbinic ruling invoked the argument of pursuit to allow the separation of the twins and the "killing" of one to allow the other to live.[16] In addition the following analogy was offered by Rabbi Moshe Tendler: "Two men jump out of a burning airplane and the parachute of the first man opens and he falls slowly and safely to earth. The parachute of the second man does not open. As he plunges past his friend, he manages to grab onto his foot and hold on. But the parachute is too small to support both of them. Now they are both plunging to their deaths." It is morally justified, concluded Tendler, for the first man to kick his friend away because they would both die if he did not, and it was the second man who was designated for death, since it was his parachute that did not open. This analogy does not seem applicable to the multiple pregnancy situation, however, since all the fetuses are equal and no single one has been designated for death. However, all will die if nothing is done.

What if three of the six fetuses suffer from an incurable disease? Is it then permissible to abort the three diseased fetuses to allow the three healthy ones to be born and thrive? Perhaps not, because the diseased fetuses are not endangering the healthy fetuses because of their disease per se. Rather the situation of six fetuses in a single womb at the same time is medically incompatible with the normal birth and survival of all six.

Abortion of one or more fetuses is never allowed in Judaism for the sake of the fetus. Abortion is permissible and even mandated only where the pregnancy, single or multiple, is posing a serious danger to the mother's physical or mental health or constitutes a threat to her life. Since multiple pregnancies are associated with a high rate of serious maternal complications, such as pre-eclampsia, eclampsia, bleeding, uterine atony, and urinary tract infections,[17] it might be permissible to destroy one or more fetuses in a multiple gestation situation to reduce or eliminate these serious risks to the mother.

Pregnancy Reduction Before Forty Days Post-Conception

As discussed above, Jewish sources, including the Talmud and Maimonides,[18] consider the fertilized zygote prior to forty days after conception to represent "mere fluid," since form and shape of the fetus have not yet taken place.[19] Many rabbis are lenient during this time period and permit abortion even without a threat to the mother's health or life. Thus, Drimmer states that a fetus less than forty days old is not fully formed and has no life at all, and there is no prohibition to prevent a Jew or a Gentile from aborting it.[20] Grodzinski, Rosen, and others are also of the opinion that there is no biblical prohibition forbidding the destruction of a pre-forty-day-old fetus by a Jew or a Gentile.[21] Plotzki supports his view allowing abortion prior to forty days by citing the talmudic commentator Rabbenu Tam, who states that a woman is allowed to douche after coitus, thereby discarding the "seed" even if it is a fertilized zygote, because it is before forty days post-conception.[22]

Weinberg allows abortion during the first forty days of pregnancy if the mother was exposed to rubella.[23] On the other hand, Unterman does not allow abortion for rubella exposure even during the first forty days because the fetus is a potential person even during that early period, and one must desecrate the Sabbath on its behalf if necessary if its "life" is in danger.[24] Unterman expresses a minority view, however.

In multiple pregnancies, medical technology using ultrasonic guidance is sufficiently sophisticated today to allow the gynecologist to successfully perform pregnancy reduction prior to forty days after conception. Therefore, since most rabbis permit termination of pregnancy during this period even without a strong maternal medical indication, it seems likely that they will be lenient and allow the destruction of some pre-forty-day-old embryos in order to allow the others to mature and be born healthy.

One can also argue that the "potential person" or "partial person" status of the unborn fetus, as described above in the abortion discussion (see chap. 11), may not apply even after forty days to multiple fetuses of a single pregnancy, since none of the fetuses will likely survive if the pregnancy is allowed to proceed to term without intervention.[25] This situation may, therefore, be viewed differently in Jewish law from the case of a single or twin pregnancy, where the unborn fetus or fetuses, if left undisturbed, have an excellent chance of surviving and may, therefore, not be aborted except to save the life of the mother.

Summary and Conclusion

The recent advent of *in vitro* fertilization and the induction of ovulation by hormones has resulted in the more-than-occasional occurrence of multiple gestations in which pregnant women may be carrying up to seven or eight fetuses at one time. The incidence of maternal morbidity and mortality is much higher in multiple pregnancy than in single pregnancy. Pregnancy reduction, i.e., the intrauterine destruction of some of the fetuses so that the others might live, is an option frequently suggested to the prospective parents. This option is offered to reduce the high risk of maternal complications as well as to reduce the high fetal morbidity and mortality associated with multiple pregnancy.

Judaism does not sanction termination of pregnancy for the sake of the fetus. Therefore, grounds for the permissibility of pregnancy reduction must rest on the consideration that continuation of a multiple pregnancy constitutes a significant hazard to the health and/or life of the mother. Another area of leniency in Jewish law might be the first forty days after conception, during which time considerable rabbinic opinion permits abortion, even in the absence of a clear threat to the mother's health or life, because prior to forty days the small embryo is technically considered to represent "mere fluid."

To accentuate the positive, it seems that a more appropriate term for "selective pregnancy reduction" is "enhanced survival of multifetal pregnancies in the first trimester,"[26] since that is the whole goal of the procedure. The other consideration, as already mentioned, is enhanced safety for the mother, in whom post-partum hemorrhage and eclampsia are far less common in single than in multiple gestations.

Notes

1. J. G. Schenker, S. Yarkoni, and M. Granat, "Multiple Pregnancies Following Induction of Ovulation," *Fertility and Sterility* 35 (1981): 105–125.

2. D. Feldberg, N. Laufer, D. Dicker, et al., "Quadruplet Pregnancy in IVF," *European Journal of Obstetrics, Gynecology, and Reproductive Biology* 23 (1986): 101–106.

3. C. H. Syrop and M. W. Varner, "Triplet Gestation: Maternal and Neonatal Implications," *Acta Genet Med Gemellol* 34 (1985): 81–88.

4. J. C. Hobbins, "Selective Reduction—a Perinatal Necessity?" *New England Journal of Medicine* 318 (1988): 1062–1063.

5. B. J. Botting, I. M. Davies, and A. J. Macfarlane, "Recent Trends in the Incidence of Multiple Births and Associated Mortality," *Archives of Diseases of Children* 62 (1987): 941–950.

6. E. M. Walker and N. B. Patel, "Mortality and Morbidity in Infants Born Between 20 and 28 Weeks Gestation," *British Journal of Obstetrics and Gynaecology* 94 (1987): 670–674.

7. R. L. Berkowitz, L. Lynch, U. Chitkara, I. A. Wilkins, K. E. Mehalek, and E. Alvarez, "Selective Reduction of Multifetal Pregnancies in the First Trimester," *New England Journal of Medicine* 318 (1988): 1043–1047.

8. H. H. H. Kanhai, E. J. C. van Rijssel, R. J. Meerman and J. B. Gravenhorst, "Selective Termination in Quintuplet Pregnancy during First Trimester," *Lancet* 1 (1986): 1447.

9. Hobbins, op. cit.

10. F. O. Redwine and P. M. Hays, "Selective Birth," *Seminars Perinatology* 10 (1986): 73–81.

11. Z. J. Hagay, M. Mazor, J. R. Leiberman, and Y. Biale, "Management and Outcome of Multiple Pregnancies Complicated by the Antenatal Death of One Fetus," *Journal of Reproductive Medicine* 31 (1986): 717–720; E. P. Sakala, "Intrauterine Demise of Two Fetuses in an Unsuspected Triplet Pregnancy: A Case Report," *Journal of Reproductive Medicine* 31 (1986): 1055–1060.

12. D. G. Gallup and W. E. Lucas, "Heparin Treatment of Consumption Coagulopathy Associated with Intrauterine Fetal Death," *Obstetrics and Gynecology* 35 (1970): 690–694; H. Skelly, M. Marivate, R. Norman, et al., "Consumptive Coagulopathy Following Fetal Death in Triplet Pregnancy," *American Journal of Obstetrics and Gynecology* 142 (1982): 595–596; R. Romero, T. P. Duffy, R. L. Berkowitz, and et al., "Prolongation of a Preterm Pregnancy Complicated by Death of a Single Twin in Utero and Disseminated Intravascular Coagulation: Effects of Treatment with Heparin," *New England Journal of Medicine* 310 (1984): 772–774.

13. M. Melnick, "Brain Damage in Survivor After In Utero Death of Monozygous Co-Twin," *Lancet* 2 (1977): 1287.

14. Terumot 8:12.

15. M. Maimonides, *Mishneh Torah, Hilchot Yesodei HaTorah* 5:5.

16. D. C. Drake, "One Must Die So the Other Might Live," *Philadelphia Inquirer,* Oct. 16, 1977.

17. R. C. Benson, "Multiple Pregnancy," in *Current Obstetric and Gynecological Diagnosis and Treatment,* ed. M. L. Pernoll and R. C. Benson, (Norwalk, Conn.: Appleton & Langer, 1987), pp. 321–331.

18. Yebamot 69b; M. Maimonides, *Mishneh Torah, Hilchot Terumot* 8:3.

19. Ibid., *Hilchot Issurei Biyah* 10:1.

20. S. Drimmer, Responsa *Bet Shlomo, Choshen Mishpat,* no. 132.

21. Ch. O. Grodzinski, Responsa *Achiezer,* pt. 3, no. 65; J. Rosen, Responsa *Tzofnat Pane'ach,* pt. 1, no. 49; Schneur Zalman of Lublin, Responsa *Torat Chesed, Even Haezer* 42:32–33.

22. M. D. Plotzki, Responsa *Chemdat Yisrael,* p. 886, citing Rabbenu Tam on Yebamot 12b.

23. Y. Weinberg, Responsa *Seridei Aish,* pt. 3, no. 127.

24. I. Y. Unterman, "Abortion in Jewish Law," *Noam* (1963): 1–11.

25. M. D. Tendler, Personal Communication, Oct. 25, 1988.

26. S. L. Romney, "Selective Reduction of Multifetal Pregnancies," *New England Journal of Medicine* 319 (1988): 949.

13

Fetal Therapy and Fetal Surgery

There is an emerging consensus in tort law of a mother's responsibilities to her unborn fetus. There is also an increasing legal recognition of the right of viable fetuses. Legal and ethical issues arise when the mother's constitutional rights of autonomy, liberty, and privacy conflict with the fetus's right to be born healthy or to be healed from a life-threatening condition by medical or surgical intervention in the mother. Reconciliation of these opposing rights in specific situations is a problem under active discussion in medical, ethical, and legal circles.

Fetal therapy and fetal surgery can correct a variety of disorders and malformations, such as hydronephrosis and hydrocephalus. The International Fetal Surgery Registry reported that between 1982 and 1985, seventy-three placements of catheter shunts for fetal obstructive uropathy and forty-four drainage procedures for obstructive hydrocephalus were performed.[1] The attempts to decompress the obstructed fetal urinary tracts resulted in the survival of thirty fetuses (41 percent). Pulmonary hypoplasia was the major cause of death in both treated and untreated fetuses.

Fletcher points out four ethical issues in fetal therapy and fetal surgery.[2] The first is the conflict between the perceived interests of the fetus with a correctable defect and the interests of the parents, especially the mother, who must give consent for the fetal medical or surgical intervention. The second ethical issue concerns the apparent inconsistency of encouraging fetal therapy on the one hand by considering the fetus as a "patient" and respecting parental choice about abortion on the other. The third ethical issue concerns the proper conditions for learning about the fetus as an object of therapy, i.e., ethical guidelines for fetal research. The final issue is the question of the social and economic priority that should be assigned to investigations of the risks and benefits of fetal therapy.

In a later paper, Fletcher asserts that informed consent by the parents may be more difficult to obtain for fetal therapy than in other health care situations.[3] The affected fetus is nearly always a wanted child. Many parents are morally opposed to abortion, especially when fetal therapy is offered as an alternative, however risky the procedure. Thus, a careful consent process should be designed and implemented.

Fletcher also discusses two long-term issues. What is society's obligation to protect the treatable, nonviable human fetus? The ethics of abortion and the ethics of fetal therapy will collide. The former (i.e., abortion) gives the mother's interests precedence when these are in conflict with those of a nonviable fetus. The ethics of fetal therapy, however, require society to protect the treatable viable fetus. Further, is fetal therapy worth the costs of development for wide use? Will the correction of fetal disorders simply preserve more genetic disorders in the population and add to the burden of suffering? Fletcher concludes that the benefits to society are indeed richer than the economic savings of not performing fetal therapy.

Elias and Annas discuss the enhanced status of the fetus in light of developments in fetal therapy and surgery.

> These innovations raise complex ethical questions about the rights of the mother and fetus as patients. If both are really patients, do both need their own physician? Is the obstetrician to view the fetus or the mother as his patient? Usually, there is no need to make a distinction, but what if the physician believes a procedure [such as fetal surgery] is indicated and the mother refuses to consent?[4]

One of the most difficult legal and ethical issues we currently face is how to balance the rights of the mother and the medical needs of the fetus when they conflict. The basic issue is whether the fetus is a patient separate from its mother. Although many obstetricians view the mother and fetus as a single biological entity, this perception is bound to be altered in light of advances in fetal care, which clearly differentiate the fetus from its mother for treatment purposes. Moreover, most perinatologists are advocates on behalf of the fetus. Thus, advances in fetal surgery are accentuating the potential and actual conflict between maternal interests and the interests of the fetus as a patient.

Some people interpret court-ordered obstetrical interventions such as cesarean sections to imply that "a woman's only function is to produce healthy babies." Many women (and men) may be offended by this unwarranted conclusion. Should women be allowed to decide with impunity on a course of action (e.g., refusal of a relatively safe intervention such as a cesarean section) that may seriously injure their offspring? Does a woman not have a moral obligation not to harm her unborn child? Should a pregnant woman be allowed to drink alcohol, smoke cigarettes, or take cocaine or crack, knowing full well that such behavior has serious deleterious effects on her fetus? Who speaks for the fetus? Why should the mother be the only one who decides on what is or is not done on behalf of her unborn baby?

Blanck discusses women's rights and responsibilities during gestation.[5] He points out that the mother's right to autonomy and privacy in reproduction is fundamental, but like all other constitutional rights, it is not absolute. He quotes Robertson, who said:

> The mother has, if she conceives and chooses not to abort, a legal and moral duty to bring the child into the world as healthy as is reasonably possible. She has a duty to avoid actions or omissions that will damage the fetus and child; just as she has a duty to protect the child's welfare once it is born until she transfers this duty to another. In terms of fetal rights, a fetus has no right to be conceived—or, once conceived, to be carried to viability. But once the mother decides not to terminate the pregnancy, the viable fetus acquires rights to have the mother conduct her life in ways that will not injure it.

Robertson writes that neither law nor ethics presents any barrier to the resolution of the novel legal and ethical problems posed by fetal therapy, such as in utero surgery.[6] Doctors and parents acting in good faith may use an experimental in utero intervention on a fetus that would be at great risk without it, but they are not legally or morally obligated to do so. When the therapy is established, a duty to use it may arise, and a mother's refusal of the intervention may be overriden by the courts.

Johnsen points out that our legal system has historically treated the fetus as part of the mother and has afforded it no independent rights.[7] In recent years, however, courts and state legislatures have increasingly granted fetuses rights traditionally enjoyed by persons. Johnsen concludes that any law granting fetal rights should not disadvantage women or in any way infringe on the autonomy of pregnant women.

The emerging rights of the unborn, where they conflict with the health and personal interests of the mother, present complex questions, especially where the rights pertaining to viability conflict with the choices of the pregnant woman.[8] The American College of Obstetricians and Gynecologists' Committee on Ethics issued a statement in 1987 asserting that "the maternal-fetal relationship remains a unique one, requiring a balance of maternal health, autonomy, and fetal needs. Every reasonable effort should be made to protect the fetus, but the pregnant woman's autonomy should be respected."[9] The statement recommends consultation with an institutional ethics committee when appropriate. "The use of the courts to resolve these conflicts is almost never warranted."

From the Jewish viewpoint, the position of the fetus vis-à-vis the mother has been described in the chapter on abortion. If the risk to the mother is very small, she is obligated to allow her fetus to be treated for a correctable medical or surgical condition. If the risk is substantial, the mother is not obligated to endanger her life to save that of her unborn fetus, because her life takes precedence over that of the fetus.

Notes

1. F. A. Manning, M. R. Harrison, and C. Rodeck, "Catheter Shunts for Fetal Hydronephrosis and Hydrocephalus: Report of the International Fetal Surgery Registry," *New England Journal of Medicine* 315 (1986): 336–340.

2. J. C. Fletcher, "The Fetus as Patient: Ethical Issues," *Journal of the American Medical Association* 246 (1981): 772–773.

3. J. C. Fletcher, "Ethical Considerations in and Beyond Experimental Fetal Therapy," *Seminars in Perinatology* 9 (1985): 130–135.

4. S. Elias and G. J. Annas, "Perspectives on Fetal Surgery," *American Journal of Obstetrics and Gynecology* 145 (1983): 807–812.

5. R. H. Blanck, "Emerging Notions of Women's Rights and Responsibilities during Gestation," *Journal of Legal Medicine* 7 (1986): 441–469.

6. J. A. Robertson, "The Right to Procreate and In Utero Fetal Therapy," *Journal of Legal Medicine* 3 (1982): 333–366.

7. D. E. Johnsen, "The Creation of Fetal Rights: Conflicts with Women's Constitutional Rights to Liberty, Privacy, and Equal Protection," *Yale Law Journal* 95 (1986): 599–625.

8. E. Raines, Editorial, *Obstetrics and Gynecology* 63 (1984): 598–599.

9. Committee on Ethics, *Parent Choice: Maternal-fetal Conflict*, ACOG Committee Opinions no. 55 (Washington: American College of Obstetricians and Gynecologists, 1987).

14

Tay-Sachs Disease: To Screen or Not to Screen

Medical Aspects

In 1881, the British ophthalmologist Warren Tay first described degeneration of the macular region of the eye in a one-year-old child. Six years later, the American neurologist Bernard Sachs published the clinical and pathological findings. Sachs noted the familial nature of the condition, which he called amaurotic familial idiocy. There are six different types, including infantile, late infantile, and adult forms.

The term Tay-Sachs disease refers to the congenital disorder that occurs primarily but not exclusively in Jewish families from Eastern Europe. The disease is characterized by weakness beginning at about six months of age, progressive mental and motor deterioration, blindness, paralysis, dementia, seizures, and death usually by three years of age. The "cherry-red spot" in the macula of the eye is the clinical sign most frequently associated with Tay-Sachs disease.

Pathologically, there is a ballooning of nerve cells throughout the nervous system due to accumulation of lipid material. By electron microscopy, cytoplasmic nerve cell lipid bodies are visible. The lipid that accumulates is ganglioside GM_2, and the specific enzymatic defect responsible for the widespread deposition of this lipid is the absence of hexosaminidase A. The diagnosis of Tay-Sachs disease requires the identification of the accumulated lipid material and documentation of the specific enzymatic defect.

Since hexosaminidase A is deficient in all tissues of patients with Tay-Sachs disease, and since carriers on the average have 50 percent of normal hexosaminidase A activity, the assay for this enzyme can be performed on serum, fibroblasts, or other easily available tissue, including leukocytes and tears.

The inheritance of Tay-Sachs disease follows the laws of Mendelian genetics. The transmission appears to be autosomal recessive, since both parents of patients are clinically normal, sex ratios are equal, and both parents have enzyme levels that are intermediate between those of patients and normal controls. Thus a child who inherits one recessive gene from only one parent is a carrier or has the trait, but is clinically completely normal. Only a child who inherits two Tay-Sachs genes, one from each parent, will have the fatal disease. If two carriers marry, there is a 25 percent chance with each pregnancy that the child will have the disease and a 50 percent chance that the child, like the parents, will be a carrier. There is also a 25 percent chance that the child will be totally free of the disease as well as of the carrier state. If a carrier marries a noncarrier, none of the children can have the fatal disease, but half the children will be carriers.

Concerning the gene frequency, it has been estimated that one in thirty Ashkenazi Jews and one in three hundred non-Jews is a carrier of the Tay-Sachs gene. If a Jew (one-in-thirty risk) marries another Jew (one-in-thirty risk), the chance that both husband and wife are carriers is one in nine hundred. Therefore, one in nine hundred Jewish couples is at risk for having children with Tay-Sachs disease. For such a couple, each pregnancy has a 25 percent chance of producing a child with the fatal disease. Hence, the incidence of Tay-Sachs disease in the Jewish population (assuming there is no intermarriage with non-Jews) is one in thirty-six hundred births. The disease is one hundred times less common in non-Jews. In view of the high rates of intermarriage between Jews and non-Jews in the United States, the incidence of Tay-Sachs births is probably much less than one in thirty-six hundred.

Intrauterine diagnosis of Tay-Sachs disease in an unborn fetus is possible by the procedure called transabdominal amniocentesis, in which a small quantity of amniotic fluid which bathes the developing embryo is removed from the mother's uterus. The fetal cells in this fluid are grown in the laboratory and tested for the presence or absence of hexosaminidase A. Amniotic fluid itself or uncultured cells can also be used for enzyme assay. The incidence of unfavorable side effects of amniocentesis to mother or fetus is low, and accidents of major significance are unusual.

Amniocentesis to detect the disease and screening programs to detect the carrier state of Tay-Sachs will be unnecessary if and when the cure for this disease is developed. Since the specific enzymatic deficiency in Tay-Sachs disease is now known, it seems theoretically possible to prepare, purify, and administer this enzyme as replacement therapy to patients afflicted with the disease. The disease may not be cured, but the clinical symptomatology may be controlled and the patient enabled to lead a nearly normal life. Preliminary attempts at such replacement therapy for Tay-Sachs disease seem to be forthcoming in the not too distant future. Furthermore, genetic engineering may also in the future be able to effect a cure.

Screening for Tay—Sachs Carriers

There have been and continue to be debates concerning the screening of large populations of Jewish people for the carrier state of Tay-Sachs disease and the performance of amniocentesis for the prenatal detection of the fatal disease. Many private organizations and governmental agencies have published pamphlets and other descriptive material relating to various aspects of Tay-Sachs disease. The Tay-Sachs Foundation offers screening for the carrier state and amniocentesis for prenatal diagnosis of the disease. With rare exceptions, articles, pamphlets, and booklets relating to Tay-Sachs disease not only offer but recommend abortion if the amniocentesis reveals an affected child. To eliminate Tay-Sachs disease by "selective termination of affected pregnancies"[1] may not be acceptable in Judaism, although some rabbis might sanction such a procedure. Although local rabbinical support for Tay-Sachs screening programs may be active, such support is usually limited to detecting the carrier state and does not include the performance of amniocentesis with the sole aim of abortion if the fetus is found to have Tay-Sachs disease.

There are other reasons to make one think twice before undertaking mass screening programs. The major reason for the decision of an advisory committee of physicians to recommend against organizing a mass screening program for Tay-Sachs disease was the potential psychic burden on the young people discovered to be heterozygotes.[2] A study of the behavior of physicians and clients in a voluntary program of testing for the Tay-Sachs gene showed a 15 percent anxiety reaction to the discovery of the carrier state.[3]

Another group of physicians specifically discourages unmarried people from being tested because of the possible social problems that carrier identification might create.[4] What are the psychological problems created by the information that one is a carrier for a fatal genetic disease? Should a known carrier refuse to marry a mate who has not been tested? Should two carriers break up an engagement or a marriage if they learn they are both carriers as a result of a screening program? Should a young person inquire about the Tay-Sachs status of a member of the opposite sex prior to meeting that individual on a social level? When should a person who knows he or she is a carrier tell this fact to an intended spouse? Should one sacrifice primary prevention of Tay-Sachs disease by mate selection to avoid psychosocial consequences? Is this method of disease prevention an attractive aspect of genetic screening for recessives?

One must remember that twenty-nine of thirty people tested for the carrier state are found to be free of the Tay-Sachs gene. It is certainly desirable for these twenty-nine of each thirty tested to have peace of mind. Is the anxiety of the thirtieth person on learning that he or she is a carrier sufficiently great to warrant not testing at all? Obviously not! However, one cannot minimize the possible psychosocial trauma to such an individual.

The social stigma of being a carrier of the Tay-Sachs gene is not fully appreciated. Misinformed and/or uninformed people may look at carriers in the same manner as patients with epilepsy and leprosy were looked at half a century ago, i.e., as individuals afflicted with a "taboo" disease, to be shunned and ostracized from normal social contact. Discrimination against carriers of Tay-Sachs disease may also occur in a variety of areas, if the experience of sickle cell screening is repeated. Individuals found to have sickle cell trait were dismissed from their jobs. Several life insurance companies charge higher premiums for individuals with sickle cell trait or refuse to insure them at all. Several airlines reject flight attendants from employment in that capacity if they have sickle cell trait. The United States Air Force, until recently, did not train black recruits with sickle cell trait to become pilots. Job seeking is thus made more difficult for carriers of this hemoglobinopathy. The National Association of Sickle Cell Clinics compiled a list of major insurance companies that discriminate against blacks and others with sickle cell trait. Maryland was the first state to pass a law banning discrimination in employment, life, accident, and health insurance against those who possess the sickle cell trait. Is this fate also to be suffered by people who, on screening, are found to be carriers of the Tay-Sachs gene? Total confidentiality in screening might avoid such problems and should be an essential part of all such programs.

The selection of target groups to be screened for the Tay-Sachs gene, the planning, organization, and implementation of such screening events, the educational activities that must precede screening, the laboratory aspects of the testing, and the referral of people for counseling are beyond the scope of this essay. Suffice it to say that compliance with screening for Tay-Sachs disease is dependent not only on the motivation of the client, his or her perception of the susceptibility to and seriousness of the inherited condition, the possible consequences of noncompliance, and the potential benefits from participation, but also on the moral, ethical, and religious background of the Jewish people who are the clients at risk.

If the purpose of Tay-Sachs screening is to provide eligible clients with genetic counseling about reproductive and mating options, few will argue against screening. If the purpose, however, is to introduce couples at risk to the benefits of prenatal diagnosis by amniocentesis with the specific intent of recommending abortion of affected fetuses, a procedure that may be contrary to the religious dictates of the client, then screening should not be performed. The religious teachings of the Jewish people must be considered if cooperation from the rabbinate and compliance from the clients is to be obtained in any screening program. A plan for the screening of heterozygotes for Tay-Sachs disease in Israel specifically includes the rabbinate, although the portion of the plan that dictates abortion for homozygote fetuses is obviously not acceptable to the Chief Rabbinate.[5]

There is little doubt that screening for hypertension and diabetes and other common conditions, which, although not curable, can be controlled by medical therapy, is highly desirable and should be done. There is less certainty that the benefits of Tay-Sachs screening outweigh the disadvantages, although a qualified affirmative answer on this matter is my position. It is not sufficient to know whether screening is feasible and/or effective; it is also important to know whether it is moral.

Legal Aspects

Some bitter lessons were learned from the laws passed in regard to sickle cell screening. Georgia had a law that required sickle cell screening of all newborns unless the parents objected on religious grounds. In California, all black people admitted to hospitals must be screened by law. In Illinois, mandatory premarital screening for sickle cell trait was enacted "if the physician indicates that it is needed." In New York, premarital testing only of blacks is required, as is screening of all newborns for sickle cell disease and a variety of other genetic diseases and other abnormalities, such as hypothyroidism and phenylketonuria. Many other states passed mandatory screening laws, but few, if any, enforce them.

Most of these laws were challenged on constitutional grounds. Obligatory screening of any age group for any genetic disease seems to be an unconstitutional invasion of the rights of the individual. As a result, many of the laws pertaining to sickle cell screening have been or are being repealed or amended. In some states, such as Virginia and Kentucky, premarital screening is now voluntary, the mandatory provision of the original law having been amended.

In the famous *Jacobsen* decision in 1905, the United States Supreme Court upheld the law of mandatory smallpox vaccination on the basis of the needs of society to protect its citizens from smallpox. However, neither sickle cell disease nor Tay-Sachs disease is a contagious illness, and therefore they do not constitute a danger to others. Although there may be a financial burden on society to care for such patients and/or to support the screening, education, and counseling of potential carriers of either disease, mandatory screening laws still seem to be unconstitutional when weighed against the right of individual privacy.

Discriminatory screening along racial or ethnic lines is also unconstitutional. To pass a law mandating sickle cell screening only for blacks or Tay-Sachs screening only for Jews is clearly discriminatory and underinclusive. Screening must be offered to all, although not all ethnic or racial groups need participate in the screening if they so choose.

If any law is to be passed in regard to Tay-Sachs disease, it must indicate that screening is completely voluntary and that the results will remain confidential. Not only is the preservation of confidentiality an essential component of the doctor-patient relationship and a patient's constitutional right, but a repetition of discriminatory practices that occurred in the sickle cell screening experience must be avoided. Finally, any proposed law concerning Tay-Sachs screening may not require abortion, sterilization, or prohibition of marriage but must preserve the fundamental rights of marriage and procreation.

The Jewish View

Rabbi Moshe Feinstein was asked whether or not it is advisable for a boy or girl to be screened for Tay-Sachs disease, and if it is proper, at what age the test should be performed. He was further asked whether screening should be performed as part of a publicized screening program or only as a private test. His answer was:

> . . . it is advisable for one preparing to be married, to have himself tested. It is also proper to publicize the fact, via newspapers and other media, that such a test is available. It is clear and certain that absolute secrecy must be maintained to prevent anyone from learning the result of such a test performed on another. The physician must not reveal these to anyone. . . . these tests must be performed in private, and, consequently, it is not proper to schedule these test in large groups as, for example, in Yeshivas, schools, or other similar situations.[6]

Rabbi Feinstein also points out that most young people are quite sensitive to nervous tension or psychological stress and, therefore, young men (below age twenty) or women (below age eighteen) not yet contemplating marriage should not be screened for Tay-Sachs disease. Finally, Rabbi Feinstein strongly condemns abortion for Tay-Sachs disease[7] and even questions the permissibility of the amniocentesis which proves the presence of a Tay-Sachs fetus, since amniocentesis is not without risk, albeit small.

Rabbi Feinstein was also asked about the use of contraceptives by a woman who had already given birth to two Tay-Sachs babies, both of whom died in infancy. He disallows the use of a contraceptive diaphragm but permits the use of spermicidal foams and jellies.[8] Feinstein also allows the use of spermicidal foams and jellies by a woman who should not become pregnant because of danger to life.[9] However, he does not allow sterilization of a woman with mental anguish who had previously given birth to two physically defective children,[10] nor for a woman who has given birth to two blind children.[11] Instead he suggests that she practice contraception.[12]

Rabbi J. David Bleich indicates that the elimination of Tay-Sachs disease is, of course, a goal to which all concerned individuals subscribe.[13] He points out, however, that

> the obligation with regard to procreation is not suspended simply because of the statistical probability that some children of the union may be deformed or abnormal. While the couple may quite properly be counseled with regard to the risks of having a Tay-Sachs child, it should be stressed that failure to bear natural children is not a *halakhically* [Jewish legal] viable alternative.

> Of at least equal if not graver concern is the proposal that fetal monitoring be performed with a view toward termination of the pregnancy if the fetus be identified as a victim of Tay-Sachs disease.
>
> The fear that a child may be born physically malformed or mentally deficient does not in itself justify recourse to abortion. . . . Since the sole available medical remedy following diagnosis of severe genetic defects is abortion of the fetus, which is not sanctioned by *Halakhah* [Jewish law] in such instances, amniocentesis, under these conditions, does not serve as an aid in treatment of the patient and is not *halakhically* permissible.

Rabbi Bleich concludes that screening programs for the detection of carriers of Tay-Sachs disease "are certainly to be encouraged." He suggests that the most propitious time for such screening is childhood or early adolescence, since early awareness of a carrier state, particularly as part of a mass screening program, is advantageous.

At its seventieth-anniversary biennial convention in 1974, the Union of Orthodox Jewish Congregations of America adopted a resolution concerning Tay-Sachs screening that essentially echoes the opinion of Rabbi Bleich cited above. The Union suggests that "the Orthodox community can extend support to programs of genetic screening *only* when competent *Halachic* guidance is provided for all participants." The Union called upon its constituent synagogues to work for such programs in every Jewish community but emphasized that all Tay-Sachs screening programs must be accompanied by adequate and competent rabbinic counseling.

The Association of Orthodox Jewish Scientists issued a statement in 1973 outlining its position in regard to Tay-Sachs screening as follows:

> We endorse voluntary screening of young adults of an age in which marriage has become a serious consideration but before definite marital commitments have been made. The screening of younger individuals, years before marriage, yields no immediate benefits and might result in a longer period of anxiety in carriers than is warranted. We feel that all screening must be linked to both genetic and religious personal counseling. Emotionally immature individuals may be traumatized psychologically if they learn of their carrier state, and these individuals must be provided with the opportunity for additional professional psy-

chological support. Genetic counseling must be in consonance with Torah principles.

The Association is unalterably opposed to amniocentesis, whose natural and logical consequence is abortion. It likewise feels that screening of married couples or those whose marriage is imminent and who are not committed to disruption of their mutual marital commitments, were both partners to be discovered to be Tay-Sachs carriers, is unwise, again because virtually the only consequences would be abortion or a childless marriage. We are also concerned that any program be absolutely voluntary, and that the nature of any educational drive be informational rather than coercive. There must also be absolute assurance that the confidentiality of all carriers will be safeguarded.[14]

Rabbi Eliezer Yehudah Waldenberg allows abortion following amniocentesis during the first trimester if the fetus is determined to have Tay-Sachs disease. His words are very expressive: "if there is a strong suspicion that the fetus will be born physically deformed and suffer greatly, one can allow abortion prior to forty days of conception and perhaps even up to three months of the pregnancy before the fetus begins to move."[15]

Waldenberg relies in part on the ruling of Rabbi Jacob Emden, who sanctions abortion for a "grave need," which includes even the abortion of a bastard fetus to relieve the mother from the mental pain and anguish involved.[16] More recently, Waldenberg allows termination of pregnancy for Tay-Sachs disease up to the seventh month of pregnancy because "the defect, the anguish, the shame, the physical and mental pain and suffering of the parents are inestimable."[17] Rabbi Bleich points out that Waldenberg rules contrary to the vast majority of rabbinic opinions and contrary to the decisions of other contemporary rabbinic scholars and contrary to his own previously expressed position.[18]

The Jewish view on abortion is presented in detail elsewhere in this book (see Chap. 12). Essentially, abortion is not only allowed but mandated where the mother's life is at stake or where there is a serious threat to her physical or mental health by the continued pregnancy.

The various objections to amniocentesis and abortion in Jewish law are predicated on considerations surrounding the fetus. Extreme emotional stress in the mother leading to suicidal intent might constitute one of the situations in which abortion would be sanctioned by most rabbis. If a woman who suffered a nervous breakdown following the birth (or death) of a child with Tay-Sachs disease becomes pregnant again, and is so distraught with the knowledge that she may be carrying another child with the fatal disease that she threatens suicide, Jewish law would allow amniocentesis. If this procedure reveals an unaffected fetus, the pregnancy continues to term. If the result of the amniocentesis indicates a homozygous fetus with Tay-Sachs disease, rabbinic consultation regarding the decision of whether or not to perform an abortion should be obtained. No general rule of permissiveness or prohibition can be enunciated in regard to abortion in Jewish law. Each case must be individualized and evaluated on the basis of its merits, taking into consideration all the prevailing medical, psychological, social, and religious circumstances.

Notes

1. L. R. Glazermann, "Screening for Genetic Disease," *New England Journal of Medicine* 289 (1973): 754–755.

2. M. D. Kuhr, "Doubtful Benefits of Tay-Sachs Screening," *New England Journal of Medicine* 292 (1975): 371.

3. E. Beck, S. Blaichman, C. R. Scriver, and C. L. Clow, "Advocacy and Compliance in Genetic Screening: Behavior of Physicians and Clients in a Voluntary Program of Testing for the Tay-Sachs Gene," *New England Journal of Medicine* 291 (1974): 1166–1170.

4. M. M. Kaback, R. S. Zeiger, L. W. Reynolds, et al., "Tay-Sachs Disease: A Model for the Control of Recessive Genetic Disorders," *Proceedings of the Fourth International Conference on Tay-Sachs Disease. Vienna, Sept. 2–8, 1973* (Amsterdam: Excerpta Medica, 1974), pp. 218–262.

5. B. Padeh, "A Screening Program for Tay-Sachs Disease in Israel," *Israel Journal Of Medical Sciences* 9 (1973): 1330–1334.

6. Responsum kindly provided by Rabbi Feinstein's son-in-law, Rabbi Dr. Moshe D. Tendler.

7. M. Feinstein, in *Halachah Urefuah* 1 (1980): 304–306.

8. M. Feinstein, Responsa *Iggrot Moshe, Even Ha'ezer*, no. 62.

9. Ibid., *Even Ha'ezer*, pt. 3, no. 21.

10. Ibid., no. 12.

11. Ibid., no. 13.

12. See above, chap. 8.

13. J. D. Bleich, "Tay-Sachs Disease," *Tradition* 13 (1973): 145–148; and in *Or HaMizrach* 21 (1972): 216–218.

14. Personal communication from the President of the Association of Orthodox Jewish Scientists.

15. Waldenberg, Responsa *Tzitz Eliezer*, vol. 9, no. 51:3.

16. Emden, Responsa *She'elat Yavetz*, no. 43.

17. Waldenberg, op. cit., vol. 13, no. 102, and in *Assia* 13 (March 1976): 8–10.

18. J. D. Bleich, *Contemporary Halakhic Problems* (New York: Ktav, 1977), pp. 109–115.

15

Genetic Engineering

Introduction

The nucleus of every cell in the human body contains twenty-three pairs of chromosomes. One chromosome of each pair is derived from the maternal egg and the other from the paternal sperm. Each chromosome is composed of thousands of genes, which are the functional units of heredity. The science of genetics is the study of heredity, or the transmission of genes for particular traits or characteristics from parent to offspring.

Primitive attempts by man to change the genetic makeup of certain lower forms of life involved the removal of the nuclei from frog cells and their transplantation into fertilized frog eggs whose nuclei had been previously removed. Viable tadpoles have developed, all of whom had the precise features of the original frog from whom the nuclei were obtained. This process is called nuclear cloning because a whole clone of genetically identical creatures is produced. The technical problems surrounding nuclear cloning by nuclear transplantation in man have not yet been surmounted.

On a more basic level, the genetic material within the nucleus, DNA, can be enzymatically cut into smaller sequences of genes, and these small segments can be spliced or recombined. This recombinant DNA technology has now made it possible to transfer genes to totally unrelated hosts. A vector (usually a virus) is needed to transfer this DNA material into the animal, plant, or bacterial cell of choice. Hereditary material from virtually any plant or animal cell can now be propagated in bacteria, and bacterial genes can be inserted into animal cells. Various terms have been used to describe these revolutionary methods including "gene splicing," "gene grafting," "gene cloning," "gene transplantation," "genetic manipulation," and "genetic meddling." The two most widely accepted terms are "recombinant DNA research" and the broader phrase "genetic engineering." Medical science now has the capacity to rearrange the genetic heritage of thousands of years.

The potential advantages of recombinant DNA research are several. Some genes can now be copied, and, thus, their precise structure can be more easily studied. Bacteria can be directed by the gene transplanted into it to assemble a protein valuable to man. Insulin, antibiotics, antiviral agents, and numerous other drugs, chemicals, and vaccines might be synthesized in large quantities by the technology of genetic engineering. Patients with absent or defective genes, suffering from such genetic disorders as Tay-Sachs disease, hemophilia, sickle-cell anemia, and the like, might be given a replacement gene. Clones of nitrogen-producing bacteria might be useful for agriculture. Bacteria that concentrate trace elements, such as uranium or platinum, could be cloned to increase the supply of such elements. Other commercial applications of recombinant DNA research, such as the manufacture of methane gas and the production of pollution-eating bacteria, also exist. Specially engineered bacteria are thus envisioned as "factories" for the production of numerous important substances for medicine and industry.

On the other hand, potential hazards of recombinant DNA research exist. Genes for pathogenic products might be transplanted into bacteria deliberately or inadvertently. Unexpected alterations may occur. One must contemplate the possibility of accidental release into the environment of organisms carrying extraneous genetic material and/or the infection of plant or animal life with these bacteria. Recombinant DNA may be taken up by human cells in such a way as to produce cancer or other diseases. One writer in a popular magazine cautions that "pollution-gobbling bugs might go on uncontrolled binges, eating every chemical in sight; nitrogen-fixing bacteria could possibly devastate soil ecology. Possibly worst of all is the fact that, once created, the new bugs cannot be destroyed."

Legal Aspects

With the launching of recombinant DNA technology in 1973, scientists at the Gordon Conference, a meeting on nucleic acids held in New England in the summer of that year, expressed their concerns and requested the National Academy of Sciences to recommend specific actions or guidelines in the light of potential hazards.

The scientists also asked their colleagues to voluntarily defer action on certain experiments because of the possible hazards. Individual investigators responded by voluntarily halting such research pending further discussion and the development of adequate guidelines, but this moratorium was not observed everywhere.

A meeting was held subsequently at the Asilomar Conference Grounds, Pacific Grove, California, in 1975, where 150 international scientists discussed the future of recombinant DNA research. A provisional statement was issued that proposed a tentative classification of experiments by risk, and specified appropriate safeguards for low-, moderate-, and high-risk experiments. Research continued, although adherence to the recommendations was voluntary.

In July 1976, the National Institutes of Health (NIH) issued a comprehensive set of guidelines governing recombinant DNA research. Compliance was mandatory for NIH laboratories and all projects supported by NIH grants and contracts. The regulations attempted to reduce the risks associated with such investigation by means of stringent safeguards that prohibited certain types of experimentation, and imposed standards for physical and biologic containment of possibly dangerous organisms. The guidelines, however, did not apply to research performed in the private sector that was not funded by NIH.

Revised guidelines were proposed two years later, adopted in 1978, and went into effect early in 1979. The stringencies of the original guidelines were relaxed. In February 1982, the federal Recombinant DNA Advisory Committee recommended additional relaxation of the existing safety guidelines. At its previous meeting in September 1981, the committee voted a recommendation that would have changed the entire set of federal guidelines into a nonbinding code of good laboratory practice. The reasons for these relaxations relate in part to the fact that, over the years, no known hazards have materialized but several potentially valuable medical products have been produced through gene-splicing techniques.

Early concern about the possible deleterious effects on society of genetic-engineering research and application was voiced by many scientific bodies and governmental agencies. The New York Academy of Sciences and the Institute of Society, Ethics and the Life Sciences cosponsored a conference on Ethical and Scientific Issues Posed by Human Uses of Molecular Genetics.[1] The First Annual Congress of Recombinant DNA Research was held in February 1981 in San

Francisco. By the time the National Institute for Child Health and Human Development held a public forum on gene therapy in November 1983 in Bethesda, Maryland, the discussion reflected the change of attitude and lack of substantial opposition to such biomedical activities. There was recognition of the fact that the preponderance of evidence to date supports the conclusion that recombinant DNA research poses no serious hazards to public health, laboratory workers, or the environment. According to one writer, "The benefits reaped and projected for humanity surpass all unsubstantiated risks, and without question, justify continuation of the research. Debate was protracted because scientists exercised their responsibility for discreet transmission of conjectural information to an alarmed public."[2]

Moral and Ethical Issues

In 1980, Dr. Martin J. Cline, a professor at the UCLA (University of California at Los Angeles) School of Medicine and his colleagues conducted two controversial gene therapy experiments on human beings overseas.[3] A review board at UCLA had not yet granted permission for the experiments, saying more animal research was needed. Early the next year, Dr. Cline was reprimanded by the National Institute of Health, which later stripped him of $200,000 in federal research grants.

Gene therapy refers to the process of introducing a properly functioning gene in somatic cells to correct the effect of a defective one in order to cure hereditary diseases that are caused by gene mutations. Diseases such as sickle cell anemia, thalassemia, Tay-Sachs disease, and the like, might be cured by gene therapy. Suppose we could eliminate diabetes, cancer, and heart disease by genetic engineering? Would we not grasp the opportunity?

Is it ethical to attempt to insert new genetic information into humans to alleviate or cure a serious or lethal disease in a patient before the probable benefits and risks have been determined in tissue culture systems and in animals? If not, at what point is it ethical to begin trying such new treatments? Some ethicists argue that before such experiments are performed in human beings, there should be reasonable evidence from animal studies that the new gene can be put into the target cells and remain in them, that the new gene can be regulated appropriately, and that the presence of the new gene does not harm the cell.[4]

The technical aspects and the potentials of gene therapy are reviewed by Mercola and Cline, who consider the following points paramount because of the ethical considerations involved:

> Initial trials should be conducted in patients with limited alternative options [i.e., advanced disease unresponsive to conventional therapy]; the trial should be of potential benefit to the patient [i.e., a genuine chance of ameliorating disease must exist]; the patient or responsible guardian should understand the study and its uncertainties as thoroughly as possible; and the study should be designed so that useful information will be obtained to aid in design of future trials.[5]

The ethical principles governing human experimentation also apply to gene therapy and genetic engineering.[6] These principles dictate the approach that before any gene is manipulated or inserted in a human being, animal studies must ensure that the new gene has a reasonable chance of producing the desired result and that there is a reasonable expectation that it will not produce a harmful result. These principles are presented in greater detail by Grobstein and Flower, who suggest that medical science "proceed with caution" in regard to gene therapy.[7] The power to cure a genetic defect is an awesome one, but since the goal of biomedical research is the alleviation of human suffering, gene therapy "is a proper and logical part of that effort."[8]

Related issues of genetic screening and counseling, embryo transfer, *in vitro* fertilization, host mothers, artificial insemination, sex organ transplants, sex preselection and predetermination and manipulation, are discussed elsewhere in this book.

Cloning of man raises yet other moral and ethical issues. Are we encroaching on the Creator's domain? Is man allowed to tamper with his very essence in an attempt to duplicate himself in creating an "artificial" man? Is man permitted to alter humanhood or humanity or both by genetic manipulations? Some horrifying thoughts come to mind, eloquently expressed by a popular writer:

> Professional athletic organizations might well be attracted to the idea of making direct multiple copies of their basketball stars . . . military leaders with billions of dollars available for research might well be interested in mass-producing humans high in endurance, strength, or proneness to obedience. . . . If a

> husband and wife were in deep distress because a greatly beloved child was dying, they could arrange to create another child that would be genetically identical. . . .
>
> People interested in personal immortality could assure themselves of at least a start. They could arrange, through cell banking, to have persons of their exact genotype live on. . . . There would be problems right from the start. Who would decide what individuals were to be mass-produced by cloning? Would it be left to the free enterprise market mechanism? Or would the state take over? If so, there would probably be black-marketing. Or would a nervous world set up the International Commission for Genetic Control to license clonists? A new set of human ethics would seem to be required.[9]

Cloning and recombinant DNA research have been compared to a Dr. Frankenstein producing biological monsters[10] and characterized as a Faustian bargain.[11] The eugenic aspects of cloning are beyond the scope of this essay but must also be considered. Critics as well as proponents of such research all agree that regulation of some type is necessary, since the technology of genetic engineering is so potent that even a slight deviation from the intended path might cause grievous consequences to society and to the individuals concerned. The social and ethical issues of genetic engineering were reviewed in detail by the President's Commission for the Study of Ethical Problems in Medicine and Biomedical and Behavioral Research.[12]

A new area of ethical concern relates to the fact that genetic engineering is creating a new world of financial opportunities.[13] Late in 1983, Harvard University granted exclusive licensing on a genetic engineering process it had patented to a biotechnology firm whose chairman, a former Harvard professor, had invented the process. Several months earlier, Harvard's faculty had adopted a comprehensive set of rules to limit the ability of commercial companies to influence research they sponsor on the campus. These seemingly contradictory actions by Harvard again raise the issue of the link between the genetics and other biomedical industries and universities.

In 1981, the Du Pont Company of Wilmington, Delaware, announced a $6 million grant for genetic research at Harvard Medical School. The Massachusetts General Hospital accepted a $60 million grant for similar research from the West German chemical conglomerate Hoechst-Roussel Pharmaceuticals. The Massachusetts Institute of Technology was awarded $120 million by the Edwin C.

Whitehead Foundation for the construction and operation of an independent biomedical research institute capable of conducting research in recombinant DNA. Stanford University and the University of California at Berkeley cooperated with six private companies on a $10 million genetic engineering project and the formation of a new company.

Also in 1981, Emory University in Atlanta and Hybridoma Sciences jointly created a new corporation to fund an immunobiology research center to be wholly a part of the university. The corporation in turn receives first licensing rights to all commercially useful developments arising from research at the center. Ownership of the developments remains with the university and the discovering scientists, and royalties to the university are to be negotiated individually for each licensed discovery. In 1982, Washington University in St. Louis and the Monsanto Chemical Company formed a partnership with a $24 million grant from the company for biomedical research. The university holds the patents and receives royalties for inventions, but Monsanto has the exclusive licensing rights. Although the researchers are free to publish all the results, Monsanto has the right to review potentially patentable findings and delay their publication.

The sudden interest in the financial aspects of genetic engineering and other biotechnology, coupled with the fact that universities are a rich source of knowledgeable researchers in this field, has created unprecedented moral and ethical problems and has brought enormous pressures on universities and their faculties. One of the major concerns is the potential threat to the open and free exchange of ideas and information. Another concern is the potential for conflict of interest where professors have financial interests in the companies that sponsor their academic research. Should the professors and the university share in the profits? Should the companies that support and convert the research into marketable products be entitled to the lion's share of the profits? This new ethical issue is of much broader dimensions than genetic engineering alone, since it concerns the world of commerce and industry and its involvement in the academic medical center, and is beyond the scope of this presentation.

The Jewish View

To Jews life is of infinite value; one moment of life is equal to living seventy years. Thus Jews are permitted to desecrate the Sabbath to save the life of one who will live only for a short while. All biblical and rabbinic commandments are set aside for the overriding consideration of saving a life.

Since man was created in the image of God, human beings are holy and must be treated with dignity and respect, both during life and after death. Our bodies are God-given, for only God gives and takes life. Recent developments in medicine and science threaten our observing these fundamental Jewish principles. When scientists master genetic engineering, are we tampering with life itself? Nature was created by God for man to use to his advantage and benefit. Hence, animal experimentation is permissible in Jewish law.[14] The production of hormones in animals for man's benefit by recombinant DNA techniques also seems perfectly permissible. Gene therapy, such as the replacement of the missing or defective gene in Tay-Sachs disease or hemophilia, is also probably sanctioned in Jewish law because it can restore health and preserve and prolong life.

Ancient Jewish writings, including the Bible and Talmud, are not devoid of source material relating to genetics. A recent writer describes in some detail how the laws of Mendelian genetics were applied by Jacob in the biblical narrative of the speckled and spotted sheep.[15] The Talmud and subsequent rabbinic writings describe the precise sex-linked genetics of hemophilia.[16]

The literature on cloning, recombinant DNA technology, and genetic engineering, as viewed in Jewish law, is very sparse indeed.[17] A lengthy article entitled "Legal and Halachic Aspects of Genetic Engineering" is, in fact, devoted mostly to artificial insemination, *in vitro* fertilization, and "test-tube" babies, with only brief mention of cloning.[18]

The medical problems of removing the ovum, modifying some of its genes by microsurgical techniques, and replacing the viable ovum in the mother have not yet been surmounted. However, assuming such surgery can be successfully performed, one rabbi contends that gene surgery would be permissible in Jewish law because genes are submicroscopic particles and no process invisible to the naked eye is forbidden in Jewish law.[19] For example, laws of forbidden foods do not apply to microorganisms. Further, the priest only declares ritually unclean that which his eyes can see.

Another argument for the permissibility of gene surgery is the fact that the ovum (or sperm) is not a person, since conception has not yet taken place. Thus, gene manipulation would not be considered as tampering with an existing human being but only with a potential one. Some authorities, however, would argue that the destruction of even a potential human being (either the unborn fetus or the unfertilized human seed) is prohibited in Jewish law.[20]

One can also argue that any surgery performed on a live human being must certainly be permitted on an ovum (or sperm) before conception. For example, if a surgical cure for hemophilia or Tay-Sachs disease were possible, it would surely be permissible; hence, it would certainly be permissible to cure hemophilia or Tay-Sachs disease by gene surgery.

If it were possible to perform gene transplants by transplantation of genes from one person into the ovum or sperm of another, the following Jewish legal questions would arise: Are gene transplants considered to be a type of perverted sex act between the gene donor and the recipient? Would such transplants be forbidden, in particular, if donor and recipient were close relatives? Would a child conceived from such a manipulated ovum or sperm be regarded as related to the gene donor? Can one draw parallels from rabbinic responsa dealing with ovarian transplants and conclude that since no sex act is involved in a gene transplant, the recipient is not forbidden to marry the donor's relatives, and the child conceived and born following a gene transplant is not related to the gene donor? In most organ transplants (kidney, cornea, heart, ovary, "gene") the organ becomes an integral part of the recipient.

Rabbi Moshe Hershler writes that we should not blind ourselves to the potential of genetic engineering and gene therapy, which is no longer a dream or a fantasy but becoming a medical and scientific reality.[21] Hershler raises the question of the permissibility (or lack thereof) of experimenting with gene therapy to try to save the life of a child with thalassemia or Tay Sachs disease if the unsuccessful outcome of the experimentation would be a shortening of the child's life.[22] Hershler is of the opinion that gene therapy and genetic engineering may be prohibited because "he who changes the [Divine] arrangement of creation is lacking faith [in the Creator],"[23] and he cites as support for his view the prohibition against mating diverse kinds of animals, sowing together diverse kinds of seeds, and wearing garments made of wool and linen.[24] However, genetic engineering does not seem to be comparable to the grafting of diverse types of animals or seeds. The main purposes of gene therapy are to cure disease, restore health, and prolong life, all goals within the physician's Divine license to heal.[25] Why is "gene grafting" any different than an "organ graft," such as a kidney or corneal transplant, which nearly all rabbis conclude is permissible?[26]

Conclusion

Increased medical knowledge and technological advances in the past decade have made organ transplants, genetic engineering, cloning, *in vitro* fertilization, and host mothers a reality. The potential risks, potential benefits, and ethical considerations of such research and its applications must be carefully considered. Tampering with the very essence of life and encroaching upon the Creator's domain are considerations worthy of extensive discussion from the Jewish standpoint. Are we creating artificial human beings bordering on *golems* (artificial men), an example of which is described in the Talmud as having been created by Raba?[27] Is such a *golem* human? Elsewhere, the Talmud tells us:

> There are three partners in man: the Holy One, blessed be He, his father, and his mother. His father supplies the semen of the white substance out of which are formed the child's bones, sinews, nails, the brain in his head, and the white of his eye. His mother supplies the semen of the red substance out of which is formed his skin, flesh, hair, blood, and the black of his eye. And the Holy One, blessed be He, gives the spirit and the breath, beauty of features, eyesight, the power of hearing, the ability to speak and walk, understanding and discernment.[28]

The spiritual and theological aspects of genetic engineering and DNA recombinant research also require exploration. Rabbis must examine these issues from the Jewish standpoint and offer legal guidance to the medical and lay communities. In the meanwhile, Rabbi Immanuel Jakobovits expresses sentiments which we should all take to heart.

> It is indefensible to initiate uncontrolled experiments with incalculable effects on the balance of nature and the preservation of man's incomparable spirituality without the most careful evaluation of the likely consequences beforehand. . . . "Spare-part" surgery and "genetic engineering" may open a wonderful chapter in the history of healing. But without prior agreement on restraints and the strictest limitations, such mechanization of human life may also herald irretrievable disaster resulting from man's encroachment upon nature's preserves, from assessing human beings by their potential value as tool-parts, sperm-donors or living incubators, and from replacing the

matchless dignity of the human personality by test-tubes, syringes and the soulless artificiality of computerized numbers.

Man, as the delicately balanced fusion of body, mind and soul, can never be the mere product of laboratory conditions and scientific ingenuity. To fulfill his destiny as a creative creature in the image of his Creator, he must be generated and reared out of the intimate love joining husband and wife together, out of identifiable parents who care for the development of their offspring, and out of a home which provides affectionate warmth and compassion.[29]

Notes

1. M. Lappé, and R. S. Morison, eds., "Ethical and Scientific Issues Posed by Human Uses of Molecular Genetics," *Annals of the New York Academy of Sciences* 265 (1976): 1–208.

2. V. W. Franco, "Ethics of Recombinant DNA Research and Technology: An Assessment of Its Risks and Benefits," *New York State Journal of Medicine* 81 (1981): 1035–1044.

3. K. E. Mercola and M. J. Cline, "The Potential of Inserting New Genetic Information," *New England Journal of Medicine* 303 (1980): 1297–1300.

4. W. F. Anderson and J. C. Fletcher, "Gene Therapy in Human Beings: When Is It Ethical to Begin?" *New England Journal of Medicine* 303 (1980): 1293–1296.

5. Mercola and Cline, op. cit.

6. Rosner, F. Modern Medicine, Religion and Law. Human Experimentation *New York State Journal of Medicine* 75 (1975): 758–764.

7. C. Grobstein and M. Flower, "Gene Therapy: Proceed with Caution," *Hastings Center Report* 14 (1984): 13–17.

8. Anderson and Fletcher, op. cit.

9. V. Packard, *The People Shapers* (Boston: Little, Brown, 1977), p. 141.

10. W. Gaylin, "The Frankenstein Factor," *New England Journal of Medicine* 297 (1977): 665–667.

11. P. Siekevitz, "Recombinant DNA Research: A Faustian Bargain," *Science* 194 (1976): 256.

12. President's Commission for the Study of Ethical Problems in Medicine and Biomedical and Behavioral Research, *Splicing Life: A Report on the Social and Ethical Issues of Genetic Engineering with Human Beings* (Washington, D.C., November 1982).

13. F. Rosner, "Is Academia Going into Business?" *Cancer Investigation*, 1984, vol. 2, 493–495.

14. See below, chap. 25.

15. Y. Flicks, "Torsha Usevivah Bema'aseh Yaakov Batzon Laban" [Heredity and environment: Genetics in Jacob's handling of Laban's flock], *Techumin* 3 (1982/5742): 461–472. The biblical incident is recounted in Genesis 3:32 ff.

16. F. Rosner, "Hemophilia in the Talmud and Rabbinic Writings," *Annals of Internal Medicine* 70 (1969): 833–837.

17. F. Rosner, "Recombinant DNA, Cloning, Genetic Engineering, and Judaism," *New York State Journal of Medicine* 79 (1979): 1439–1444.

18. M. Drori, "Hahandassah Hagenetis: Iyun Reeshoni Behibatim Mishpatiyim Vehabilihatim," *Techumin* 1 (1980/5740): 280–296.

19. A. Rosenfeld, "Judaism and Gene Design," *Tradition* 13 (1972): 71–80.

20. See above chap. 11.

21. M. Hershler, "Handassah Genetis Behibatim Hilchatim" [Genetic engineering in Jewish law], *Halachah Urefuah* 2 (1981): 350–353.

22. See below, chap. 17.

23. Hershler, op. cit.

24. Leviticus 19:19. See also Pesachim 54b.

25. See above chap. 1.

26. See below chap. 21.

27. Sanhedrin 65b.

28. Niddah 31a.

29. I. Jakobovits, *Jewish Medical Ethics* (New York: Bloch, 1975), pp. 261–266.

PART III
The End of Life

16

Euthanasia

Introduction

The word *euthanasia* is derived from the Greek *eu*, meaning "well, good, or pleasant," and *thanatos*, meaning "death." Webster's dictionary defines euthanasia as the mode or act of inducing death painlessly or as a relief from pain. The popular expression for euthanasia is mercy killing. Perusal of the medical literature of the last three decades reveals a host of books, articles, editorials, and letters to editors of journals dealing with this subject. These writings are exclusive of the legal, theologic, psychologic, and social literatures. Even the lay press is replete with writings on euthanasia, from the withholding of treatment from a handicapped newborn to the withdrawal of life-support systems from a terminally ill patient.

There is thus little doubt as to the tremendous interest in euthanasia. This chapter is an attempt to briefly review the subject by providing classification and terminology, citing selected examples, describing the legal attitude toward euthanasia in various countries, discussing the arguments put forth for and against euthanasia, briefly mentioning the Catholic and Protestant viewpoints on euthanasia, and finally presenting in detail the Jewish attitude toward euthanasia.

Classification and Terminology

A euphemistic term used by euthanasia societies for mercy killing is "merciful release"[1] or "liberating euthanasia."[2] Some people classify euthanasia into three types: eugenic, medical, and preventive.[3] A more meaningful classification speaks of eugenic, active medical, and passive medical euthanasia.[4] Eugenic euthanasia encompasses the "merciful release" of handicapped newborns and socially undesirable individuals, such as the mentally retarded and psychiatrically disturbed. Perhaps an extreme example of this method of extermination was the Nazi killing of all the socially unacceptable or socially unfit, including Jews. To many, this German practice as well as all eugenic euthanasia is considered nothing less than murder; there are very few proponents of this type of euthanasia.

Active medical euthanasia is exemplified by the case where a drug or other treatment is administered, and death is thereby hastened. This type of euthanasia may be voluntary or involuntary, that is, with or without the patient's consent.

Passive medical euthanasia is defined as the situation in which therapy is withheld so that death is hastened by omission of treatment. This type of euthanasia has also been called automathanasia,[5] meaning automatic death, such as without therapeutic heroics. This passive form of euthanasia can also be voluntary or involuntary.

Exemplification of the Problem

Many a physician has had to wrestle with the problem of an incurably ill, suffering patient. Such physicians fully realize that "whereas life is lengthened, man's period of usefulness is not always lengthened."[6] Some are of the opinion that advanced medicine should "serve only to improve the condition of human life as it increases the life span and not the useless prolongation of human suffering."[7] Thus, a general practitioner in Manchester, New Hampshire, ended a cancer patient's suffering by injecting into the patient a substantial quantity of air intravenously. He was acquitted.[8] A Stamford, Connecticut, woman shot and killed her father who was dying of incurable cancer. She was acquitted.[9]

The problem is far from localized to the shores of the United States. Giuseppe F., having settled in France, was struck with an incurable disease. He summoned his brother Luigi and convinced the latter to kill him, which Luigi did. The jury acquitted Luigi.[10]

One of the most famous instances exemplifying many of the problems surrounding euthanasia is the case of the physician son of the founder of the British Euthanasia Society, who told a Rotary meeting: "To keep her from pain . . . I gave her an injection to make her sleep."[11] His objective, as specifically stated, was to relieve pain, not to put an end to the patient's life. An outcry in the British press followed, labeling the incident "a mercy killing." Even the British Euthanasia Society admitted that from a strictly legal sense mercy killing is murder, but it backed the physician by insisting that "every doctor must be guided by his own conscience." Many physicians disagreed, saying euthanasia is legalized murder. Others cited the Hippocratic oath, which states: "I will give no deadly medicine to anyone if asked, nor suggest any such counsel." Still others were of the opinion that the Hippocratic oath refers only to premeditated murder. The medical council refused to act against the physician unless the family of the deceased lodged a formal complaint. However, the family consented to the physician's actions. Thus, all the ingredients to emphasize the problem of euthanasia are present in this case: the incurable patient in great pain, the request for euthanasia by patient and family, and the physician's acquiescence and participation.

The list of examples one could cite is endless. The aforementioned illustrative cases serve as background for the ensuing discussion.

Legal Considerations

Although suicide is not legally a crime in most American jurisdictions, aiding and abetting suicide is a felony. Euthanasia, even at the patient's request, is legally murder in the United States. In England the Suicide Act of 1961 states that it is not a criminal offense for a person, whether in sickness or in health, to take his own life or to attempt to do so. However, any individual who helps him to do so becomes liable to a charge of manslaughter. Euthanasia per se does not exist in the law books of France and Belgium, and in both countries it is considered premeditated homicide. However, a bill to legalize euthanasia for some "damaged" children came before the Belgian government following the famous Liège trial involving parents, relatives, and a physician charged with murdering a thalidomide-damaged child.[12]

In Italy, euthanasia is only a crime if the victim is under eighteen years of age, mentally retarded, or menaced or under the effect of fear. More tolerant attitudes also exist in Denmark, Holland, Yugoslavia, and even Catholic Spain. In the Soviet Union, euthanasia is considered "murder under extenuating circumstances" and punishable with three to eight years in prison.[13] Switzerland seems to have the most lenient legislation.[14] The Swiss penal code, as revamped in 1951, distinguishes between killing with bad intentions, that is, murder, and killing with good intentions, that is, euthanasia. In addition, in 1964 in Sweden, passive euthanasia was legalized. Even in countries where euthanasia is legally murder, "the sympathies of juries towards mercy killings often cause the law to be circumvented by various methods, making for great inequities of the legal system."[15]

In 1935 the first Euthanasia Society was founded in England for the purpose of promoting legislation which would seek to "make the act of dying more gentle." In 1936, one year after the founding of the society, a bill was introduced into the House of Lords which sought to permit voluntary euthanasia in certain circumstances and with certain safeguards. Following a rather heated debate, it was decided that "in view of the emergence of so many controversial issues, it would be best to leave the matter for the time being to the discretion of individual medical men . . . the bill was rejected by 35 votes to 14."[16]

Three years after the inception of the British group, the Euthanasia Society of America, Inc., was founded. This nonsectarian, voluntary organization, rather than seeking to have legislation enacted to legalize euthanasia, attempts to achieve a more enlightened public understanding of euthanasia through dissemination of information through discussions in medical societies and other professional groups, research studies and opinion polls, dissemination of literature, a speaker's bureau, and other responsible media of communication.

Other euthanasia societies have been founded in other countries. Support for these societies and their work comes from various other groups, such as the American Humanist Association and the Ethical Culture Society. Opposition to euthanasia is also strong, however. The Academy of Moral and Political Sciences of Paris passed a motion completely outlawing, forbidding, and rejecting euthanasia in all its forms.[17] In addition, the Council of the World Medical Association, meeting in Copenhagen in April 1950, recommended that the practice of euthanasia be condemned.

The debate continues. The problem has been well stated by Fibey: "When a tortured man asks: 'For God's sake, doctor, let me die, just put me to sleep,' we have yet to find the answer as to whether to comply is for God's sake, the patient's sake, our own, or possibly all three."[18] Even if the moral issue of euthanasia could be circumvented, other questions of logistics would immediately arise: Who is to initiate euthanasia proceedings? The patient? The family? The physician? Who is to make the final decision? The physician? A group of physicians? The courts? Who is to carry out the decision if it is affirmative? The physician? Others?

Arguments For and Against

The arguments in favor of and against euthanasia are numerous and will only be briefly summarized. Opponents of euthanasia say that if voluntary, it is suicide. Although in British law suicide is no longer a crime, Christian and Jewish religious teachings certainly outlaw suicide. The answer offered to this argument is that martyrdom, a form of suicide, is condoned under certain conditions. However, the martyr primarily seeks not to end his life but to accomplish a goal, death being an undesired side product. Thus martyrdom and suicide do not seem comparable.

It is also said that euthanasia, if voluntary, is murder. Murder, however, usually connotes premeditated evil. The motives of the person administering euthanasia are far from evil. On the contrary, such motives are commendable and praiseworthy, although the methods may be unacceptable. A closely related objection to euthanasia says that it transgresses the biblical injunction *Thou shalt not kill.*[19] To overcome this argument, some modern biblical translators substitute "Thou shalt not commit murder," and, as just mentioned, murder usually represents violent killing for purposes of gain or treachery or vendetta and is dissimilar to the "merciful release" of euthanasia.

That God alone gives and takes life[20] and that one's life span is divinely predetermined is not denied by the proponents of euthanasia. The difficulty with this point, seems to be the question of definition as to whether euthanasia represents shortening of life or shortening of the act of dying.

It is also said that suffering is part of the Divine plan, with which man has no right to tamper. This phase of faith remains a mystery and is best exemplified by the story of Job.

It is further argued by opponents of euthanasia that since physicians are only human beings, they are liable to error. There is no infallibility in a physician's diagnosis of an incurably ill patient, and mistakes have been made. They may be exceedingly rare, but they do occur. The same is true of spontaneous remission of cancer: it has been reported, but only in very rare instances.

The need for euthanasia today is minimized by some because of the availability of hypnotics, narcotics, anesthetics, and other analgesic means to keep a patient's pain and distress at a tolerable level. This fact, in general, may be true, but occasional patients develop severe pain which is refractory to all drugs and requires surgical interruption of nerve pathways for relief.

The Hippocratic oath or similar vow which physicians take upon graduation from medical school is conflicting. On the one hand, it states that a physician's duty is to relieve suffering, yet on the other hand, it also states that the physician must preserve and protect life. This oath is used as an argument by both proponents and opponents of euthanasia.

A valid point of debate is the suggestion that if euthanasia for incurably ill, suffering cancer patients were legalized, extension of such legislation to handicapped, deformed, psychotic, or senile patients might follow. An editorial states: "If euthanasia is granted to the first class, can it long be denied to the second? . . . Each step is so short; the slope so slippery; our values in this age, so uncertain and unstable . . ."[21]

Further questions are the sincerity of patients and/or family in requesting euthanasia. A patient racked with pain may make an impulsive but ill-considered request for merciful release which he will not be able to retract or regret after the *fait accompli.* The patient's family may not be completely sincere in its desire to relieve the patient's suffering. The family also wishes to relieve its own suffering. Enemies or heirs of the patient may request hastening of the patient's death for ulterior motives. These and further arguments both for and against euthanasia continue to be discussed and debated.

Catholic Attitude

In at least five places the New Testament contains the biblical admonition *Thou shalt not kill.*[22] Based thereon, the attitude of the Catholic church in this matter is cited as follows:

> The teaching of the Church is unequivocal that God is the supreme master of life and death and that no human being is allowed to usurp His dominion so as deliberately to put an end to life, either his own or any one else's without authorization . . . and the only authorizations the Church recognizes are a nation engaged in war, execution of criminals by a Government, killing in self defense. . . . The Church has never allowed and never will allow the killing of individuals on grounds of private expediency;

for instance . . . putting an end to prolonged suffering or hopeless sickness.[23]

Thus we see a blanket condemnation of active euthanasia by the Catholic church as murder and, therefore, a mortal sin. The reasons behind this teaching include the inviolability of human life, or the supreme dominion of God over His creatures, and the purposefulness of human suffering.[24] Man suffers as penance for his sins, perhaps an earthly purgatory; man endures pain for the spiritual good of his fellowman, and suffering teaches humility.

Passive medical euthanasia is treated quite differently. The church distinguishes between "ordinary" and "extraordinary" measures employed by physicians when certain death and suffering lie ahead. In this day of artificial and auxiliary hearts, artificial kidneys, respirators, pacemakers, defibrillators, and similar instruments, the definition of "extraordinary" is unclear. Pope Pius XII issued an encyclical not requiring physicians to use heroic measures in such circumstances.[25] Thus, passive euthanasia seems to be sanctioned by the Catholic church. In an address to the congress of Italian anesthetists on February 24, 1957, the Pope further stated: "Even if narcotics may shorten life while they relieve pain, it is permissible."[26]

Protestant Attitude

In the Protestant churches there are "all possible colors in the spectrum of attitudes toward euthanasia."[27] Some condemn it, some favor it, and many are in between, advocating judgment of each case individually. Perhaps the greatest Protestant advocate of legalized euthanasia is the Anglican minister Joseph Fletcher. His three main reasons are the following: (a) suffering is purposeless, demoralizing, and degrading; (b) human personality is of greater worth than life per se; and (c) the New Testament phrase "Blessed are the merciful, for they shall obtain mercy" is as important as the biblical *Thou shalt not kill.*

Jewish Attitude

BIBLICAL SOURCES

In the Bible we find: *Whoso sheddeth man's blood, by man shall his blood be shed.*[28] In the second book of the Pentateuch it is stated: *Thou shalt not murder,*[29] and in the next chapter, *And if a man come presumptuously upon his neighbor, to slay him with guile: thou shalt take him from Mine altar, that he may die.*[30] In the next book is the phrase *And he that smiteth any man mortally shall surely be put to death,*[31]and four sentences later, *And he that killeth a man shall be put to death.*[32] In Numbers it states: *Whoso killeth any person, the murderer shall be slain at the mouth of witnesses.*[33] Finally, the sixth commandment of the Decalogue is repeated: *Thou shalt not murder.*[34] Thus, in every book of the Pentateuch, we find at least one reference to murder or killing. Accidental death or homicide is dealt with separately in the Bible and represents another subject entirely.

Probably the first recorded instance of euthanasia concerns the death of King Saul in the year 1013 B.C.E. At the end of the First Book of Samuel, we find the following:

> Now the Philistines fought against Israel, and the men of Israel fled from before the Philistines and fell down slain in Mount Gilboa. And the Philistines pursued hard upon Saul and upon his sons; and the Philistines slew Jonathan and Abinadab and Malchishua, the sons of Saul. And the battle went sore against Saul, and the archers overtook him, and he was greatly afraid by reason of the archers. Then said Saul to his armor-bearer: "Draw thy sword, and thrust me through therewith, lest these uncircumsised come and thrust me through and make a mock of me." But his armor-bearer would not; for he was sore afraid. Therefore, Saul took his sword and fell upon it. And when the armor-bearer saw that Saul was dead, he likewise fell upon his sword and died with him. So Saul died and his three sons, and his armor-bearer, and all his men, that same day together.[35]

From this passage it would appear as if Saul committed suicide. However, at the beginning of the Second Book of Samuel, when David is informed of Saul's death, we find the following:

> And David said unto the young man that told him: "How knowest thou that Saul and Jonathan his son are dead?" And the young man that told him said: "As I happened by chance upon Mount Gilboa, behold, Saul leaned upon his spear; and lo, the chariots and the horsemen pressed hard upon him. And when he looked behind him, he saw me, and called unto me.

> And I answered: Here am I. And he said unto me: Who art thou? And I answered him: I am an Amalekite. And he said unto me: Stand, I pray thee, beside me, and slay me, for the agony hath taken hold of me; because my life is just yet in me. So I stood beside him, and slew him, because I was sure that he would not live after that he was fallen . . ."[36]

Many commentators consider this a case of euthanasia. Rabbi David Kimchi *(Radak)* specifically states that Saul did not die immediately on falling on his sword but was mortally wounded and in his death throes asked the Amalekite to hasten his death. Rabbi Levi ben Gerson *(Ralbag)*, Rabbi Shlomo ben Isaac *(Rashi)*, and Rabbi David Altschul *(Metzudat David)* also support this viewpoint. Some modern scholars think that the story of the Amalekite was a complete fabrication.

TALMUDIC SOURCES

The Talmud states as follows: "One who is in a dying condition *(goses)* is regarded as a living person in all respects."[37] This rule is reiterated by the codifiers of Jewish law, including Maimonides and Karo, as described below. The Talmud continues:[38]

> One may not bind his jaws, nor stop up his openings, nor place a metallic vessel or any cooling object on his navel until such time that he dies, as it is written: *Before the silver cord is snapped asunder.*[39]
>
> One may not move him, nor may one place him on sand or on salt until he dies.
>
> One may not close the eyes of the dying person. He who touches them or moves them is shedding blood because Rabbi Meir used to say: This can be compared to a flickering flame. As soon as a person touches it, it becomes extinguished. So too, whosoever closes the eyes of the dying is considered to have taken his soul.

Other laws pertaining to a *goses*, or dying person, such as the preparation of a coffin, inheritance, marriage, and so forth, are then cited.

The Talmud also mentions: "He who closes the eyes of a dying person while the soul is departing is a murderer [lit. he sheds blood].

This may be compared to a lamp that is going out. If a man places his finger upon it, it is immediately extinguished."[40] *Rashi* explains that this small effort of closing the eyes may slightly hasten death.

The most famous talmudic passage concerning euthanasia is the story of Rabbi Chanina ben Teradion, who was wrapped by the Romans in a Scroll of the Law (Torah), with bundles of straw around him which were set on fire.[41] The Romans also put tufts of wool which had been soaked in water over his heart so that he should not die quickly. His disciples pleaded with him to open his mouth "so that the fire enter into thee" and put an end to his agony. He replied: "Let Him who gave me [my soul] take it away" but no one is allowed to injure himself or hasten his death.

CODES OF JEWISH LAW

The twelfth-century code of Maimonides treats our subject matter as follows:

> One who is in a dying condition is regarded as a living person in all respects. It is not permitted to bind his jaws, to stop up the organs of the lower extremities, or to place metallic or cooling vessels upon his navel in order to prevent swelling. He is not to be rubbed or washed, nor is sand or salt to be put upon him until he expires. He who touches him is guilty of shedding blood. To what may he be compared? To a flickering flame, which is extinguished as soon as one touches it. Whoever closes the eyes of the dying while the soul is about to depart is shedding blood. One should wait a while; perhaps he is only in a swoon.[42]

Thus, we again note the prohibition of doing anything that might hasten death. Maimonides does not specifically forbid moving such a patient, as does the Talmud, but such a prohibition is implied in Maimonides' text. Maimonides also forbids rubbing and washing a dying person, acts which are not mentioned in the Talmud. Finally, Maimonides raises the problem of the recognition of death, a problem becoming more pronounced as scientific medicine improves the methods for supporting respiration and heart function.

The sixteenth-century code of Rabbi Joseph Karo devotes an entire chapter to the laws of the dying patient.[43] The individual in whom death is imminent is referred to as a *goses*. Karo's code begins, as do Maimonides and the Talmud, with the phrase "A *goses* is considered as a living person in all respects," and then Karo enumerates various acts that are prohibited. All the commentaries use the concept "lest they hasten the patient's death" to explain these prohibitions. One of the forbidden acts not mentioned by Maimonides or the Talmud is the removal of the pillow from beneath the patient's head. This act had already been prohibited two centuries earlier by Rabbi Jacob ben Asher, known as *Tur*.[44] Karo's text is nearly identical to that of *Tur*. The latter, however, has the additional general explanation: "the rule in this matter is that any act performed in relation to death should not be carried out until the soul has departed." Thus, not only are physical acts on the patient, such as those described above, forbidden, but one should also not provide a coffin or prepare a grave or make other funeral or related arrangements lest the patient hear of this and his death be hastened. Even psychological stress is prohibited.

On the other hand, thirteenth-century Rabbi Judah ben Samuel the Pious states: "if a person is dying and someone near his house is chopping wood, so that the soul cannot depart, then one should remove the [wood] chopper from there."[45]

Based on this ruling, Rabbi Moses Isserles, known as *Rema*, in his famous gloss on Karo's code, asserts:

> if there is anything which causes a hindrance to the departure of the soul, such as the presence near the patient's house of a knocking noise, such as wood chopping, or if there is salt on the patient's tongue, and these hinder the soul's departure, it is permissible to remove them from there because there is no act involved in this at all but only the removal of the impediment.[46]

Furthermore, Rabbi Solomon Eger, in his commentary on Karo's code,[47] quotes another rabbinic authority, who states "it is forbidden to hinder the departure of the soul by the use of medicines."[48] Other rabbinic authorities, however, disagree with the latter view.[49] Rabbi Joshua Boaz Baruch, known as *Shiltei Gibborim*, pleads for the abolition of the custom of those who remove the pillow from beneath the dying person's head, following the popular belief that the bird feathers contained in the pillow prevent the soul from departing.[50] He further states that Rabbi Nathan of Igra specifically permitted this act. *Shiltei Gibborim* continues: "After many years I found in the *Sefer Chasidim* support for my contentions, as it is written there that if a person is dying but cannot die until he is put in a different place, he should not be moved."[51] This law is not contradictory to the earlier statement in the *Sefer Chasidim*, as both *Shiltei Gibborim* and *Rema* explain: To do an act which prevents easy death, such as chopping wood, is forbidden, and on the contrary, such impediments to death should be removed. On the other hand, it is definitely forbidden to perform any act which hastens death, such as moving the dying person from one place to another.

RECENT RABBINIC RULINGS

This discussion of the Jewish attitude toward euthanasia is summarized by Jakobovits, who states that

> any form of active euthanasia is strictly prohibited and condemned as plain murder . . . anyone who kills a dying person is liable to the death penalty as a common murderer. At the same time, Jewish law sanctions the withdrawal of any factor—whether extraneous to the patient himself or not—which may artificially delay his demise in the final phase.[52]

Jakobovits is quick to point out, however, that all the Jewish sources refer to an individual called a *goses* in whom death is imminent, three days or less in rabbinic references. Thus, passive euthanasia in a patient who may yet live for weeks or months is not condoned. Furthermore, in the case of an incurably ill person in severe pain, agony, or distress, the removal of an impediment which hinders his soul's departure, although permitted in Jewish law, as stated by *Rema*, may not be analogous to the withholding of medical therapy that is perhaps sustaining the patient's life unnaturally. The impediments spoken of in the codes of Jewish law, whether far removed from the patient, as exemplified by the noise of wood chopping, or in physical contact with him, such as the case of salt on the patient's tongue, do not constitute any part of the therapeutic armamentarium employed in the medical management of the patient. For this reason, such impediments may be removed. However, the discontinuation of life-support systems which are specifically designed and utilized in the treatment of incurably ill patients might only be permissible if one is certain that in doing so one is shortening the act of dying and not interrupting life.

Rabbi Eliezer Yehudah Waldenberg reiterates that physicians and others are obligated to do everything possible to save the life of a dying patient, even if the patient will only live for a brief period, and even if the patient is suffering greatly.[53] Any action that results in hastening of the death of a dying patient is forbidden and considered an act of murder. Even if the patient is beyond cure and is suffering greatly and requests that his death be hastened, one may not do so or advise the patient to do so.[54] A terminally ill incurable patient, continues Waldenberg, may be given oral or parenteral narcotics or other powerful analgesics to relieve his pain and suffering, even at the risk of depressing his respiratory center and hastening his death, provided the medications are prescribed solely for pain relief and not to hasten death.[55] Waldenberg also states that it is not considered interference with the Divine will to place a patient on a respirator or other life-support system.[56] On the contrary, all attempts must be made to prolong and preserve the life of a patient who has a potentially curable disease or reversible condition.[57] Thus, one must attempt resuscitation on a drowning victim who has no spontaneous respiration or heartbeat because of the possibility of resuscitation and reversibility.[58] One is not obligated or even permitted, however, to initiate artificial life support and/or other resuscitative efforts if it is obvious that the patient is terminally and incurably and irreversibly ill with no chance of recovery. One is also allowed to disconnect and discontinue life-support instrumentation, according to Waldenberg[59] and others, if one can establish that the patient is dead according to Jewish legal criteria,[60] that is, if the patient has no independent brain function or spontaneous cardiorespiratory activity.[61] If it is not clear whether the respirator is keeping the patient alive or only ventilating a corpse, the respirator must be maintained. It may not be turned off to test whether the patient has spontaneous respiratory activity because that small act may be the one that causes the patient's death, similar to the flickering lamp which may be extinguished if someone touches it (see above). Therefore, from a practical standpoint, Waldenberg advises that one use respirators with automatic time clocks set for a twelve or twenty-four hour period.[62] When the respirator shuts itself off, one can observe the patient for signs of spontaneous respiration. If none are present and if the heart is not beating and the brain is irreversibly damaged, one does not reconnect the respirator. Finally, Rabbi Waldenberg asserts that blood transfusions, oxygen, antibiotics, intravenous fluids, oral and parenteral nutrition, and pain-relief medications must be maintained for a terminally ill patient till the very end.[63]

Rabbi Shlomo Zalman Auerbach also states that a terminally ill patient must be given food and oxygen even against his will.[64]

However, one may withhold, at the patient's request, medications and treatments which might cause him great pain and discomfort. Rabbi Gedaliah Aharon Rabinowitz reviews the laws pertaining to the care of the terminally ill and the criteria for defining the moment of death.[65] He also states that experimental chemotherapy for cancer patients is permissible but not obligatory.[66] Such therapy must have a rational scientific basis and be administered by expert physicians. Untested and unproven remedies may not be used on human beings. Dr. A. Sofer Abraham quotes Rabbi Auerbach as distinguishing between routine and nonroutine treatments for the terminally ill.[67] For example, a dying cancer patient must be given food, oxygen, antibiotics, insulin, and the like, but does not have to be given painful and toxic chemotherapy which offers no chance of cure but at best temporary palliation. Such a patient may be given morphine for pain even if it depresses his respiration. An irreversibly ill terminal patient whose spontaneous heartbeat and breathing stop does not have to be resuscitated.

Rabbi Moshe Hershler opines that withholding food or medication from a terminally ill patient so that he dies is murder.[68] Withholding respiratory support is equivalent to withholding food, since it will shorten the patient's life. Every moment of life is precious, and all measures must be taken to preserve even a few moments of life. However, if the physicians feel that a comatose patient's situation is hopeless, they are not obligated to institute life-prolonging or resuscitative treatments.

Hershler also states that if only one respirator is available and two or more patients need it, the physicians should decide which patient has the best chance of recovery. However, a respirator may not be removed from a patient who is connected thereto for another, even more needy patient, since one is prohibited from sacrificing one life to save another. Only if the patient has no spontaneous movement, reflexes, heartbeat, and respiration can the respirator be removed.

Rabbi Zalman Nechemiah Goldberg discusses the question of whether or not a physician may leave a dying patient to attend another patient.[69] Rabbi Avigdor Nebenzahl describes the permissible use of narcotics for terminally ill patients.[70] The treatment of the terminally ill and the definition of a *goses* are reviewed by Levy and Abraham.[71] Rabbi Nathan Friedman reiterates that euthanasia in any form is prohibited as an act of murder even if the patient asks for it.[72] A person is prohibited from taking his own life even if he is in severe pain and suffering greatly.[73] Even if the patient cries out, "Leave me be and do not help me because I prefer death," everything possible must be done for the support and comfort of the patient, including the use of large doses of pain relief medications.[74]

Rabbi J. David Bleich affirms that although euthanasia in any form is forbidden, and the hastening of death, even by a matter of moments, is regarded as tantamount to murder, there is one situation in which treatment may be withheld from the moribund patient in order to provide for an unimpeded death.[75] While the death of a *goses* may not be hastened, there is no obligation to perform any action which might lengthen the life of such a patient. Bleich emphasizes, however, that "the distinction between an active and a passive act applies to a *goses* and a *goses* only." Among the criteria which indicate that the patient has become terminally ill and can be classified as a *goses* is the observation that he has the death rattle in his throat, probably representing "secretions in his throat on account of the narrowing of his chest."[76] Bleich cites some authorities who not only sanction withholding of treatment but prohibit any action which may prolong the agony of a *goses*. Other authorities insist that the life of a *goses* may not be shortened even passively by withdrawal of medication. Even the permissive rulings only sanction acts of omission for a *goses* in whom death is expected in less than seventy-two hours but not for a terminally ill patient who may yet survive weeks or months.

Conclusion

Bleich has succinctly summarized the Jewish attitude toward euthanasia.

> The practice of euthanasia—whether active or passive—is contrary to the teachings of Judaism. Any positive act designed to hasten the death of the patient is equated with murder in Jewish law, even if the death is hastened only by a matter of moments. No matter how laudable the intentions of the person performing an act of mercy-killing may be, his deed constitutes an act of homicide. . . .
>
> In discharging his responsibility with regard to prolongation of life, the physician must make use of any medical resources which are available. However, he is not obligated to employ procedures which are themselves hazardous in nature and may potentially foreshorten the life of the patient. Nor is either the physician or the patient obligated to employ a therapy which is experimental in nature.

> . . . The attempt to sustain life, by whatever means, is naught but the expression of the highest regard for the precious nature of the gift of life and of the dignity in which it is held.
>
> . . . Only the Creator, who bestows the gift of life, may relieve man of that life, even when it has become a burden rather than a blessing.[77]

Since the decisions about withholding specific therapy for a terminally ill patient, about the discontinuation of life-support systems, about whether or not to employ resuscitative measures in a given situation are complex and not free of family and/or physician personal and emotional involvement and even bias, it seems advisable to consult with a competent rabbinic authority for adjudication on a case-by-case basis.

Notes

1. E. E. Fibey, "Some Overtones of Euthanasia," *Hospital Topics* 43 (1965): 55 ff.
2. C. P. Delhaye, "Euthanasie ou mort par pitié," *Union Médicale de Canada* 90 (1961): 613 ff.
3. J. Crinquette, "L'euthanasie," *Journale de Sciences Médicales de Lille* 81 (1963): 522 ff.
4. Fibey, op. cit.
5. F. Monnerot-Dumaine, "Les notions d'euthanasie et d'automathanasie," *Presse Médicale* 72 (1964): 1458.
6. A. A. Levisohn, "Voluntary Mercy Deaths: Sociolegal Aspects of Euthanasia," *Journal of Forensic Medicine* 8 (1961): 57 ff.
7. Ibid.
8. Delhaye, op. cit.
9. Ibid.
10. P. R. Archambault, "Le problème d'euthanasie considerée par un médecin Catholique," *Union Médicale de Canada* 91 (1962): 543 ff.
11. Levisohn, op. cit.
12. L. Colebrook, "The Liège Trial and the Problem of Voluntary Euthanasia," *Lancet* 2 (1962): 1225.
13. Delhaye, op. cit.
14. Crinquette, op. cit.
15. G. A. Friedman, "Suicide, Euthanasia and the Law," *Medical Times* 85 (1957): 681 ff.
16. *A Plan for Voluntary Euthanasia* (London: Euthanasia Society, 1962), p. 28.
17. Delhaye, op. cit.
18. Fibey, op. cit.
19. Exodus 20:13 and Deuteronomy 5:17.
20. See Deuteronomy 32:39, *I kill and I make alive*, and Ezekiel 18:4, *Behold, all souls are Mine.*
21. Editorial, "Euthanasia," *Lancet* 2 (1961): 351.
22. Matthew 5:21 and 19:18, Mark 10:19, Luke 18:20, and Romans 13:9.
23. I. M. Rabinowitch and H. E. McDermot, "Euthanasia," *McGill Medical Journal* 19 (1950): 160 ff.
24. E. F. Torrey, "Euthanasia: A Problem in Medical Ethics," *McGill Medical Journal* 30 (1961): 127 ff.
25. Archambault, op. cit.; J. H. McClanahan, "The Patient's Right to Die: Moral and Spiritual Aspects of Euthanasia," *Memphis Medical Journal* 38 (1963): 303 ff.
26. Archambault, op. cit.
27. Torrey, op. cit.
28. Genesis 9:6.

29. Exodus 20:13.
30. Ibid. 21:14.
31. Leviticus 24:17.
32. Ibid. 24:21.
33. Numbers 35:30.
34. Deuteronomy 5:17.
35. I Samuel 31:1–6.
36. II Samuel 1:5–10.
37. Semachot 1:1.
38. Ibid. 1:2–4.
39. Ecclesiastes 12:6. The Midrash interprets the silver cord to refer to the spinal cord.
40. Shabbat 151b.
41. Avodah Zarah 18a.
42. Maimonides, *Mishneh Torah, Hilchot Avel* 4:5.
43. Karo, *Shulchan Aruch, Yoreh Deah* 339.
44. *Tur, Yoreh Deah* 339.
45. Judah the Pious, *Sefer Chasidim*, no. 723.
46. *Rema* on *Shulchan Aruch, Yoreh Deah* 339:1.
47. Eger, Commentary *Gilyon Maharsha* on *Shulchan Aruch, Yoreh Deah* 339:1.
48. Jacob ben Samuel, Responsa *Bet Yaakov*, no. 59.
49. J. Reischer, Responsa *Shevut Yaakov*, pt. 3, no. 13.
50. Baruch, Commentary *Shiltei Gibborim* on Moed Katan, end of chap. 3.
51. See Judah the Pious, op. cit.
52. I. Jakobovits, "The Dying and Their Treatment in Jewish Law: Preparation for Death and Euthanasia," *Hebrew Medical Journal* 2 (1961): 251 ff. See also idem, *Jewish Medical Ethics* (New York: Bloch, 1959), pp. 123–125.
53. Waldenberg, Responsa *Tzitz Eliezer*, vol. 5, *Ramat Rachel*, no. 28:5.
54. Ibid., no. 29, and vol. 10, no. 25:6.
55. Ibid, vol. 13, no. 87.
56. Ibid., vol. 15, no. 37.
57. Ibid., vol. 13, no. 89.
58. Ibid., vol. 14, no. 81.
59. Ibid., vol. 13, no. 89.
60. Ibid., vol. 9, no. 46, and vol. 10, no. 25:4.
61. See below, chap. 20.
62. Waldenberg, op. cit., vol. 13, no. 89.
63. Ibid., vol. 14, no. 80.
64. S. Z. Auerbach, in *Halachah Urefuah* 2 (1981): 131.
65. G. A. Rabinowitz, in *Halachah Urefuah* 3 (1983): 102–114.
66. Ibid., pp. 115–118.
67. A. S. Abraham, in *Halachah Urefuah* 2 (1981): 185–190.

68. M. Hershler, in *Halachah Urefuah* 2 (1981): 30–52.

69. Z. N. Goldberg, in *Halachah Urefuah* 2 (1981): 191–195.

70. A. Nebenzahl, "The Use of Narcotics for Terminally Ill Patients," *Assia* 4 (1983): 260–262.

71. Y. Levy, in *Noam* 16 (1973): 53–63; A. S. Abraham, "Treatment of the Terminally Ill *(Goses)* and the Determination of Death," *Assia* 3 (1983): 467–473.

72. N. Friedman, Responsa *Netzer Matta'ai*, no. 30.

73. Asher ben Yechiel, known as *Rosh*, Responsa *Besamim Rosh*, no. 348; M. Schreiber, Responsa *Chatam Sofer*, *Even Ha'ezer*, pt. 1, no. 69. See also below, chap. 1:9.

74. Waldenberg, op. cit., vol. 9, no. 47:5.

75. J. D. Bleich, *Judaism and Healing* (New York: Ktav, 1981), pp. 134–145.

76. M. Isserles, Commentary *Rema* on Karo's *Shulchan Aruch*, *Even Ha'ezer* 121:7 and *Choshen Mishpat* 211:2. Bleich also refers the reader to Maimonides' *(Rambam)* and Yom Tov Lippman Heller's *(Tosafot Yom Tov)* commentaries on Arachin 1:3.

77. Bleich, op. cit.

17

Heroic Measures to Prolong Life

Introduction

Because of advances in medical technology, some people who in an earlier era would have died are today alive and well. Others who would have died are now alive but in a coma or a vegetative state. Medical technology has created as many problems as it has solved.

The cover of the November 3, 1975, issue of *Newsweek* had a small picture of Karen Ann Quinlan and in large letters, the phrase "A Right to Die?" This patient was then lying in a "persistent vegetative state" in a hospital in New Jersey, her life being maintained by a Bennett respirator. Some physicians openly said they would "pull the plug" to end her life.[1] She did not have a flat electroencephalogram. Even the states, such as California, Kansas, and Maryland, that base their definitions of death on brain activity would not define Miss Quinlan as dead. Yet Superior Court Judge Robert Muir, Jr., was asked by Miss Quinlan's parents to order an end to the use of artificial life supports that had kept the girl alive, but in coma, for years. The court ruled that to turn off the respirator would be considered murder. Stirred in part by the Karen Ann Quinlan controversy, "right to die" movements gained much momentum in the United States and in Europe.[2]

In Switzerland, a prominent physician was accused of murder in the deaths of elderly hospitalized patients because he allowed them to die and did not force-feed and otherwise treat those in irreversible coma.[3]

From a hospital room in New York, Charles Lindbergh asked to be flown home to Maui in Hawaii to die of his malignant lymphoma, which was resistant to radiotherapy and chemotherapy.[4] He wanted no respirator, defibrillator, or other artificial machinery. None was provided. He received excellent, prompt, responsive nursing care, oxygen when needed, a minimum of analgesia, and a great deal of love and consideration from his family and medical staff.

By contrast, an eighty-year-old professor of medicine who was hospitalized for intense back pain permitted only simple tests and X-ray examinations without contrast media. All complicated, fatiguing, and expensive procedures he considered unnecessary and consequently refused to undergo them. He regarded himself as too old for radical therapy and concluded that to aim at an accurate diagnosis was useless. As he was very determined, he got his way. He refused transfusions, antibiotics, and intensive care. He was allowed to be ill and die according to his wishes. Autopsy disclosed metastatic cancer of the prostate.[5] A correspondent rightly pointed out that despite the professor's age of more than eighty years, the metastatic cancer of the prostate could have been treated, resulting in relief of pain and rehabilitation.[6] A few simple diagnostic tests and a few milligrams of estrogenic hormone could have avoided this tragic and probably premature loss of a life. These measures are certainly not "heroic" or "extraordinary" in any sense.

At the other extreme of life is the physically deformed or mentally deficient infant. A recent report enumerates forty-three deaths in a special-care nursery associated with discontinuance of treatment for children with multiple anomalies, trisomy, cardiopulmonary disease, meningomyelocele and other central nervous system disorders, and the short bowel syndrome.[7] After careful consideration of each case, parents and physicians in a group decision concluded that prognosis for meaningful life was extremely poor or hopeless and, therefore, rejected further treatment. Is allowing such hopelessly ill patients to die accepted medical practice? Critical issues in a newborn intensive care unit include the following questions: Is it ever right not to resuscitate an infant at birth? Is it ever right to withdraw life support from a clearly diagnosed poor-prognosis infant? Is it ever right to intervene directly to kill the dying infant? Is it ever right to displace a poor-prognosis infant in order to provide intensive care to a better-prognosis infant?[8] Certain guidelines have been suggested, but they are far from adequate in providing complete answers to these questions.[9] The recent Baby Jane Doe controversy is beyond the scope of this chapter.[10]

Ethical Considerations

The cases cited above illustrate some of the problems faced by the physician today. There is a great confusion between euthanasia and sound medical practice. One writer states that the sound medical care of the dying patient lies somewhere between mercy killing and the inexcusable prolongation of death and suffering.[11] He further says that it is sound medical practice, not positive or negative euthanasia, to discontinue treatment that no longer affects the patient's disease and to use pain-relieving measures in adequate amount. He also believes that it is not the physician's right to decide when a patient should die. The physician is not obligated to keep the patient alive or to kill him, but to treat his terminal illness as best he can. How crude to assert: "The earlier he is killed, the more pain he is spared, the easier it is on the physician and relatives, and the less the cost of hospitalization. Why keep the patient alive when there are so many advantages in killing him?" The suffering patient may well ask for death, but it is relief from mental and physical suffering that he seeks, not death.

It has been bluntly stated that in the late twentieth century, "most Americans can expect to go through the tortures of the damned before they are allowed to die of cancer, heart or lung failure, or pure senile decay."[12] Everyone would agree that the process of dying should be as pleasant as possible. Many patients prefer the warm surroundings of their own homes in the last days of their lives. They feel more secure and "more in control of forces acting on them in their dependent state than they would in the hospital."[13] Patients need to feel dignified enough during their dying to participate in decision-making and to feel esteemed enough to interact supportively with their family and friends.[14]

Often, however, dying occurs in the lonely, mechanical, dehumanized atmosphere of the hospital rather than the privacy of one's own home, surrounded by friends and family. The physician should perhaps make "terminal illness rounds" just as he makes medical or surgical or chart rounds. Such rounds would not solve all the moral dilemmas surrounding death and dying, including the physician's reactions to dying patients.[15] The new technology denies the physician a simple physiological end point for death. When is a donor dead, so that his organs can be removed for organ transplantation? Is it ethical to infuse mannitol into a patient dying of head injury to preserve his kidneys for grafting? Dare we remove kidneys from a donor whose heart is still beating? Is it "cruel" in the presence of a fatal disease, in the agonal hours, to prolong life (or death) by the use of machines?

Does the age of a patient play a role in the decision whether to use "ordinary" or "extraordinary" (to be defined below) measures to prolong life? The medical definitions of "ordinary" and "extraordinary" are different from those of the ethicist. To the latter, the terms are relative and depend on time, place, and situation circumstances. How does one approach a five-year-old child with terminal acute leukemia? Is an eighty-year-old man with terminal prostatic cancer to be treated differently from the child with leukemia?

What should be done and what should not be done for a terminally ill patient? Who is to weigh the value of a few more days of life? Who is to decide when the end should come? The physician? The patient? Should the decision be put upon the family? Should the patient have the option to choose a peaceful death without exposure to the seemingly relentless application of medical technology? Should one discuss this option with the patient? The basic question seems to be the extent to which any individual owns his own death. Does a person have the right to select how and when he will die? Is such a decision by the patient akin to suicide? What is an individual's responsibility to his life and health? Judeo-Christian teaching is that life is a gift of God to be held in trust. One is duty bound to care for one's life and health. Only God gives life, and hence only God can take it away. This individual responsibility for the preservation of one's life and health is apart from the duty of one person (including a physician) toward another's life and health and society's responsibility concerning the life and health of its citizens.

Not only have man's birth and death moved from his home to the hospital, but the physician has often replaced the clergyman. Many terminal patients lack religious faith, yet they desperately need emotional support; but by whom? The busy physician? The busy nurse? Many physicians shy away from dying patients. Is the hospital, during this era of advanced technology, a place where illness and organs, rather than people, are treated? The emotional support and reassurance to the dying patient are usually provided by the family and clergy where appropriate, in addition to the medical team.

Although the patient may not be best suited or morally or religiously allowed to decide for himself about life and death, he probably does have personal inalienable rights. Pope Pius XII said that the physician has no separate and independent rights of his own and can act only with the patient's request and permission. The physician should not impose his will on the patient. If the Pope's statement is true, then the judge's decision in the Karen Quinlan case was wrong, since the latter said that the physician's obligation extends beyond the wishes of the patient. The judge further said that since a patient places his trust in the physician, the latter must do all in his human power to save the life of the patient.

The doctor-patient relationship is no longer what it used to be because of a variety of factors. There are legal forces, such as the medical malpractice issue, that may interfere with the physician's best clinical and ethical judgment. There are psychological forces pushing the physician to "do something." There are professional forces that may force a physician to act to protect himself from peer review. Patients are beter informed and becoming more vocal. The physician's own religious and ethical values, his own experiences, his teachings by preceptors all play a role in deciding how he approaches a dying patient. Factors such as the values of the medical profession in general, the expectations of the patient, the family, and the institution where the patient is hospitalized may also modify the physician's decision to use or not to use "heroic measures," however one defines that phrase. Ultimately, to whom is the physician responsible? To himself? To the patient? To society? Or to God?

Should the care of the dying be no different from that of any patient? One must always consider the therapeutic goal. One goal may be appropriate to the disease and another appropriate to the patient. For some diseases, such as tuberculosis, the goals are identical, i.e., eradicate the disease, thus curing the patient. Even if the disease cannot be cured, food, analgesics, and good nursing care can and should be given. It is often easy to treat the disease purely medically. It is much harder to treat the patient as a person with a disease. In a terminally ill patient, penicillin may be considered by the ethicist but not by the physician to be "extraordinary" treatment. Yet the physician may not administer the penicillin because the goal may not be to cure the pneumonia in an incurably ill cancer patient.

The terms "heroic" and "extraordinary" will be discussed further later. It is indeed unfortunate that confusing and ambiguous slogans such as "Death with Dignity,"[16] "Beneficent Euthanasia,"[17] and "Quality of Life"[18] have emerged. The promotion of death with dignity is but one manifestation of what appears to be a current literary obsession with death in both lay and professional writings.[19] There has even developed a backlash against medical ethics;[20] a major lecture during the 1975 annual session of the American

College of Physicians was entitled "The Unethical in Medical Ethics."[21] One writer even went so far as to assert that "the most inflated non-issue currently absorbing time and energy in the health community and its governmental command posts is the loose amalgamation of anxieties and passions that comes under the banner of medical ethics."[22]

Be that as it may, the physician at the bedside of a critically or terminally ill patient is faced with moral and ethical dilemmas to which there are no easy solutions. Need everything be done to prolong life at all costs? Should patients be spared painful and expensive therapy by the cessation or nonapplication of such therapy? Is it ethically permitted to intervene actively to terminate life?

Legal Considerations

Black's law dictionary defines death as the cessation of life and the absence of respiration and pulse. To the ordinary observer, in the majority of cases death was and still is a phenomenon recognized through visible and palpable manifestations, such as the cessation of respiration and heartbeat.[23] Since the law must be precise, not only the fact of death but the time of death must be clearly established. Death is not a continuing event but one that occurs at a precise time. This is most important for transplantation surgery, in addition to a variety of legal questions, such as guilt of murder, inheritance laws, and the like.

In 1968, a Uniform Anatomical Gift Act was proposed and adopted by many states. It specifies procedures whereby a living person can donate an organ or his entire body. A close relative can also give such consent. The act, however, does not define death. It says that death shall be determined by the physician.

Among physicians and medical groups there is no unanimity of opinion or uniformity in defining death; religious definitions may be at variance with those of either the medical or the legal profession.

The criteria for defining death acceptable to many physicians include complete bilateral, pupillary dilatation with no reaction to local constricting stimuli, complete abolition of reflexes, complete cessation of spontaneous respiration, absence of measurable blood pressure, and a flat electroencephalogram.[24]

One neurologist requires that

> there can be no induced or spontaneous purposeful movements, and reflex responses should be consistent with a decorticate or

decerebrate state. Pupillary light responses should be absent and dilation present. The electroencephalogram should be isoelectric, or flat, indicating no cortical potentials are being produced. To further substantiate the degree of central nervous system damage, and its irreversibility, the neurovegetative reaction of respiration should be absent as evidenced by the lack of spontaneous respiration for at least two minutes. Finally these observations of the brain and lower nervous system functions should be consistently present for a minimum of two or three days, after resolution of the process which induced cerebral death.[25]

These criteria may seem quite strict. However, they are not much less rigid than the criteria proposed by a special commission consisting of surgeons, neurosurgeons, anesthesiologists, and medicolegal experts formed by the German Society of Surgery. This commission proposed that

> if the patient is unconscious for at least 12 hours and if spontaneous respiration ceases, bilaterial mydriasis sets in, pupils do not react to light, all reflexes are extinct, and the encephalographic tracing shows an isoelectric line for at least one hour without interruption, then the patient can be considered dead notwithstanding the fact that the heart may still respond to artificial stimulation.[26]

At the 1968 national meeting of the American Medical Association, guidelines for organ transplants were approved by the House of Delegates. One of the major guidelines states:

> When a vital single organ is to be transplanted, the death of the donor shall have been determined by at least one physician other than the recipient's physician. Death shall be determined by the clinical judgment of the physician. In making this determination, the ethical physician will use all available, currently accepted scientific tests.[27]

How does one ascertain the irreversibility of the process of life? The Ad Hoc Committee of the Harvard Medical School to Examine the Definition of Brain Death arrived at a definition of irreversible coma that essentially requires unresponsiveness to external stimuli, absence of movements or spontaneous breathing, absence of reflexes and fixed dilated pupils, and a flat electroencephalogram, if available. All the tests are to be repeated at least twenty-four hours later.[28]

At what point need a physician no longer attempt resuscitation? The Twenty-second World Medical Association meeting in Australia, on August 8, 1968, adopted a statement, known as the Declaration of Sydney, that states in part that a physician's determination of death "should be based on clinical judgment, supplemented if necessary by diagnostic aids, of which the electroencephalograph is the current most helpful single one." Drafters of the statement admitted its indefiniteness and stressed that there are no precise scientific criteria or definition for what is the moment of death.

When is the dying patient beyond help? When is the physician guilty of a grave moral and religious sin by not doing everything possible to "maintain" his patient? Just as one cannot properly define health as the absence of disease, it seems totally inappropriate to define death as the absence of life. Society in general and the medical and legal professions in particular are struggling to come up with an acceptable definition of death.

In 1970, the state of Kansas passed a law defining death as the absence of spontaneous respiration and circulation where resuscitation is considered hopeless *and* the absence of spontaneous brain function. Death is to be pronounced before artificial means are stopped and before organs are removed. Neither the Harvard criteria nor the Kansas statute speak of the informed consent of the patient or the next of kin for the removal of organs for transplantation or the cessation of artificial life-support systems.

In 1974, the state of California adopted a statute recognizing brain death as a valid criterion for establishing death. The law *mandates* a physician to pronounce a patient dead if brain death has occurred. It states:

> A person *shall* be pronounced dead if it is determined by a physician that the person has suffered a total and irreversible cessation of brain function. There shall be independent confirmation of the death by another physician.
>
> Nothing in this chapter shall prohibit a physician from using other usual and customary procedures for determining death as the exclusive basis for pronouncing a person dead.[29]

Brain death as a criterion of when death has occurred was supposed to be a refinement of, and complement to, the traditional methods of detection.[30] The California statute mandating brain death *alone* as a definition of death seems to nullify this hope.

Similar legislation including the cessation of brain function as *one* of the criteria for death has been passed in many other states, including New York.[31] One must be very cautious in the legislative approach to defining death. If a statute is not well drafted or is too restrictive or too lenient, it can do more harm than good. It can create more problems than it solves. We do not want the patient-family-doctor context of health care to be invaded so that the physician "becomes increasingly a tool of technology dictated by law."[32] Highly undesirable is the flood of laws, bureaucratic ordinances, and judicial decisions that tend to restrict even more the freedom of the physician in the practice of medicine.[33] More laws involving medicine have been passed in the last decade than in all the rest of United States history.

But what is becoming glaringly evident is that the proliferation of controls and safeguards in the medical area threatens the very possibility of even conducting medical care as we have hitherto known it. The incredible complexity of the medical system and the inability of legislators and bureaucrats alike to foresee the consequences of their interventions are reasons for this threat.

How, then, is the physician in a hospital to conduct himself? When, if ever, does he decide whether or not emergency life-saving or life-prolonging procedures should be withheld from a patient? Is it proper for the physician to write a "do not resuscitate" order in the medical record of a hospitalized patient? Should this be controlled by federal, state, or local law? There is no established legal precedent in this country to provide definitive or specific guidelines governing the institution or withholding of life-saving or life-prolonging procedures. From a legal viewpoint, there is no rule that a physician must always use every available means to prolong a patient's life.[34]

Religious Considerations

Confronted with ethical dilemmas, the physician of bygone days would generally follow familiar guidelines provided by the canons of his faith.[35] Today, many physicians and patients do not feel firmly bound by religious precepts. Religious guidance is available, however, to those who seek it.

In 1957, Pope Pius XII enunciated that a person has the duty to care for his life and health, thereby fulfilling his duty toward God. Life is subordinated to spiritual health, however. The proper love of oneself requires only ordinary means, such as all medicines and treatments without excessive pain or inconvenience. Extraordinary means would include situations of severe physical pain, inconvenience, financial hardship, or absence of reasonable hope for success of the treatment. Life is a relative good, and the duty to preserve it is a limited one.

The categories of ordinary and extraordinary are relative ones, varying according to circumstances of persons, places, times, and culture. How much of an expense is considered excessive? One writer suggests $2,000.[36] How about a rich person? What is considered excessive pain? Pain thresholds vary from patient to patient. What is excessive inconvenience? Is moving to another climate to preserve one's health to be so considered? Some measures that might have been considered extraordinary five years ago are today routine and thus ordinary.

Catholic teaching seems to embody within it the concept of the quality of life. Life is valued but without absolute value. Not everything needs to be done to prolong life at all costs. Patients may be spared painful and expensive treatment by the cessation of that treatment. It seems acceptable for the physician to admit that the patient is incurably ill and to give up his therapeutic efforts at some point. The wishes of the patient and the family should have high priority. Good nursing care, food, and analgesics should be provided. However, there is no moral obligation to use artificial life supports if no reasonable expectation for cure exists. "Extraordinary means" of treatment need not be started, or may be stopped. Strong sedatives and analgesics may be given even though they may shorten life. Letting die, including the cessation of machines, is permissible and is not the same as mercy killing, although some philosophers and theologians reject this distinction.[37] Most Catholic ethicists insist on the distinction between "killing" and "letting die", since omission and commission may not be morally identical.

Jewish tradition views death as inevitable and just. It differentiates between the body and the soul, acknowledging resurrection for the former and immortality for the latter. Respect for death is mandated.[38] Jewish law requires the physician to do everything in his power to prolong life, but prohibits the use of measures that prolong the act of dying.[39] The value attached to human life in Judaism is far greater than that in Christian tradition or in Anglo-Saxon common law.[40] To save a life, all Jewish religious laws are automatically suspended, the only exceptions being idolatry, adultery, and murder. In Jewish law and moral teaching, "the value of human life is infinite and beyond measure, so that any part of life—even if only an hour or a second—is of precisely the same worth as seventy years of it, just as any fraction of infinity, being indivisible, remains infinite. Accordingly, to kill a decrepit patient approaching death constitutes exactly the same crime of murder as to kill a young, healthy person who may still have many decades to live".[41]

"However much Judaism cares about the mitigation of pain, what it does not sanction is the purchase of relief from suffering at the cost of life itself. Any sanction of euthanasia would cheapen life by making its preservation contingent upon considerations of expediency or relative merit."[42] How does Judaism resolve the conflict between the sanctity of life and the relief of human suffering? The concern for the patient's physical and mental welfare remains supreme to the end, and everything must be done to preserve both.

Euthanasia is opposed without qualification in Jewish law, which condemns as sheer murder any active or deliberate hastening of death, whether the physician acts with or without the patient's consent. Some rabbinic views do not allow any relaxation of efforts, however artificial and ultimately hopeless, to prolong life. Others, however, do not require the physician to resort to "heroic" methods, but sanction the omission of machines and artificial life-support systems that only serve to draw out the dying patient's agony, provided, however, that basic care, such as food and good nursing, is provided. An organ may not be removed for transplantation until the patient has been pronounced dead, defined in Judaism as the cessation of spontaneous respiration and heartbeat in a patient where resuscitation is deemed impossible.[43] Specifically questioned about the Karen Ann Quinlan case, most rabbis offered the opinion that in Jewish law we are not required to utilize heroic measures to prolong the life of hopelessly sick patients, but we are forbidden to terminate the use of such measures once they have been begun.

Concluding Remarks

Man does not possess absolute title to his life or to his body. Man is charged with preserving, dignifying, and hallowing that life.[44] The modern phrases "quality of life" and "quality of existence" embody within them a concept of worthiness with connotations of personal character and social status.

Should a decision as to whether life is worth living be determined on the basis of pain, suffering, and, as some today suggest, from a consideration of its deviancy from normal? When a person's intellect ceases to function because he is in coma, that person is intellectually dead. When a person cannot function in society because he is mentally deficient or physically malformed, he is socially dead. Should such individuals not be allowed to live because they lack "worthiness"?

Emotional and financial burdens are frequently cited as justification for decisions about "heroic" measures or life-support systems for a defective infant, a vegetative adult, or a terminally ill cancer patient. Social costs should remain divorced from such decision-making. The public should rightly assume the fiscal burden associated with maintaining incompetent patients such as Karen Ann Quinlan whose lives are being preserved.

Suffering of the family is another reason offered for allowing a patient such as Karen Ann Quinlan to die by removing artificial life supports. Precisely because of their closeness to the situation, the family is not capable of reaching a detached, dispassionate, and objective decision. On this basis, the sanctity of life as a preeminent value is being threatened. Evil has small beginnings. When the quality of life replaces the sanctity of life, society has done itself irreparable harm.

Notes

1. A. E. Hellegers, "Problem in Bioethics: I Would Have Pulled the Plug If . . .," *Internal Medicine News* 8 (1975): 10.

2. "Right to Die" movements springing up in Europe," *New York Times*, Dec. 7, 1975, p. 10.

3. B. J. Culliton, "The Haemmerli Affair: Is Passive Euthanasia Murder?" *Science* 190 (1975): 1271–1275.

4. M. M. Howell, "The Lone Eagle's Last Flight," *Journal of the American Medical Association* 232 (1975): 715.

5. I. Kerpolla-Sirola, "The Death of an Old Professor," *Journal of the American Medical Association* 232 (1975): 728–729.

6. B. J. Kennedy, "Pleasures and Tragedies of Death," *Journal of the American Medical Association* 234 (1975): 24.

7. R. S. Duff and A. G. M. Campbell, "Moral and Ethical Dilemmas in the Special Care Nursery," *New England Journal of Medicine* 289 (1973): 890–994.

8. A. R. Jonson, R. H. Phibbs, W. H. Tooley, and M. J. Garland, "Critical Issues in Newborn Intensive Care: A Conference Report and Policy Proposal," *Pediatrics* 55 (1975): 756–768.

9. R. A. McCormick, "To Save or Let Die: The Dilemma of Modern Medicine," *Journal of the American Medical Association* 229 (1974): 172–176. F. R. Harrison, III, "Dilemmas and Solutions," *Journal of the American Medical Association* 230 (1974): 401–403.

10. R. Weir, *Selective Non-treatment of Handicapped Newborns* (New York and Oxford: Oxford University Press, 1984), 292 pp.

11. C. P. Harrison, "Euthanasia, Medicine, and the Law," *Canadian Medical Association Journal* 113 (1975): 833–834.

12. W. Dock, "Dysthanasia: The Lot of the Shackled Sick," *New York State Journal of Medicine* 75 (1975): 842.

13. M. J. Krant, "The Patient Who Wants to Die at Home," *Journal of the American Medical Association* 234 (1975): 1068.

14. M. J. Krant, "Dying: A Meaningful Summation of Life," *Medical Insight* 5 (1973): 27–29.

15. E. Kubler-Ross, S. Wessler, and L. V. Avioli, "On Death and Dying," *Journal of the American Medical Association* 221 (1972): 174–179.

16. P. Ramsay, "The Indignity of 'Death with Dignity,' " *Hastings Center Report* 2 (1974): 47–62.

17. M. Kohl, *Beneficent Euthanasia* (Buffalo: Prometheus Books, 1975).

18. J. K. Luce, and J. J. Dawson, "Quality of Life," *Seminars in Oncology* 2 (1975): 323–327; W. B. Patterson. "The Quality of Survival in Response to Treatment," *Journal of the American Medical Association* 233 (1975): 280–281.

19. F. J. Ingelfinger, "Empty Slogan for the Dying," *New England Journal of Medicine* 291 (1974): 845–846.

20. K. D. Clouser, "Medical Ethics: Some Uses, Abuses, and Limitations," *New England Journal of Medicine* 293 (1975): 384–387.

21. F. J. Ingelfinger, "The Unethical in Medical Ethics," *Annals of Internal Medicine* 83 (1975): 264–269.

22. D. S. Greenberg, "Ethics and Nonsense," *New England Journal of Medicine* 290 (1974): 977–978.

23. "A report by the Task Force on Death and Dying of the Institute of Society, Ethics and the Life Sciences. Refinement in Criteria for the Determination of Death: An Appraisal," *Journal of the American Medical Association* 221 (1972): 48–53.

24. J. Z. Appel, "Ethical and Legal Questions Posed by Recent Advances in Medicine," *Journal of the American Medical Association* 205 (1968): 513–516.

25. J. J. McCutchen, "A Neurologist Looks at Death," *Journal of the American Medical Association* 204 (1968): 1197–1198.

26. International Comments, "When Is a Person Dead?" *Journal of the American Medical Association* 203 (1968): 998.

27. "Ethical Guidelines for Organ Transplantation," *Journal of the American Medical Association* 205 (1968): 341–342.

28. "A Definition of Irreversible Coma. Report of the Ad Hoc Committee of the Harvard Medical School to Examine the Definition of Brain Death," *Journal of the American Medical Association* 205 (1968): 337–340.

29. D. H. Mills, "More on Brain Death," *Journal of the American Medical Association* 234 (1975): 838.

30. Editorial, "Harvard Criteria: An Appraisal," *Journal of the American Medical Association* 221 (1972): 65.

31. New York State Court of Appeals ruling on October 30, 1984 in the companion cases *People v. Eulo* and *People v. Bonilla.*

32. R. M. McCormick, "The Karen Ann Quinlan Case," *Journal of the American Medical Association* 234 (1975): 1057.

33. H. Schwarz, "Will Medicine Be Strangled in Law?" *New York Times*, Feb. 25, 1975.

34. D. P. Wilcox, "Propriety of No Mayday Orders," *Journal of the American Medical Association* 231 (1975): 1087.

35. S. Vaisrub, "Be Your Own Philosopher," *Journal of the American Medical Association* 230 (1974): 443.

36. E. F. Healy, *Medical Ethics* (Chicago: Loyola University Press, 1956), p. 68.

37. J. Rachels, "Active and Passive Euthanasia," *New England Journal of Medicine* 292 (1975): 78–80; J. Fletcher, *Morals and Medicine* (Boston: Beacon Press, 1954), pp. 172–210.

38. S. I. Spector, "The End of Days: The Jewish Concept of Death," *Omega* 5 (1974): 267–275.

39. See above, chap. 16.

40. J. D. Bleich, "Theological Considerations in the Case of Defective

Newborns, in *Decision Making and the Defective Newborn*, ed. C. A. Swinyard (Springfield, Ill.: C. C. Thomas Co., 1978).

41. I. Jakobovits, "Medical Experimentation on Humans in Jewish Law," in *Jewish Bioethics*, ed. F. Rosner and J. D. Bleich (New York: Hebrew Publishing Co., 1979), pp. 377–383.

42. I. Jakobovits, *Jewish Medical Ethics* (New York: Bloch, 1959), pp. 123 ff.

43. See also chap. 16, 20 and 21.

44. Bleich, op. cit.

18

Rabbi Moshe Feinstein on the Treatment of the Terminally Ill

Introduction

In March, 1986, a landmark statement regarding its policy on terminating treatment was issued by the American Medical Association's Council on Ethical and Judicial Affairs. It announced that physicians may ethically withdraw artificial feeding and hydration from terminal or permanently comatose patients, provided certain conditions are satisfied, including the accuracy of the diagnosis, the irreversibility of the coma, and the knowledge of the patient's wishes. The AMA suggests that the physician weigh the benefits to be gained from continued treatment, including nutrition and hydration, against the burdens of continued treatment.

The AMA is thus clearly on record as concluding that nutrition and hydration by intravenous lines or nasogastric tubes constitute medical treatment no different from antibiotics, transfusions, or other forms of medical intervention, including respirators or other mechanical means of life support, and that such treatment should be used only if it benefits the patient. Why the sudden "about-face" in our ethical, medical, and legal thinking? Where does one draw the line? Can oral feeding and hydration also be withheld from patients who are able to eat and drink? What about ice sucking or lip moistening? Why is the practice of withdrawing or withholding fluids and nutrition gaining support from bioethicists, physicians, nurses, and other health care providers? Why is this practice no longer considered to be morally objectionable? Why is this practice no longer considered to be morally objectionable? Why is feeding a patient different from alcohol rubs, turning him to avoid bedsores, and other general supportive measures?

Is withdrawing nutritional life support a constitutional right of the patient and ethically justifiable, or is it an act of moral or legal murder by the hastening of the patient's death? Judaism views nutrition and hydration by feeding tubes or intravenous lines not as medical treatments but as supportive care, no different from washing, turning, or grooming a dying patient. This essay presents a Jewish approach to the treatment of the terminally ill as presented in the responsa of the renowned Rabbi Moshe Feinstein, with references to other rabbinic sources and responsa.

On purely philosophical or logical grounds one can argue that the denial of food and fluids to a terminally ill patient is not the same as the withholding of medical and surgical therapy.[1] First, the denial of food and fluids is biologically final in that it will certainly and directly lead to the patient's death, since survival without food and fluids is impossible, whereas life can continue without medication. Second, food and fluids are universal human needs, whereas modern medical and surgical therapy are not. Third, the doctor-patient relationship may be seriously harmed, since the patient's presumption is that physicians always aim to preserve life and never to induce death. Fourth, to permit physicians to deny food and fluid to patients who are capable of receiving and utilizing them directly attacks the very foundation of medicine as an ethical profession. Fifth, the denial of foods and fluids administered by "artificial" means is no different from such denials when food can be administered in a "normal" manner. The food that is provided is not transformed into an exotic medical substance by the simple act of pouring it into a gastrostomy tube. Sixth, the food and fluid given to a handicapped person or dying patient does not become medical therapy because another person is needed to provide it.

Classic Jewish Sources

To hasten the death of a terminally ill patient is prohibited in Judaism. The Talmud states that a terminally ill person (*goses*) is regarded as a living person in all respects.[2] One may not do any of the things customarily performed after the soul has departed, such as closing the eyes, for he who touches or moves the eyes of one who is dying is considered to have taken his soul. Other laws pertaining to a *goses*, such as the preparation of a coffin, inheritance, marriage, and so forth, are then cited.

The Talmud also says that "he who closes the eyes of a dying person while his soul is departing is a murderer [lit. he sheds blood]. This may be compared to a lamp that is going out. If a man places his finger upon it, it is immediately extinguished."[3] *Rashi* explains that this small effort of closing the eyes may slightly hasten death. A famous talmudic passage is the story of Rabbi Chanina ben Teradion, whom the Romans wrapped in a Scroll of the Law (Torah) with bundles of straw around him which were then set on fire. The Romans also put tufts of wool which had been soaked in water over his heart so that he should not die quickly. His disciples pleaded with him to open his mouth "so that the fire enter into thee" and put an end to his agony, but he replied: "Let Him who gave me [my soul] take it away" but no one is allowed to injure himself or hasten his death.[4]

Maimonides reiterates the fact that a dying person is regarded as a living one in all respects and it is prohibited to do anything to him that might hasten death.[5] A similar pronouncement is found in Karo's famous code.[6]

On the other hand, thirteenth-century Rabbi Judah the Pious states: "If a person is dying and someone near his house is chopping wood, so that the soul cannot depart, one should remove the [wood] chopper from there."[7] Based on this ruling, Rabbi Moshe Isscrles, known as *Ramo*, in his famous gloss on Karo's code, asserts that

> if there is anything which causes a hindrance to the departure of the soul, such as the presence near the patient's house of a knocking noise, such as wood chopping, or if there is salt on the patient's tongue, and these hinder the soul's departure, it is permissible to remove them from there because there is no act involved in this at all but only the removal of the impediment.[8]

Based on the aforementioned classic Jewish sources, Rabbi Immanuel Jakobovits, in his pioneering monograph on Jewish medical ethics, states

> that any form of active euthanasia is strictly prohibited and condemned as plain murder. . . . anyone who kills a dying person is liable to the death penalty as a common murderer. At the same time, Jewish law sanctions the withdrawal of any

> factor—whether extraneous to the patient himself or not—which may artificially delay his demise in the final phase.[9]

Jakobovits is quick to point out, however, that all of the Jewish sources refer to a *goses* in whom death is imminent—three days or less in rabbinic references. Thus, passive euthanasia in a patient who may yet live for weeks or months is not condoned. Furthermore, in the case of an incurably ill person in severe pain, agony, or distress, the removal of an impediment which hinders his soul's departure, although permitted in Jewish law, as stated by *Ramo*, may not be analogous to the withholding of medical therapy that is perhaps sustaining the patient's life unnaturally. The impediments spoken of in the codes of Jewish law, whether far removed from the patient, as exemplified by the noise of wood chopping, or in physical contact with him, such as the case of salt on the patient's tongue, do not constitute any part of the therapeutic armamentarium employed in the medical management of the patient. For this reason, such impediments may be removed. However, the discontinuation of life-support systems which are specifically designed for and utilized in the treatment of incurably ill patients might be permissible only if one were certain that doing so would shorten the act of dying and not interrupt life.

Rabbi J. David Bleich has succinctly summarized the Jewish view of the treatment of the dying as follows:

> Any positive act designed to hasten the death of the patient is equated with murder in Jewish law, even if the death is hastened only by a matter of moments. No matter how laudable the intentions of the person performing an act of mercy-killing may be, his deed constitutes an act of homicide. . . . In discharging his responsibility with regard to prolongation of life, the physician must make use of any medical resources which are available. However, he is not obligated to employ procedures which are themselves hazardous in nature and may potentially foreshorten the life of the patient. Nor is either the physician or the patient obligated to employ a therapy which is experimental in nature.
>
> The attempt to sustain life, by whatever means, is naught but the expression of the highest regard for the precious nature of the gift of life and of the dignity in which it is held.
>
> Only the Creator, who bestows the gift of life, may relieve man

of that life, even when it has become a burden rather than a blessing.[10]

The Teaching of Rabbi Moshe Feinstein

The most extensive discussion in the recent rabbinic literature of the treatment of the terminally ill is that of Rabbi Moshe Feinstein,[11] who, in the seventh volume of his famous responsa, *Iggrot Moshe*, states that, for a patient with pain and suffering who cannot be cured and cannot live much longer, it is not obligatory for physicians to administer medications briefly to prolong his life of pain and suffering, but nature may be allowed to take its course.[12] However, it is prohibited to give the patient any medication or do any act to hasten his death by even a moment. Pain-relief medications, however, should be administered even if the patient is not yet considered a *goses* where death is imminent.[13] A seriously ill patient with respiratory difficulties should be given oxygen, even if he can not be cured, because oxygen relieves discomfort, continues Feinstein.[14] There are times, however, when it is appropriate to pray for the death of a suffering dying patient,[15] when it is clear that prayers for his cure are of no avail, similar to the case of Rabbi Judah the Prince as described in the Talmud[16] and codified by Rabbenu Nissan.[17]

Rabbi Feinstein then discusses priorities in treating the terminally ill.[18] If a patient who is dying needs emergency treatment to relieve pain and suffering, and another patient, who is potentially curable, needs urgent treatment but only one bed is available, the potentially curable patient takes priority. However, if the incurable patient already occupies the bed, he should not be "bumped" in favor of the other patient, irrespective of whether either patient is paying for his own care. Rabbi Feinstein continues by saying[19] that priorities in Judaism are described in the Talmud.[20] In medicine, a physician should see the patient who calls or comes first, because the physician's obligation to him has already begun. However, if the second patient is sicker than the first, the physician should give priority to him. Similarly, if the physician is able to heal patient B but only to palliate A, he should care for B first unless A is in pain and discomfort, in which case he should first relieve the pain of A.

Rabbi Feinstein also points out that care must be exercised not to touch a dying patient unnecessarily, as discussed earlier in this essay, lest this act hastens the patient's death.[21] Many Jewish as well as non-Jewish physicians are either not aware of, or are not concerned about, this prohibition, decries Feinstein. However, in Jewish law, hastening a person's death by even a moment is considered an act of murder, but touching the patient as part of his medical or supportive care is obviously not only permissible but mandatory.

Rabbi Feinstein then addresses the issue of a terminally ill patient who refuses treatment,[22] and he says that if such a one refuses to accept medical treatment for his illness because he has no faith in his physicians, one should seek out another physician in whom the patient does have trust. If none is readily available or if the patient refuses treatment because of discomfort or because he has "given up," one should attempt to persuade him to accept the treatment. However, if the coercion might distress him and worsen his condition, he should not be forced to accept the treatment lest the coercion harm him and even cause his death. Physicians should consider very carefully whether or not to force a patient to accept a treatment if it is highly likely that the treatment will be of no avail, especially if it is associated with some risk, albeit less risk than the illness itself.

If a patient of sound mind refuses life-saving surgery, such as an amputation, because he would thereby be left with a handicap, one should strongly convince, and even force, him to accept the surgery.[23] Although refusal of such treatment is not comparable to the prohibition of actively wounding oneself,[24] every patient is obligated to seek healing even if such healing includes major surgery.

If a patient is suffering from advanced cancer and cannot be cured, and medications can only prolong his life of painful suffering, he should be so informed and asked if he wishes to receive such medications. If he refuses, one need not administer them, because the prolongation of his life would be with suffering.[25]

The use of dangerous medications for the terminally ill is discussed by Rabbi Feinstein as follows: Although the danger of a medication may be far less than the danger of an illness, physicians should carefully weigh whether this is true not only for relatively strong patients, or for those with non-dangerous illnesses, but also for those who are gravely ill. Only if physicians know that the risk of the side-effects of a medication is minimal in a gravely ill patient, or that more than half such patients are cured, should they administer that medication, and then only with the patient's consent. Such difficult decisions should be discussed among, and be made by, a group of physicians and not by a single one.[26]

Palliative medication for the terminally ill is again described by

Rabbi Feinstein as follows: If physicians have no medication to heal a patient and no medication even to relieve his pain, but they do have medications that will briefly prolong the patient's life without relieving the pain, they should not administer such medications.[27] This position is clearly supported by Rabbi Moshe Isserles, cited earlier in this essay, who permits, and even requires, the withdrawal of any impediment to the departure of the soul even if one thereby causes the patient to die a little sooner. The reason is obviously because of the patient's pain and suffering, since if the patient has no pain, it would not be permissible to remove such an impediment.[28]

Rabbi Feinstein continues by saying that if there is no cure available for the patient's illness and no medication to relieve pain or to strengthen the patient, then none should be given. However, one should not rely solely on one or more physicians who claim that there is no medication available to help the patient. Rather, one should consult with other physicians, even if they are younger or less experienced, to seek out possible therapeutic approaches for the terminally ill, including medications to relieve pain and suffering.

Rabbi Feinstein further points out that the Talmud states that one may (or must) set aside the certainty of a patient living a short while without any medical intervention and undertake even a dangerous and life-threatening but potentially curative medical or surgical therapy.[29] Elsewhere, Feinstein had said that if the chances of success are about 50 percent, it is permissible, but if they are greater than 50 percent, it is obligatory to administer the medication or perform the surgery by the most experienced physician.[30]

If the patient refuses the dangerous therapy, one need not force him to accept it unless there is a better than 50 percent chance that the treatment may arrest or reverse the disease process. If the physicians are not sure of the chances for success, the decision is up to the patient. If the patient is a child or an adult who cannot decide for himself, the decision can be made by the parents or next of kin, respectively.

Thus, concludes Feinstein, major surgery should not be undertaken in a terminally ill patient unless there is a chance for cure, as in Ketubot 77b, where patients with *raatan* had their skulls opened to remove some kind of growth (lit. creeping thing).[31] This operation was very dangerous but necessary because of the potential for cure. In a case where physicians suggest a therapy that has a 40 percent chance of killing the patient, that does not mean that the other 60 percent are cured, and therefore it is prohibited to give such therapy unless there is a chance that the therapy may cure the patient; then it is permitted. If 60 percent (or even only 50 percent or fewer) are cured and 40 percent killed, it would certainly be permitted.

The treatment of an intercurrent illness in a terminally ill patient is addressed by Rabbi Feinstein as follows: If a patient with a painful incurable illness (such as metastatic cancer) develops an intercurrent illness which is treatable and often completely reversible (such as pneumonia or urinary tract infection), it is obligatory to treat the intercurrent illness. However, if the underlying incurable disease is very painful and the patient refuses additional palliative therapy, it is not obligatory to administer medications that will only prolong the life of suffering without any chance of cure. If the patient is unable to voice his own opinion in this matter, one can consult with members of the immediate family about what the patient's wishes would be if he were able to express them. Such decisions should be made in consultation with a competent rabbi and the most expert physicians.[32] Later, Rabbi Feinstein reiterates that a patient who has seven days or less of life expectancy and develops another life-threatening illness, such as pneumonia, *must* be treated for the pneumonia. One should not hesitate unless the therapy for the intercurrent illness might aggravate the primary illness.[33]

Finally, specifically addressing the issue of intravenous feedings for terminally ill patients, Rabbi Feinstein says that

> for an incurably ill patient who had difficulty breathing, I have already stated that one must give him oxygen to relieve his suffering. It is also clear that such a patient who cannot eat normally must be fed intravenously, since such feeding strengthens the patient somewhat even if the patient does not feel anything [i.e., is comatose]. Food is not at all comparable to medication, since food is a natural substance which all living creatures require to maintain life.[34]

The patient should be fed (orally or intravenously) only at the direction of the physician. However, one need not force-feed an adult competent patient if he refuses food, especially if he feels that the food might harm him. If a patient's perception is that something is harmful to him, and if, nevertheless, it is applied, it may be dangerous for him. However, one should try to convince the patient to accept, and not refuse, the physician's recommendation.[35]

Feinstein concludes that, even in the final stages, the patient should be fed good things to maintain his strength for the little time that he has to live.[36] Every patient is benefited somewhat in his dying moments by maintenance of his strength. Thus, one must do all that is good for the patient (e.g., supportive care) including emotional support and pain relief and even the use of placebos to calm the patient's mind. This rule applies even to a very old man who becomes ill and claims that he has lived long enough.[37]

Elsewhere, Rabbi Feinstein permits a patient who will die without dangerous surgery to submit to the surgery even though it may hasten death because of the potential, however small, of the operation being successful, thereby adding years of life to the patient.[38]

Rabbi Feinstein also discusses the topic of the removal of life-support systems from a terminally ill patient.[39] A respirator or other life-support instrument may be removed only if it has been definitively established that the patient is dead, by criteria which Rabbi Feinstein previously cited,[40] including the absence of spontaneous respiration. If the intravenous injection of a radioactive isotope shows no circulation to the brain, including the brain stem, the patient can be considered to be physiologically decapitated, and if all other signs of death are present (e.g., no reflexes, absent caloric responses, flat electroencephalogram, etc.), the respirator may be removed. If the respirator has to be removed to allow the patient to be suctioned or to service the instrument, and if, while the respirator is disconnected, the patient shows no signs of life as above, including the absence of respiration, the respirator need not be reconnected because the patient is dead.[41]

Conclusion

Jewish tradition views death as inevitable and just. It differentiates between the body and the soul, acknowledging resurrection for the former and immortality for the latter. Jewish law requires the physician to do everything in his power to prolong life, but prohibits the use of measures that prolong the act of dying. The value attached to human life in Judaism is far greater than that in Christian tradition or in Anglo-Saxon common law. To save a life, all Jewish religious laws are automatically suspended, the only exceptions being idolatry, adultery, and murder. In Jewish law and moral teaching,

> the value of human life is infinite and beyond measure, so that any part of life—even if only an hour or a second—is of precisely

> the same worth as seventy years of it, just as any fraction of infinity, being indivisible, remains infinite. Accordingly, to kill a decrepit patient approaching death constitutes exactly the same crime of murder as to kill a young, healthy person who may still have many decades to live.[42]

Euthanasia is opposed without qualification in Jewish law, which condemns as sheer murder any active or deliberate hastening of death, whether the physician acts with or without the patient's consent. Some rabbinic views do not allow any relaxation of efforts, however artificial and ultimately hopeless, to prolong life. Others, however, do not require the physician to resort to "heroic" methods, but sanction the omission of machines and artificial life-support systems that only serve to draw out the dying patient's agony, provided, however, that basic care, such as food and good nursing, is provided.

Jewish teaching proclaims the sanctity of human life. The physician is given Divine license to heal but not to hasten death. When a physician has nothing further to offer a patient medically or surgically, the physician's license to heal ends and he becomes no different than a lay person. Every human being is morally expected to help another human in distress. A dying patient is no exception. The physician, family, friends, nurses, social workers, and other individuals close to the dying patient are all obligated to provide supportive, including psychosocial and emotional, care until the very end. Fluids and nutrition are part and parcel of that supportive care, no different than washing, turning, talking, singing, reading, or just listening to the dying patient. There are times when specific medical and/or surgical therapies are no longer indicated, appropriate, or desirable for a terminal, irreversibly ill dying patient. There is no time, however, when general supportive measures can be abandoned, thereby hastening the patient's demise.

Many legal jurisdictions and state medical and legal societies have enacted, or are considering the adoption of, guidelines on forgoing (i.e., withdrawing or withholding) life-sustaining treatment. The slippery slope has now reached the point where we are reclassifying basic supportive care such as fluids and nutrition as medical treatment to justify withholding or withdrawing it in certain cases. Where will the trend end? Will we soon consider active hastening of a person's death by a lethal injection to be acceptable legally and/or medically? At present, the courts have offered opposing rulings. Even if the courts legally sanction the withdrawal or withholding of fluids and nutrition in some instances, legal permissibility is not synonymous with moral license. What is legal is not always moral.

Since the decisions about withholding specific therapy for a terminally ill patient, about the discontinuation of life-support systems, about whether or not to employ resuscitative measures in a given situation, about the withholding or withdrawal of fluids, nutrition, and oxygen are complex and not free of family and/or physician personal and emotional involvement and even bias, it seems advisable to consult with a competent rabbinic authority for adjudication on a case-by-case basis.

Notes

1. P. G. Derr, "Why Food and Fluids Can Never Be Denied," *Hastings Center Report* 16 (February 1986): 28–30.
2. Semachot 1:1 ff.
3. Shabbat 151b.
4. Avodah Zarah 18a.
5. *Mishneh Torah, Hilkhot Avel* 4:5.
6. *Shulhan Arukh, Yoreh Deah* 339.
7. *Sefer Chasidim* 723.
8. *Ramo* on *Yoreh Deah* 339:1.
9. I. Jakobovits, *Jewish Medical Ethics* (New York: Bloch, 1959), pp. 123–125.
10. J. D. Bleich, *Judaism and Healing* (New York: Ktav, 1981), pp. 134–145.
11. M. Feinstein, Responsa *Iggrot Moshe, Choshen Mishpat,* pt. 2, no. 73:1.
12. In support of the Feinstein view is Rabbi Eliezer Yehuda Waldenberg (Responsa *Tzitz Eliezer*, vol. 5, *Ramat Raḥel,* no. 28:5), who reiterates that physicians and others are obligated to do everything possible to save the life of a dying patient, even if the patient will live only for a brief period, and even if the patient is suffering greatly. Any action that results in hastening of the death of a dying patient is forbidden and considered an act of murder. Even if the patient is beyond cure and is suffering greatly and requests that his death be hastened, one may not do so or advise the patient to do so (ibid., no. 29, and vol. 10, no. 25:6).
13. Rabbi Waldenberg continues (see previous note) that a terminally ill, incurable patient may be given oral or parenteral narcotics or other powerful analgesics to relieve his pain and suffering, even at the risk of depressing his respiratory center and hastening his death, provided the medications are prescribed solely for pain relief and not to hasten death (ibid., vol. 13, no. 87).
14. Dr. A. Sofer Abraham quotes Rabbi Auerbach as distinguishing between routine and non-routine treatments for the terminally ill (A. S. Abraham, in *Halakhah Urefuah* 2 [1981]: 185–190). For example, a dying cancer patient must be given food, oxygen, antibiotics, insulin, and the like, but does not have to be given painful and toxic chemotherapy which offers no chance of cure but, at best, temporary palliation. Such a patient may be given morphine for pain even if it depresses his respiration. An irreversibly ill terminal patient whose spontaneous heartbeat and breathing stop does not have to be resuscitated.
15. Feinstein, Responsa *Iggrot Moshe, Ḥoshen Mishpat,* pt. 2, no. 74:4.
16. Ketubot 104a.
17. *Ran* in Nedarim 40.
18. Feinstein, op. cit., No. 73:2.

19. Ibid., no. 74:1.
20. Horayot 13a.
21. Feinstein, op. cit., no. 73:3.
22. Ibid., no. 73:5.
23. Ibid., no. 74:5.
24. Baba Kamma 91a.
25. Feinstein, op. cit., no. 75:1.
26. Ibid.
27. Ibid., no. 74:1.
28. Rabbi Chaim David Halevi, in *Techumin* 2 (1981): 297–305, equates the removal of salt from a terminally ill patient's tongue with the removal of an artificial respirator. The former is considered in Jewish law to be an obstacle to the departing of the soul and is of no therapeutic benefit and may be removed to allow the person to die. So, too, claims Halevi, the artificial respirator was first attached to the patient in an attempt to maintain the patient's life. However, when it becomes obvious that there is no more therapeutic benefit to be derived from the respirator, it may be removed. Not only is it allowed to remove the respirator from a terminally, irreversibly ill patient, but it is, in fact, an obligation to do so, says Halevi.
29. Feinstein, op. cit., no. 74:5, referring to Avodah Zarah 27b.
30. Feinstein, op. cit., pt. 3, no. 36.

Rabbi Gedaliah Aharon Rabinowitz reviews the laws pertaining to the care of the terminally ill and the criteria for defining the moment of death (in *Halachah Urefuah* 3 [1983]: 102–114). He also states that experimental chemotherapy for cancer patients is permissible but not obligatory (ibid., pp. 115–118). Such therapy must have a rational scientific basis and be administered by expert physicians. Untested and unknown remedies may not be used on human beings.

31. Feinstein, op. cit., pt. 2, no. 75:3.
32. Ibid., no. 74:2.
33. Ibid., no. 75:4.
34. Ibid., no. 74:3.
35. Rabbi Shlomo Zalman Auerbach states that a terminally ill patient must be given food and oxygen even against his will (in *Halachah Urefuah* 2 [1981]: 131). However, one may withhold, at the patient's request, medications and treatments which might cause him great pain and discomfort. Rabbi Moshe Hershler holds that withholding food or medication from a terminally ill patient so that he dies is murder (in *Halachah Urefuah* 2 [1981]: 30–42). Withholding respiratory support is equivalent to withholding food, since it will shorten the patient's life. Every moment of life is precious, and all measures must be taken to preserve even a few moments of life. However, if the physicians feel that a comatose patient's situation is hopeless, they are not obligated to institute life-prolonging or resuscitative treatments.
36. Feinstein, op. cit., no. 75:6.

37. Ibid., no. 75:7.

38. Ibid., pt. 2, no. 58 and pt. 3, no. 36.

39. Ibid., pt. 3, no. 132.

40. Ibid., pt. 2, no. 146.

41. Feinstein's position on the use and discontinuation of life-support systems is supported by Rabbi Eliezer Yehudah Waldenberg, who states that it is not considered interference with the Divine will to place a patient on a respirator or other life-support systems (Responsa *Tzitz Eliezer*, vol. 15, no. 37). On the contrary, all attempts must be made to prolong and preserve the life of a patient who has a potentially curable disease or reversible condition (ibid., vol. 13, no. 89). Thus, one must attempt resuscitation on a drowning victim who has no spontaneous respiration or heartbeat because of the possibility of resuscitation and reversibility (ibid., vol. 14, no. 81). One is not obligated or even permitted, however, to initiate artificial life-support and/or other resuscitative efforts if it is obvious that the patient is terminally and incurably and irreversibly ill with no chance of recovery. One is also allowed to disconnect and discontinue life-support instrumentation, according to Waldenberg (ibid., vol. 13, no. 89) and others, if one can establish that the patient is dead according to Jewish legal criteria (ibid., vol. 90, no. 46 and vol. 10, no. 25:4), i.e., if the patient has no independent brain function or spontaneous cardiorespiratory activity. If it is not clear whether the respirator is keeping the patient alive or is only ventilating a corpse, the respirator must be maintained. Therefore, from a practical standpoint, Waldenberg advises that one uses respirators with automatic time clocks set for a twelve-hour or twenty-four-hour period (ibid., vol. 13, no. 89). When the respirator shuts itself off, one can observe the patient for signs of spontaneous respiration. If none are present and if the heart is not beating and the brain is irreversibly damaged, one does not reconnect the respirator. Finally, Rabbi Waldenberg asserts that blood transfusions, oxygen, antibiotics, intravenous fluids, oral and parenteral nutrition, and pain-relief medications must be maintained for a terminally ill patient until the very end (ibid., vol. 14, no. 80).

42. I. Jakobovits, "Medical Experimentation on Humans in Jewish Law," in *Jewish Bioethics*, ed. F. Rosner and J. D. Bleich (New York: Hebrew Publishing Co., 1979), pp. 377–383.

19

Suicide

Introduction

Every day in the United States, about sixty people kill themselves by poisoning, hanging, drowning, shooting, stabbing, jumping from high places, or other means. Although nearly 25,000 deaths from suicide are recorded annually in the United States, the actual figure, according to the National Institute of Mental Health, is probably closer to 50,000 yearly. Worldwide, more than 500,000 suicides are registered yearly, according to the World Health Organization, and there are approximately eight times as many suicide attempts.

The problem of suicide reached such proportions that the United States Public Health Service created the National Center for Studies of Suicide Prevention in October 1966. A periodical devoted exclusively to suicide is the *Bulletin of Suicidology*, published by the United States Public Health Service since 1967.

The medical, psychological, psychiatric, legal, and social literatures are replete with articles, monographs, symposia, and other publications on suicide. Factors such as age, sex, marital status, day of week, month of year, method, religion, race, motivation, living conditions, repetitive attempts, medical and psychiatric histories of patients attempting and committing suicide are amply covered in these writings as well as the many books published on this subject.

Several salient features of the problem deserve mention. Suicides are three times as frequent in men than in women, although there are more attempts by women than men. Twice as many white Americans commit suicide than do black Americans, and twice as many single people kill themselves than do married individuals. College students have a suicide rate 50 percent higher than non–college students of comparable age, sex, and race. In industrialized countries, physicians, dentists, and lawyers have a higher rate of suicide than other professionals. Although the suicide rate has remained relatively constant in the United States over the past decade or so, poisoning by drugs, especially barbiturates, has become popular as a method of choice. The age group with the highest suicide rate is that above sixty-five years. Suicide ranks third as a cause of death among teenagers. It has also been estimated that the ratio of suicide attempts to actual successes in adolescents is one hundred to one.

One phase of suicide hardly discussed at all is the religious aspect. This chapter attempts to organize and present in a systematic fashion the subject of suicide as found in Jewish sources. The closely related topic of martyrdom is discussed briefly at the end.

Suicide in the Bible

During the period of the Judges, in approximately the eleventh or twelfth century B.C.E., lived Samson of the tribe of Dan, whose story is known to all. Samson's final effort in bringing down the Philistine temple upon himself as well as his enemies is vividly described.

> And Samson said: "Let me die with the Philistines." And he bent with all his might; and the house fell upon the lords, and upon all the people that were therein. So the dead that he slew at his death were more than they that he slew in his life.[1]

Elsewhere in the Bible, we read of King Saul's final battle against the Philistines on Mount Gilboa in the eleventh century B.C.E.[2] Here, Saul saw his three sons Jonathan, Abinadab, and Malchishua and most of his army slain. Not wishing to flee or to be taken prisoner and exposed to the scorn of the Philistines, King Saul entreated his armor-bearer to kill him. The latter refused, and so the king fell upon his own sword. The biblical passage concludes: "And when his armor-bearer saw that Saul was dead, he likewise fell upon his sword and died with him."[3]

From these events it would appear as if Saul committed suicide. However, later on when David is informed of Saul's death, the Bible states:

> And David said unto the young man that told him: "How knowest thou that Saul and Jonathan his son are dead?" And the young man that told him said: "As I happened by chance upon Mount Gilboa, behold, Saul leaned upon his spear; and lo, the chariots and the horsemen pressed hard upon him. And when he looked behind him, he saw me, and called unto me. And I answered: Here am I. And he said unto me: Who art thou? And I answered him: I am an Amalekite. And he said unto me: Stand, I pray thee, beside me, and slay me, for the agony hath taken hold of me because my life is just yet in me. So I stood beside him and slew him, because I was sure that he could not live after that he was fallen . . ."[4]

Biblical commentators differ in their interpretation of this passage. Rabbi David Kimchi, known as *Radak*, explains that Saul did not die immediately when he fell on his sword but was mortally wounded. In his death throes, Saul asked the Amalekite to render the final blow of mercy to hasten his death. Rabbi Solomon ben Isaac *(Rashi)*, Rabbi Levi ben Gerson *(Ralbag)*, and Rabbi David Altschul *(Metzudat David)* all agree with Kimchi and consider the death of King Saul as a case of euthanasia. Others view the story of the Amalekite as a complete fabrication.

In any event, Saul did attempt suicide. Only the question of his success is debated. As to Saul's armor-bearer, no one disputes that he committed suicide.

King David's faithless counselor, Achitophel, committed suicide by hanging himself in his native town of Giloh. One of several reasons probably prompted suicide. First, he knew that Absalom's attempt to overthrow David was doomed and that he would die a traitor's death. Second, and less likely, is the disgust of Achitophel at Absalom's conduct in setting aside his counsel, thus wounding Achitophel's pride and disappointing his ambition.[5] Finally, David's curse may have prompted Achitophel to hang himself.[6]

> And when Achitophel saw that his counsel was not followed, he saddled his ass and arose, and got himself home unto his city, and set his house in order, and strangled himself; and he died and was buried in the sepulchre of his father.[7]

King Baasha of Israel reigned from 888 B.C.E. and was succeeded by his son Elah. The latter was addicted to idleness and drunkenness and passed the days drinking in his palace while his warriors were battling the Philistines at Gibbethon.[8] Zimri, a high-ranking officer, took advantage of the situation, assassinated Elah, and mounted the throne. His reign, however, lasted only seven days. As soon as the news of King Elah's murder reached the army on the battlefield, General Omri was elected king and laid siege to the palace. When Zimri saw that he was unable to hold out against the siege, he set fire to the palace and perished in the flames. The Bible records: "And it came to pass, when Zimri saw that the city was taken that he went unto the castle of the king's house, and he burnt the king's house over him with fire, and he died."[9]

Some biblical commentators, notably *Radak* and *Metzudat David*, to whom the thought of suicide was abhorrent, state that Omri burned the house over Zimri. Most commentators, however, interpret the biblical passage literally.

Suicide in the Apocrypha

In the Second Book of Maccabees, two acts of suicide are recorded. The first occurred when King Demetrius I of Syria (162–150 B.C.E.) escaped from his imprisonment in Rome and returned home as an invader.[10] Attempting to put down a rebellion of his Judean subjects, King Demetrius sent Nicanor, one of the warriors who had escaped with him from Rome, to Judea, to treat the insurgents with the utmost harshness. Nicanor, in order to induce surrender from the Judeans, ordered that the most respected man in Jerusalem, Ragesh (or Razis) be seized. When the arresting soldiers were forcing open the courtyard door to Ragesh's house, "he fell upon his sword, preferring to die nobly rather than to fall into the wretches' hands."[11] The ghastly tale of his lack of success in the first suicide attempt, his subsequent attempt by throwing himself down from a wall, and his final success by self-disembowelment is vividly described.[12]

The second act of suicide is that of Ptolemy, an advocate of the Judeans at the Syrian court, who was called a traitor before King Antiochus Eupator. Unable to maintain the dignity of his office, Ptolemy poisoned himself.[13]

Other Suicides and Near-Suicides in Ancient Jewish Writings

All the suicides mentioned in the Bible and Apocrypha are pyschologically understandable. Each knew what lay ahead if he remained alive, namely a prolonged, torturous martyrdom and/or disgrace to the God of Israel. All were prominent people. Except perhaps for King Saul, none could be accused of having experienced temporary insanity to excuse his act of self-destruction. Perhaps Ragesh and Ptolemy were influenced by the Greek philosophy of their times, in which suicide was highly acceptable.

There are several individuals mentioned in the Bible, Apocrypha, and other ancient Jewish writings who considered suicide and perhaps wished to attempt it, but did not.

Job, during his quest for an explanation of his wretchedness, speaks of suicide: *And my soul chooseth strangling, and death rather than these my bones.*[14] He did not attempt suicide, perhaps out of either love or fear of God, as he himself states: *Though He slay me, yet will I trust in Him.*[15]Possibly Job did not mean to even consider suicide but was remarking that he would prefer death to life. This question remains unresolved.

One of the most famous "near-suicides" is Flavius Josephus, who failed to commit suicide at Jotapata in the year 69 C.E. when all the other Zealots there did so in a mass-suicide pact. Flavius Vespasian, successor to Nero as emperor of Rome, had come to conquer Judea. Strong resistance was offered at the fortress of Jotapata. After a forty-day siege, the fortress fell. Many chose suicide by flinging themselves over the walls or falling on their weapons. Josephus, however, sought concealment in a huge cistern in which he found forty of his own soldiers. They all swore to die by their own hand in a mass-suicide pact. When his turn came Josephus reneged and surrendered to the Romans.[16] In Josephus' *Antiquities of the Jews*, there are numerous examples cited of suicide, including the mass suicide at Masada.

Suicide in the Talmud

The Talmud is replete with stories concerning suicide and martyrdom as well as discussions relating to the laws of burial and mourning for the deceased. Among the most renowned examples is the story of Rabbi Chanina ben Teradyon's death by burning at the hands of the Romans.[17] He was wrapped in a Scroll of the Law, bundles of branches were placed around him, and these were set ablaze. The Romans also brought tufts of wool which they had soaked in water, placing them over his heart to prevent a quick death. When his disciples pleaded with him to open his mouth so that the fire would consume him more quickly, he replied that one is not to accelerate one's own death. The executioner asked him: "Rabbi, if I raise the flame and remove the tufts of wet wool from your heart, will I enter the world-to-come?" "Yes," was the reply. The executioner did as he proposed, and the rabbi died speedily. The executioner then jumped into the fire and was burned to death. A voice from heaven exclaimed that Rabbi Chanina ben Teradyon and his executioner had been assigned to the world-to-come.

Another case of suicide is related of Herod the Great, who was a slave of the Hasmonean house of the Maccabees and had set his eyes on a certain maiden of that house.[18] One day he heard a voice from heaven saying that every slave that rebelled now would succeed. So he killed the entire houshold but spared the maiden. When she saw that he wanted to marry her, she ran up to the roof and cried out: "Whoever comes and says that he is from the Hasmonean house is a slave, since I alone am left of it, and I am throwing myself down from this roof." Herod loved her so much that he preserved her body in honey for seven years.

The suicide of a Roman officer who saved the life of Rabban Gamliel is portrayed as follows:[19] When Tinneius Rufus the wicked destroyed the Jewish Temple, Rabban Gamliel was condemned to death. A high officer came to the house of study to search for him, but Rabban Gamliel hid. The officer found him and asked him secretly: "If I save you, will you bring me into the world-to-come?" The answer was affirmative. After making Rabban Gamliel swear to it, the officer mounted the roof and threw himself down and died. The Romans annulled the decree against Rabban Gamliel, according to their tradition that the death of one of their leaders (i.e., the officer's suicide) was a punishment for an evil decree. Thereupon a voice from heaven was heard saying that this high officer was destined to enter the world-to-come.

Nearly identical stories are told in the Talmud in two separate discussions.[20] Because of an incident that once occurred, it was decreed that guests might not give any of the food that was set before them to the host's son or to his servant or deputy unless they had received the host's permission to do so. The incident was that in a time of scarcity a man invited three guests to his house and only had three eggs which he set before them. When the host's hungry child entered and stood before them, one of the guests took his portion and gave it to him; the second guest did the same, and so did the third. When the father came in and saw his son with one egg in his mouth and holding two in his hands, he picked him up to his full height and flung him to the ground, so that he died. When the mother saw her child dead, she went up to the roof, threw herself down, and died. On seeing this, the father also went up to the roof, threw himself down, and died. Rabbi Eliezer ben Jacob said: "Because of this, three souls perished."

A related incident that terminated in suicide concerns a man who had sent his friend a barrel of wine and there was oil floating at the mouth of the barrel, leading the recipient to believe that the whole barrel contained oil. He invited some guests to partake of it. When he came and found that it was only wine, he went and hanged himself out of shame because he had nothing else prepared to set before his guests. As a result, it was decreed that a man should not send his neighbor a barrel of wine with oil floating on top of it.

Another talmudic episode of suicide is found in the commentary of *Rashi.*[21] Rabbi Meir is said to have fled to Babylon. One of the reasons given is "because of the incident of [his wife] Beruryah." The incident concerns the fact that Rabbi Meir's wife once taunted him regarding the rabbinic adage that women are temperamentally lightheaded. He replied that one day she would testify to its truth. Subsequently she was enticed by one of her husband's disciples, proving she was too weak to resist. She then committed suicide by strangulation.

A mass suicide is described in the Talmud, where four hundred boys and girls are said to have been carried off for immoral purposes.[22] They guessed what they were wanted for and said to themselves that if they drowned in the sea they would attain the life of the future world.[23] The girls leaped into the sea first and the boys followed.

Elsewhere in the Talmud is related the story from the Second Book of Maccabees of the woman and her seven martyred sons.[24] The sons were killed one by one by Emperor Antiochus Epiphanes for refusing to serve an idol. As the last son was being led away to be killed, his mother said to him: "My son, go and say to your father Abraham: Thou didst bind one [son to the altar, i.e., Isaac], but I have bound seven altars." Then she went up on a roof and threw herself down and was killed. A voice thereupon came forth from heaven saying *A joyful mother of children.*[25]

Another incident relates to a certain student who once left his phylacteries in a hole on the side of the road before entering a privy.[26] A harlot passed by and took them. She came to the house of learning and said: "See what so-and-so gave me for hire." When the student heard this, he went to the top of a roof and threw himself down and killed himself.

The rules and regulations governing suicide are discussed in at least two places in the Talmud.[27] "No *halachah* [Law] may be quoted in the name of one who surrenders himself to meet death for the words of the Torah." Later in the same tractate we find: ". . .who is the *tanna* that maintains that a man may not injure himself? It could hardly be said that he was the *tanna* of the teaching *And surely your own blood of your souls will I require,*[28] which Rabbi Eleazar interpreted to mean 'I [i.e., God] will require your blood if shed by the hands of yourselves [i.e., suicide],' for murder is perhaps different." *Rashi* interprets this scriptural verse to mean that even though one strangles oneself so that no blood flows, still "I [God] will require it."

The major talmudic discussion of the rules governing suicide states that we do not occupy ourselves at all with the funeral rites of someone who committed suicide willfully.[29] Rabbi Ishmael said: We exclaim over him, "Alas for a lost [life]. Alas for a lost [life]." Rabbi Akiva said to him: "Leave him unmourned; speak neither well nor ill of him." Further "we do not rend garments for him, nor bare the shoulder as [signs of mourning], or deliver a memorial address over him. We do however, stand in a row for him [at the cemetery after the funeral to offer condolences] and recite the mourner's benediction for him because this is respectful for the living [relatives]. The general rule is that we occupy ourselves with anything that is intended as a matter of honor for the living."

The Talmud defines an intentional suicide.[30] It is not he who climbed to the top of a tree and fell down and died, nor he who ascended to the top of a roof and fell down and died, as these may have been accidents. Rather, a willful suicide is one who calls out: "Look, I am going to the top of the roof or to the top of the tree, and I will throw myself down that I may die." When people see him go up to the top of the tree or roof and fall down and die, then he is considered to have committed suicide willfully. A person found strangled or hanging from a tree or lying dead on a sword is presumed not to have committed suicide intentionally, and none of the funeral rites are withheld from him.

The Talmud next relates two childhood suicides and considers neither an intentional suicide.[31] One case concerns the son of Gornos of Lydda who ran away from school, and the other case is that of a child in Bene-Berak who broke a bottle on the Sabbath. In each case, the father threatened to punish the child, and out of fear each child destroyed himself in a pit. Rabbi Tarfon in the former case and Rabbi Akiva in the latter case ruled that these were not willful suicides and therefore none of the funeral rites should be withheld.

Suicide in the Midrash

In the Midrash the story is told of Rabbi Akiba walking barefoot to Rome when met by a eunuch officer of the emperor riding on a horse.[32] The officer asked him whether he was the famous rabbi of the Jews and he answered yes. In order to embarrass Rabbi Akiba, the eunuch said three things: "He who rides on a horse is a king, he who rides on a donkey is a free man, and he whose feet have shoes on is a human being; he who has none of these is worse than a dead person." Rabbi Akiba replied saying three things: "One's beard is one's majestic countenance, happiness of heart is one's wife, and the inheritance of God is to have children; woe is the man who is lacking all three. Not only that but Scripture states, *I have seen servants upon horses and princes walking as servants upon the earth.*"[33] When the eunuch officer heard these words, he knocked his head against a wall until he died.

Another case of intentional suicide is that of Yakum of Tzerorot, nephew of Rabbi Yose ben Joezer of Tzeredah.[34] Yakum taunted Rabbi Joseph Meshita and, as self-punishment, subjected himself to the four modes of execution inflicted by the courts: stoning, burning, decapitation, and strangulation. He took a post, implanted it in the earth, raised a wall of stones around it, and tied a cord to it. He made a fire in front of it and fixed a sword in the middle of the post. He hanged himself on the post, and when the cord burned through, he was strangled. Then the sword caught him, while the wall of stones fell upon him and he was burned.

Suicide in the Codes of Jewish Law

In the *Mishneh Torah*, Maimonides states:

> For one who has committed suicide intentionally we do not occupy ourselves at all with the funeral rites, and we do not mourn for him nor eulogize him. However, we do stand in a row for him, and we recite the mourner's benediction, and we do all that is intended as a matter of honor for the living.[35]

Maimonides then defines an intentional suicide exactly as defined in the Talmud. The commentators on Maimonides' code, Rabbi David ben Zimra, known as *Radvaz*, Rabbi Joseph Karo, known as *Keseph Mishneh*, and Rabbi Abraham Boton, known as *Lechem Mishneh*, all point out that Maimonides considers mourning an honor for the dead and therefore prohibited.

Rabbi Jacob ben Asher, known as *Tur*, codifies the section on suicide of the Talmud nearly verbatim.[36] He states that we do not rend garments, bare the shoulder, or eulogize the willful suicide victim. However, we do stand in a row to offer condolences to the family at the cemetery, and we utter the mourner's benediction, for these are intended as a matter of honor for the living relatives. *Tur* then continues by saying that the prohibition of rending the garments refers only to distant relatives, but the immediate relatives who have to mourn the deceased should rend their garments as a sign of mourning. This is diametrically opposed to Maimonides. Rabbi Joseph Karo, in his *Shulchan Aruch*, follows Maimonides.

Tur defines a willful suicide as it is defined in the Talmud.[37] However, a child who committed suicide even willfully is not considered to have attained his full measure of intelligence. Similarly, he continues, anyone who commits suicide in unusual circumstances, such as King Saul, is not considered a willful suicide and is entitled to all funeral rites. According to Rabbi Joel Sirkes, known as *Bet Chadash*, and Rabbi Joseph Karo, known as *Bet Joseph*, in their commentaries on Jacob ben Asher, the latter statement by *Tur* is based on Nachmanides' work entitled *Sefer ha-Adam*.

In his *Shulchan Aruch*, Rabbi Joseph Karo seems to combine the talmudic and Maimonidean regulations regarding suicide. He states that we do not occupy ourselves at all for anyone who has committed suicide willfully.[38] We do not mourn for him (contrary to Jacob ben Asher but in agreement with Maimonides) nor eulogize him nor rend garments for him nor bare the shoulder. However, all that is in honor of the living, such as standing in a row to offer condolences to the relatives of the deceased, is performed.

Several commentators on Karo, including Rabbi Zechariah Mendel of Cracow, known as *Ba'er Hetev*, Rabbi Abraham Tzvi Hirsh Eisenstadt, known as *Pischei Teshuvah*, and Rabbi Shabtai ben Meir Hakohen, known as *Sifsei Kohen* or *Shach*, point out that Jacob ben Asher's code differs from Karo's in that the former requires garment rending and mourning of close relatives of the deceased. *Sifsei Kohen* also quotes Rabbi Solomon ben Abraham Adret, who explains that "we do not occupy ourselves at all," as cited from the Talmud and Maimonides, does not refer to burial itself.[39] Rather, only the rites surrounding the funeral are withheld but the deceased must be buried.

Suicide in Recent Rabbinic Writings

Responsa literature on suicide is rather sparse. Rabbi Moses Schreiber was asked concerning a person found drowned in a river.[40] Rabbi Schreiber defines in great legal detail what a willful suicide is in Jewish law. He seeks legal technicalities, such as fear, anger, emotional instability on the part of the victim, which, if present, would remove the deceased from being considered an intentional suicide. He thus justifies the actions of Saul and Achitophel. Rabbi Schreiber concludes that laws of mourning, including the recitation of the *Kaddish* prayer, are observed even for an intentional suicide victim.

Rabbi Yechiel Michael Tukazinsky devotes an entire chapter to a discussion of suicide.[41] The person who commits willful suicide is considered a murderer. It matters not whether he kills someone else or himself, since his own soul is not his, just as someone else's soul is not his. Were we able to bring this man to justice in this world, he would be adjudicated as any murderer. In fact, he may be so judged in heaven above.

Thirteenth-century Rabbi Judah the Pious states that one who neglects the preservation of his health is guilty of partially murdering himself.[42] Rabbi Tukazinsky states that it may even be a graver sin to commit suicide than to murder someone else, for several reasons. First, by killing himself, a person removes all possibility of repentance. Second, in most circumstances death is the greatest atonement for one's sins;[43] however, in a suicide's death there has been committed a cardinal transgression rather than expiation. A third reason why Judaism abhors suicide is that the person who takes his own life asserts by this act that he denies the Divine mastery and ownership of his life, his body, and his soul. The willful suicide further denies his Divine creation. Our sages compare the departure of a soul from a human body to a Torah scroll which has been consumed by fire. Thus, a person who commits suicide can be likened to one who burns a *Sefer Torah.*

He who takes his own life is also one who denies the Judaic teaching of the immortality of the soul and the eternal existence of Almighty God. Such a person will have to answer to heavenly judgment in the world-to-come, as our rabbis of blessed memory stated: "He who willfully destroys himself has no share in the world-to-come."

Martyrdom in Judaism

The subject of suicide is intertwined with the topic of martyrdom, since many suicides are committed as an act of martyrdom. The

Jewish attitude toward martyrdom is based upon the following biblical passage: *Ye shall therefore keep My ordinances and My judgments, which if a man do, he shall live in them: I am the Eternal.*[44] The rabbis deduce from the words *he shall live* that martyrdom is prohibited save for idolatry, adultery, and murder.[45] All other commandments may be transgressed if life is in danger in order that *he shall live*. Martyrdom includes both the ending of one's own life for the sanctification of the name of God[46] and allowing oneself to be killed in times of religious persecution rather than transgress biblical commandments. Perhaps the best-known examples of martyrdom in Jewish life are the ten famous scholars executed or martyred by the Roman state at different times for their insistence on teaching the Torah.

Suicide and Modern Psychiatry

The preponderance of modern psychiatric thinking on the pathology of suicide is that, with rare exceptions, the act of suicide, whether or not successful, is *prima facie* evidence of mental illness. Most often the illness is depression or despondency but occasionally may manifest itself as a psychosis or schizophrenia. The rare exception can be illustrated by a person who has lived a full and good life and who feels he (or she) has nothing to look forward to. If this type of person attempts or commits suicide, it is not a sign of despondency.

Suicide may represent an act which expresses the fantasy reunion of a person with a departed loved one or a fantasy reunion with God. Such a psychiatric aberration of a person's mind cannot be classified as anything other than pathological. Suicide can accompany virtually all psychiatric illnesses or may occur during periods of life crisis and stress in persons without discernible mental illness.

Although physicians daily witness profound despair and tragedy in their patients, suicide attempts are an unusual event, and successful suicide is rarer still. The clinician should recognize the painful states of bitterness and desperation which so often raise the suicidal impulse.

At the other extreme of modern psychiatric thought is the American psychiatrist Thomas Szasz, who claims that suicide is rarely, if ever, a sign of mental illness. He further asserts that a person should have the right to commit suicide just as a person has many civil rights. *Halachah* (Jewish Law) would not condone such an approach because, in Judaism, we believe that the human body is not ours to do with as we please. Man was created in the image of God and was entrusted with his body, to guard it and to watch over it. This is the philosophy behind Judaism's abhorrence of suicide. Since the vast majority of suicides are assignable to emotional stress or psychiatric illness, lenient rabbinic rulings are usually enunciated.[47]

Summary and Conclusions

Judaism regards suicide as a criminal act and strictly forbidden by Jewish law. The cases of suicide in the Bible as well as those in the Apocrypha, Talmud, and Midrash took place under unusual and extenuating conditions.

In general a suicide is not accorded full burial honors. The Talmud and codes of Jewish law decree that rending one's garments, delivering memorial addresses, and other rites of mourning which are an honor for the dead are not to be performed for a suicide victim. The strict definition of a suicide for which these laws apply is one who had previously announced his intentions and then killed himself immediately thereafter by the method he announced. Children are never regarded as deliberate suicides and are afforded all burial rites. Similarly, those who commit suicide under extreme physical or mental strain, or while not in full possession of their faculties, or in order to atone for past sins are not considered as willful suicides, and none of the burial and mourning rites are withheld.

These considerations may condone the numerous acts of suicide and martyrdom committed by Jews throughout the centuries, from the priests who leaped into the flames of the burning Temple to the martyred Jews in the time of the Crusades, from the Jewish suicides during the medieval persecutions to the martyred Jews in more recent pogroms. Only for the sanctification of the name of the Lord would a Jew intentionally take his own life or allow it to be taken as a symbol of his extreme faith in God. Otherwise intentional suicide would be strictly forbidden because it constitutes a denial of the Divine creation of man, of the immortality of the soul, and of the atonement of death.[48]

Notes

1. Judges 16:23–31.
2. I Samuel 31:1–7.
3. Ibid. 31:5.
4. II Samuel 1:5–10.
5. H. Graetz, *History of the Jews* (Philadelphia: Jewish Publication Society, 1956), vol. 1., p. 143.
6. Makkot 11a.
7. II Samuel 17:23.
8. Graetz, op. cit., p. 192.
9. I Kings 16:18.
10. Graetz, op cit., pp. 482–485.
11. II Maccabees 14:41–42.
12. Ibid. 14:43–46.
13. Ibid. 10:12.
14. Job 7:15.
15. Job 13:15.
16. Graetz, op. cit., pp. 276–290.
17. Avodah Zarah 18a.
18. Bava Batra 3b.
19. Taanit 29a.
20. Chullin 94a and Derech Eretz Rabbah, chap. 9:57b.
21. Avovdah Zarah 18b.
22. Gittin 57b.
23. As portrayed in Psalms 68:23.
24. Gittin 57b.
25. Psalms 113:9.
26. Berachot 23a.
27. Bava Kamma 61a and 91b.
28. Genesis 9:5.
29. Semachot 2:1 ff.
30. Ibid. 2:2.
31. Ibid. 2:4–5.
32. Ecclesiastes Rabbah 10:7:26b
33. Ecclesiastes 10:7.
34. Genesis Rabbah 65:22:130b.
35. Maimonides, *Mishneh Torah, Hilchot Avel* 1:11.
36. *Tur, Yoreh Deah* no. 345.
37. Semachot 2:1 ff.
38. Karo, *Shulchan Aruch, Yoreh Deah* no. 345.
39. Adret, Responsa *Rashba* 763.
40. Schreiber, Responsa *Chasam Sofer, Yoreh Deah*, no. 326.
41. Tukazinsky, *Gesher HaChayim* (Jerusalem, 1960), chap. 25.
42. Judah the Pious. *Sefer Chasidim*, no. 675.

43. Yoma 86a.
44. Leviticus 18.5.
45. Sanhedrin 74a.
46. Leviticus 22:32.
47. See Tukazinsky, loc. cit.
48. See also Avodah Zarah 17b, Taanit 29a, Berachot 61b, Pesachim 50a, Bava Batra 10b, Sanhedrin 11a, 14a, 74a, 74b, 110b; I. Y. Unterman, *Shevet Mi-Yehudah* (Jerusalem, 1955), pp. 38 ff.; and I. Jakobovits, *Jewish Medical Ethics* (New York: Bloch, 1959), pp. 52–54.

20

Definition of Death

Introduction

The modern era of human heart transplantation, which began late in 1976, initiated intense debate about the moral, religious, and legal issues relating to life and death and especially the definition of death. The traditional definition of death as reflected in *Black's Law Dictionary* is the "total stoppage of the circulation of the blood, and the cessation of the animal and vital functions consequent thereon, such as respiration, pulsation . . ." With the advent of heart transplantation, this definition of death became inadequate and a new definition of death, so-called brain death, evolved. Brain death is now socially acceptable and legislatively sanctioned throughout most of the civilized world.

In a classic 1968 article on brain death, an Ad Hoc Committee of the Harvard Medical School recommended four criteria: unreceptivity and unresponsivity, no movements, no reflexes, and a flat electroencephalogram.[1] This paper was reprinted as a "landmark article" in 1984[2] with an accompanying perspective editorial which states:

> The Harvard Committee report likely spawned more medicolegal discussion and action than any other publication. Almost every legal entity has had to deal with this new concept of death, and most medical standards for death of the brain originated, with some modifications, from the criteria set forth in this article. The prescience of this committee has become even more obvious

as hundreds of clinical observations have borne out the diagnostic value of their clearly stated clinical rules.[3]

In 1981, the President's Commission for the Study of Ethical Problems in Medicine and Biomedical and Behavioral Research published its report that defined death.[4] This definition was approved by the American Bar Association and many other organizations and prominent individuals. The recommended proposal was the following:

> An individual who has sustained either (a) irreversible cessation of circulatory and respiratory functions, or (b) irreversible cessation of all functions of the entire brain, including the brain stem, is dead. A determination of death must be made in accordance with accepted medical standards.

The duration of time for observation has not been settled. The Harvard Ad Hoc Committee stated that "all of the above tests shall be repeated at least 24 hours later with no change." The President's Commission recommended an observation period of six hours if confirmatory tests are available and twelve hours if they are not. For anoxic brain damage, the Commission stated that twenty-four hours of observation is generally desirable for ascertainment of brain death, but that this period may be reduced if a test shows cessation of cerebral blood flow or if an electroencephalogram shows electrocerebral silence (i.e., a flat tracing) in an adult patient without drug intoxication, hypothermia, or shock.

At present, most statutes and judicial opinions accept the extension of the definition of death first introduced by the Harvard Ad Hoc Committee and recognize that death can be accurately demonstrated either on the traditional grounds of irreversible cessation of heart and lung functions or on the basis of irreversible loss of all functions of the entire brain. This recognition is codified in the Uniform Determination of Death "Standard," which does not specify diagnostic tests or medical procedures required to determine death but leaves the medical profession free to make use of new medical knowledge and diagnostic advances as they become available. The determination of death must thus be made in accordance with accepted medical standards.

In New York State, the governor in 1984 appointed a Task Force on Life and the Law which published its recommendations on the Determination of Death in July 1986. (Rabbi J. David Bleich, a member of the Task Force, issued the lone dissent from the group's decision.) The Task Force suggested that the New York State Department of Health promulgate a regulation which establishes that an individual is dead when the individual has suffered either (a) irreversible cessation of respiratory and circulatory function or (b) irreversible cessation of all functions of the entire brain, including the brain stem. On June 18, 1987, the State Hospital Review and Planning Council adopted a regulation recognizing the total and irreversible cessation of brain function as a basis for determining death in New York State. Shortly thereafter, the Department of Health amended its regulations to include this standard, so that either the brain death standard or the circulatory or respiratory standard may be relied on to determine that death has occurred.

The brain death standard applies to hospital and nursing home patients who have lost *all* brain function and whose breathing and circulation are artificially maintained. Under the standard, patients like Karen Ann Quinlan, who had brain stem capacity and the ability to regulate basic functions such as heartbeat and respiration, are considered alive.

It is of paramount importance not to confuse brain death with other forms of irreversible brain damage, particularly the permanent vegetative state, for a patient in such a state is alive according to all legal, moral, medical, and religious definitions. Such a patient is certainly not dead in the medical or legal sense, and his organs may not be removed for transplantation until death has been established by either classic irreversible cardiorespiratory criteria or by irreversible brain stem death criteria.

Does Judaism Recognize Brain Death?

There is at present an intense debate among rabbinic authorities as to whether or not Jewish law (halachah) recognizes brain death as a definition of death. It is our thesis that the answer is affirmative. The classic definition of death in Judaism as found in the Talmud and the codes of Jewish law is the absence of spontaneous respiration in a person who appears dead (i.e., shows no movements and is unresponsive to all stimuli). The absence of hypothermia or drug overdose must be ascertained because these conditions can result in depression of the respiratory center with absence of spontaneous respiration and even heartbeat. If resuscitation is deemed possible, no matter how remote the chance, it must be attempted.

Jewish writings provide considerable evidence for the thesis that the brain and the brain stem control all bodily functions, including respiration and cardiac activity. It, therefore, follows that if there is irreversible total cessation of all brain function including that of the brain stem, the person is dead, even though there may still be some transient spontaneous cardiac activity. Brain function is divided into higher cerebral activities and the vegetative functions of the vital centers of the brain stem. A criterion of death based on higher cerebral death alone is ethically and morally unacceptable. If a person is decapitated, his heart and lungs may still function for a brief period of time, but that person is obviously dead at the moment the brain and brain stem are severed from the remainder of the body. If one can medically establish that there is total cessation of all brain function including the brain stem, the patient is as if "physiologically decapitated."

There are a number of objective tests that can evaluate the viability of the brain stem. Brain stem death may be the preferable definition of death in Judaism since it is irreversible. Brain stem death confirms bodily death in a patient with absence of spontaneous respiration who may still have a heartbeat. Support will be provided for our position from ancient and recent Jewish sources.

Classic Definition of Death in Jewish Law

The definition of death in Jewish law is first mentioned in the Babylonian Talmud, which enumerates circumstances under which one may desecrate the Sabbath.

> . . . every danger to human life suspends the [laws of the] Sabbath. If debris [of a collapsing building] falls on someone and it is doubtful whether he is there or whether he is not there, or if it is doubtful whether he is an Israelite or a heathen, one must probe the heap of the debris for his sake [even on the Sabbath]. If one finds him alive, one should remove the debris, but if he is dead, one leaves him there [until after the Sabbath].[5]

The Talmud then comments as follows:

> How far does one search [to ascertain whether he is dead or alive]? Until [one reaches] his nose. Some say: Up to his heart. . . . life manifests itself primarily through the nose, as it is written: "In whose nostrils was the breath of the spirit of life."[6]

The renowned biblical and talmudic commentator *Rashi* explains that if no air emanates from his nostrils, he is certainly dead. *Rashi* further explains that some people suggest the heart be examined for signs of life, but the respiration test is considered of greatest import.

The rule is codified by Maimonides (*Rambam*) as follows:

> If, upon examination, no sign of breathing can be detected at the nose, the victim must be left where he is [until after the Sabbath] because he is already dead.[7]

The universally accepted code of Jewish law by Rav Joseph Karo, the *Shulchan Aruch*, states:

> Even if the victim was found so severely injured that he cannot live for more than a short while, one must probe [the debris] until one reaches his nose. If one cannot detect signs of respiration at the nose, then he is certainly dead whether the head was uncovered first or whether the feet were uncovered first.[8]

Neither *Rambam* nor Rav Karo requires examination of the heart. Cessation of respiration seems to be the determining physical sign for the ascertainment of death.

Another pertinent passage found in the *Shulchan Aruch* states:

> If a woman is sitting on the birthstool [i.e., about to give birth] and she dies, one brings a knife on the Sabbath, even through a public domain, and one incises her womb and removes the fetus, since one might find it alive.[9]

Rabbi Moses Isserles, known as *Ramo*, adds to this statement:

> However, today we do not conduct ourselves according to this [rule] even during the week [i.e., even *not* on the Sabbath], because we are not competent to recognize precisely the moment of maternal death.[10]

Several commentators explain that *Ramo* is concerned that perhaps the mother only fainted, and incising her abdomen might kill her. Maimonides, five centuries earlier, had already raised the problem of fainting complicating the recognition of death, when he wrote: "Whosoever closes the eyes of the dying while the soul is about to depart is shedding blood. One should wait awhile: perhaps he is only in a swoon."[11]

Both *Rambam* and *Ramo*, however, agree that the talmudic description of death, for all practical purposes, is the absence or cessation of respiration.

Recent Rabbinic Writings on the Definition of Death

The classic Jewish legal definition is that death is established when spontaneous respiration ceases. Rabbi Moses Schreiber (*Chatam Sofer*) asserts that if a person is motionless "like an inanimate stone" and has no palpable pulse either in the neck or at the wrist, and also has no spontaneous respiration, his soul has certainly departed, but one should wait a short while to fulfill the requirement of Maimonides, who was concerned that the patient might only be in a swoon.[12] Rabbi Sholom Mordechai Schwadron states that if any sign of life is observed in limbs other than the heart and lungs, the apparent absence of spontaneous respiration is not conclusive in establishing death.[13]

On the other hand, Rabbi Isaac Yehudah Unterman, addressing the Eleventh Congress on Jewish Law in Jerusalem in August 1968, stated that one is dead when one has stopped breathing. Thus, many talmudic and post-talmudic sages agree that the absence of spontaneous respiration is the only sign needed to ascertain death. But some would also require cessation of heart action. Thus, a patient who has stopped breathing, says Rav Unterman, and whose heart is not beating is considered dead in Jewish law.[14] (We should point out that in 1968 the Harvard criteria were new and unclear, and there was still great confusion about the definition of brain death itself.)

Rabbi Eliezer Yehudah Waldenberg also defines death as the cessation of both respiration and cardiac activity.[15] One must use all available medical means to ascertain with certainty that respiratory and cardiac functions have indeed ceased. A flat electroencephalogram in the face of a continued heartbeat is not an acceptable finding by itself to pronounce a patient dead. Even after death has been established one should wait awhile before moving the deceased.

Rabbi Immanuel Jakobovits states, in part, that "the classic definition of death as given in the Talmud and Codes is acceptable today and correct. However, this would be set aside in cases where competent medical opinion deems any prospects of resuscitation, however remote, at all feasible."[16]

Rabbi J. David Bleich traces the Jewish legal attitude concerning the definition of death from talmudic through recent rabbinic times.[17] In his opinion, brain death and irreversible coma are not acceptable definitions of death insofar as Jewish law is concerned, since the sole criterion of death accepted by Jewish law is total cessation of *both* cardiac and respiratory activity long enough to make resuscitation impossible. Rabbi Bleich also discusses the various time-of-death statutes already enacted into law in many states in this country and statutes being contemplated by other states,[18] and expresses the hope that provisions allowing for exemption from legislated definitions of death for reasons of conscience will be written into such statutes in order to preserve civil and religious liberties.

Total Brain Death in Judaism

The position that complete and permanent absence of any brain-related vital bodily function is recognized as death in Jewish law seems to be supported by Rabbi Moshe Feinstein, whose responsum on heart transplantation begins with a discussion of decapitation.[19] Rav Moshe Feinstein quotes Maimonides, who states that a person who is decapitated imparts ritual defilement to others because he is considered dead even though one or more limbs of the body may yet move spastically, temporarily.[20] The situation is comparable to the tail severed from a lizard, which may still quiver temporarily but is certainly not alive.[21] Rav Feinstein asserts that "someone whose head has been severed—even if the head and the body shake spastically—that person is legally dead." The requirement of Maimonides cited earlier in this essay, to wait awhile when death is thought to have occurred (i.e., when the patient has no spontaneous respiratory activity), according to Rav Feinstein, is to differentiate between true death and the situation "where the illness is so severe that the patient has no strength to breathe." Since only a few minutes of absent breathing is compatible with life, if the patient is observed for fifteen minutes with no spontaneous respirations, he is legally dead (unless a potentially reversible cause of respiratory absence is present, such as hypothermia or drug overdose).

In the same responsum Rav Feinstein prohibits heart transplantation if the donor's heart is removed before total brain death has occurred. The presence of any spontaneous respiratory activity, however, indicates that a person is still alive, and no matter what the clinical neurological picture, the patient may not be considered dead for any purpose, including organ transplantation.

The above responsum is dated 1968 (5728 in the Hebrew calendar). Another responsum of Rav Feinstein, dated two years later, amplifies the Jewish legal definition of death.[22] He reiterates the error of physicians who diagnose death when the patient has no cerebral function but is still breathing spontaneously. This responsum also prohibits heart transplantation as murder of the recipient because his life is thereby shortened, since (at that time) the success of cardiac transplantation in prolonging life had not been demonstrated.

On May 24, 1976, Rabbi Feinstein sent a letter to the Honorable Herbert J. Miller, who was chairman of the New York State Assembly's Committee on Health, relevant to Assembly Bill 4140/A concerning the determination of death. In his letter he said:

> The sole criterion of death is the total cessation of spontaneous respiration.
>
> In a patient presenting the clinical picture of death, i.e., no signs of life such as movements or response to stimuli, the total cessation of independent respiration is an absolute proof that death has occurred. This interruption of spontaneous breathing must be for a sufficient length of time for resuscitation to be impossible (approximately 15 min).
>
> If such a "clinically dead" patient is on a respirator, it is forbidden to interrupt the respirator. However, when the respirator requires servicing, the services may be withheld while the patient is carefully and continuously monitored to detect any signs of independent breathing no matter how feeble. If such breathing motions do not occur, it is a certainty that he is dead. If they do occur the respirator shall be immediately restarted.

A more recent responsum of Rabbi Feinstein, dated 1976, supports the acceptability of "physiologic decapitation" as an absolute definition of death.[23] Rabbi Feinstein again reiterates the classic definition of death as being the total irreversible cessation of respiration but then states that if by injecting a substance into the vein of a patient, physicians can ascertain that there is no circulation to the brain—meaning no connection between the brain and the rest of the body—that patient is legally dead in Judaism because he is equivalent to a decapitated person. Where the test is available, continues Rav Feinstein, it should be used.

We interpret Rabbi Feinstein's written responsa to indicate that Jewish law clearly recognizes that death occurs before all organs cease functioning. This is our interpretation, not necessarily accepted by others. Cellular death follows organismal death. Jewish law defines death as an organismal phenomenon involving dissociation of the correlative or coordinating activities of the body and not as individual organ death.

It is our opinion that the continued beating of the heart is not halachically critical. In the case in the Talmud where the patient is buried under debris, the interest focuses on any sign of residual life to warrant desecrating the Sabbath to dig him out. It has no relevance to a patient lying in an intensive care unit whose every function is monitored and whose status is open to full evaluation. In such a case, the issue is truly one of definition, not confirmation.

Based on the position of Rav Moshe Feinstein cited above, Rabbi M. Tendler, one of the authors of the present essay, introduced the concept of physiologic decapitation as an acceptable definition of death in Judaism even if cardiac function has not ceased.[24]

The thesis is

> that absent heartbeat or pulse was not considered a significant factor in ascertaining death in any early religious source. Furthermore, the scientific fact that cellular death does not occur at the same time as the death of the human being is well recognized in the earliest biblical sources. The twitching of a lizard's amputated tail or the death throes of a decapitated man were never considered residual life but simply manifestations of cellular life that continued after death of the entire organism had occurred. In the situation of decapitation, death can be defined or determined by the decapitated state itself as recognized in the Talmud and the Code of Laws. Complete destruction of the brain, which includes loss of all integrative, regulatory, and other functions of the brain, can be considered physiological decapitation and thus a determinant per se of death of the person.
>
> Loss of the ability to breathe spontaneously is a crucial criterion for determining whether complete destruction of the brain has occurred. Earliest biblical sources recognized the ability to breathe independently as a prime index of life . . . destruction of the entire brain or brain death, and only that, is consonant

> with biblical pronouncements on what constitutes an acceptable definition of death, i.e., a patient who has all the appearances of lifelessness and who is no longer breathing spontaneously. Patients with irreversible total destruction of the brain fulfill this definition even if heart action and circulation are artificially maintained.[25]

Thus, if it can be definitely demonstrated that all brain functions including brain stem function have ceased, the patient is legally dead in Jewish law because he is equated with a decapitated individual whose heart may still be beating. Brain stem function can be accurately evaluated by radionuclide cerebral angiography at the patient's bedside.[26] This test is a stress-free, simple, safe, highly specific, and highly reliable indicator of absence of blood flow to the entire brain, thus confirming total irreversible brain death. "The absence of cerebral blood flow is presently considered the most reliable ancillary test in diagnosing brain death."[27] There are also other tests used to confirm brain death.[28]

Extensive recent medical reviews confirm that cessation of brain flow as measured by radioisotope techniques is invariably accompanied by signs of brain cell lysis. This evidence of cellular decay, although confirmable only at post-mortem examination, is an absolute criterion of death despite the beating heart. The heart is not dependent for its stimulation on brain function. A heart completely removed from the body continues to beat as long as its nutrition is maintained. Rabbi Feinstein is of the opinion that the criterion of death in a patient who gives the clinical impression of death is cessation of spontaneous respiration. "Clinical impression of death" means "if he resembles a dead person, that is to say, he does not move any of his limbs."[29]

When a patient is on a respirator and gives all the evidence of having died, i.e., meets the Harvard criteria, he is not "brain dead"—a confusing term—but is dead as evidenced, first and foremost, by cessation of independent respiration. In addition, a careful check must be made that he meets the reservation that he appear clinically dead. This requirement is met in the fullest and most absolute measure by total unreceptivity, unresponsiveness, absence of all movements, absent cephalic reflexes, fixed dilated pupils, and persistence of all these findings for at least a twenty-four-hour period in the absence of intoxicants or hypothermia. These are the Harvard criteria.

Thus, the only valid definition of death is brain death. The classic "respiratory and circulatory death" is in reality brain death. Irreversible respiratory arrest is indicative of brain death. A brain dead person is like a physiologically decapitated individual. The requirement of Maimonides to "wait awhile" to confirm that the patient is dead is that amount of time it takes after the heart and lung stop until the brain dies, i.e., a few minutes.

Until the brain dies, one must attempt to restart the heart and respiration of a non-breathing patient. If the heart and lung functions are rapidly restored, the patient may suffer no neurological deficits. There are a number of objective tests now available that can evaluate the viability of the brain stem. A simple, non-stressful test is the radionuclide blood flow study described above. This test does not violate the prohibition against unnecessarily stressing the patient in any way and has been shown to be "nearly 100 percent" accurate. The question whether "nearly 100 percent" is accurate enough when we are dealing with the soul is an open question.

Another strong proof for our thesis that brain death is the Jewish legal definition of death is found in the *Shulchan Aruch.*[30] The author describes individuals "who are considered dead even though they are still alive" to include those whose necks have been broken and those whose bodies "are torn on the back like a fish." These people are considered dead in that they impart ritual defilement and render their wives widows even though they may still have spastic or convulsive movements and even have heartbeats. The reason is that the connection between the brain and the body has been severed by the severance of the spinal cord or by the severance of the blood supply to the brain. It thus seems clear that death of the brain is the legal definition of death in halachah.

The fifteenth-century commentator, Rabbi Yehudah Aryeh of Modinah, who was rabbi in Venice and known by the pen name of *Omar Haboneh*, states:

> All [rabbis] agree that the fundamental source of life is in the brain. Therefore, if one examines the nose first, which is an organ of servitude of the brain, and there is no [spontaneous] respiration, none of them [i.e., the rabbis] doubt that life has departed from the brain.[31]

Further support for our position can be deduced from the talmudic precedent about the woman who dies in labor but her unborn fetus is still alive,[32] which is codified in Jewish law.[33] As cited earlier, since the woman may only be in coma and not dead, we do not perform an immediate cesarean section to try to save the unborn child, "because we are not competent to recognize precisely the moment of maternal death,"[34] and thus the comatose but alive mother might be killed thereby. However, where death is certain, as for example if the mother was accidentally decapitated, an immediate cesarean section is required,[35] even if individual limbs or organs of the mother may still exhibit muscular spasms.

Rabbi Nachum Rabinowitz[36] quotes *Rambam*, who explains that the organism is no longer considered to be alive "when the power of locomotion that is spread throughout the limbs does not originate in one center, but is independently spread throughout the body."[37] Obviously, continues Rabbi Rabinowitz, "the definition of death depends upon the availability of more sophisticated techniques of resuscitation." Again citing *Rambam*,[38] he concludes that the applicability of such methods and the consequent decision as to the onset of death are determined according to the judgment of the physicians.

We believe that the sophisticated medical techniques described above, including radionuclide angiography, can definitively establish the absence of any possibility of resuscitation, equating such a physiologically decapitated patient with the hypothetical case of the decapitated woman whose death is confirmed by her decapitated status even though she may still exhibit muscular spasms.

In a later publication,[39] Rabbi Rabinowitz quotes again from Maimonides as follows: "If a person's neck is broken . . . or if his back is torn like a fish or if he is decapitated or if he is hemisected at the abdomen, he imparts ritual defilement [because he is dead] even if one of his organs is still shaking."[40] From here it can be concluded, he continues, that if the controlling center which unifies all the activities of the organism is nullified (i.e., dead), the movement of a single organ is meaningless and does not indicate that the person (i.e., the organism) is alive.

We are aware of opposition to our point of view. Rabbi Aaron Soloveichik considers our position to be a serious misinterpretation of Jewish law.[41] We maintain our position, however, that total and irreversible cessation of all brain function, as determined by the Harvard criteria, is equivalent to total destruction of the brain and, hence, tantamount to functional or physiological decapitation, which in Judaism is equated with death.

Conclusion

Judaism is guided by the concepts of the supreme sanctity of human life, and of the dignity of man created in the image of God.

The preservation of human life in Judaism is a Divine commandment. Jewish law requires the physician to do everything in his power to prolong life, but prohibits the use of measures that prolong the act of dying. To save a life, all Jewish religious laws are automatically suspended, the only exceptions being idolatry, murder, and forbidden sexual relations such as incest. In Jewish law and moral teaching, the value of human life is infinite and beyond measure, so that any part of life—even if only an hour or a second—is of precisely the same worth as seventy years of it.

When life ends is an issue which is presently being actively discussed. All rabbis agree that the classic definition of death in Judaism is the absence of spontaneous respiration in a patient with no bodily motion. A brief waiting period of a few minutes to a half hour after breathing has ceased is also required. If hypothermia or drug overdose, which can result in depression of the respiratory center with absence of spontaneous respiration and even heartbeat, are present, this classic definition of death is insufficient. Hence, wherever resuscitation is deemed possible, no matter how remote the chance, it must be attempted unless there are ethical and moral considerations for cessation of all therapy. Brain death is a criterion for confirming death in a patient who already has irreversible absence of spontaneous respiration. The situation of decapitation, where immediate death is assumed even if the heart may still be briefly beating, is certainly equated with organismal death. Whether or not total, irreversible brain stem death, as evidenced by sophisticated medical testing, is the Jewish legal equivalent of decapitation is presently a matter of debate in rabbinic circles. We are of the opinion that it is.

Notes

1. "A Definition of Irreversible Coma," Report of the Ad Hoc Committee of the Harvard Medical School to Examine the Definition of Brain Death, *Journal of the American Medical Association* 205 (1968): 337–350.
2. *Journal of the American Medical Association* 252 (1984): 677–679.
3. R. J. Joynt, "A New Look at Death," ibid., pp. 680–682.
4. President's Commission for the Study of Ethical Problems in Medicine and Biomedical and Behavioral Research, *Defining Death: Medical, Legal and Ethical Issues in the Determination of Death* (Washington, D.C.: Government Printing Office, 1981).
5. Yoma 8:6–7.
6. Ibid 85a, citing Genesis 7:22.
7. *Mishneh Torah, Hilchot Shabbat* 2:19.
8. *Shulchan Aruch, Orach Chayim* 329:4.
9. Ibid 330:5.
10. *Ramo*, gloss on *Shulchan Aruch, Orach Chayim* 330:5.
11. *Mishneh Torah, Hilchot Avel* 4:5.
12. Responsa *Chatam Sofer, Yoreh Deah*, no. 338.
13. S. M. Schwadron, Responsa *Maharsham*, vol. 4. sec. 6, no. 124.
14. I. Y. Unterman, "Points of Halachah in Heart Transplantation," *Noam* 13 (1970): 19.
15. Responsa *Tzitz Eliezer*, vol. 9, no. 46 and vol. 10, no. 25:4.
16. I. Jakobovits, Personal communication, August 1, 1968.
17. J. D. Bleich, *Contemporary Halakhic Problems* (New York: Ktav, 1977), pp. 372–393.
18. J. D. Bleich, "Time of Death Legislation," *Tradition* 16 (1977): 130–139.
19. Responsa *Iggrot Moshe, Yoreh Deah*, pt. 2, no. 174.
20. *Mishneh Torah, Hilchot Tumat Met* 1:15.
21. Oholot 1:6.
22. Responsa *Iggrot Moshe, Yoreh Deah*, pt. 2, no. 146.
23. Ibid, pt. 3, no. 132.
24. M. D. Tendler, "Cessation of Brain Function: Ethical Implications in Terminal Care and Organ Transplants," *Annals of the New York Academy of Science* 315 (1978): 394–497.
25. E. J. Veith, J. M. Fein, M. D. Tendler, et al., "Brain Death: I. A Status Report of Medical and Ethical Considerations," *Journal of the American Medical Association* 238 (1977): 1651–1655.
26. J. Kotem, P. Braunstein, A. George, et al., "Brain Death. I. Angiographic Correlation with the Radioisotopic Bolus Technique for Evaluation of Critical Deficit of Cerebral Blood Flow," *Annals of Neurology* 2 (1977): 195–205. S. H. Tsai, R. E. Cranford, G. Rockswold, S. Koehler, "Cerebral Radionuclide Angiography," *Journal of the American Medical Association* 248 (1982): 591–592. J. A. Schwartz, J. Baxter, and D. Brill, "Diagnosis of

Brain Death in Children by Radionuclide Cerebral Imaging," *Pediatrics* 73 (1982): 14–18. J. M. Goodman, L. L. Heck, and B. D. Moore, "Confirmation of Brain Death with Portable Isotope Angiography: A Review of 204 Consecutive Cases," *Neurosurgery* 16 (1985): 492–497.

27. L. A. Alvarez, R. B. Lipton, A. Hirschfeld, et al., "Brain Death Determination by Angiography in the Setting of a Skull Defect," *Archives of Neurology* 45 (1988): 225–227.

28. A. H. Ropper, S. K. Kennedy, and L. Russell, "Apnea Testing in the Diagnosis of Brain Death: Clinical and Physiological Observations." *Journal of Neurosurgery* 55 (1981): 942–946. T. V. Rowland, J. H. Donnelly, and A. H. Jackson, "Apnea Documentation for Determination of Brain Death in Children," *Pediatrics* 74 (1984): 505–508. W. Trojaborg, and E. O. Jorgensen, "Evoked Cortical Potentials in Patients with Isolectric EEG," *Electroencephalography and Clinical Neurophysiology* 35 (1973): 301–309. A. H. Ropper, S. M. Kehne, and L. Wechsler, "Transcranial Doppler in Brain Death," *Neurology* 37 (1987): 1733–1735. J. Darby, H. A. Yonas, and R. P. Brenner, "Brainstem Death with Persistent EEG Activity: Evaluation by Xenon-Enhanced Tomography," *Critical Care Medicine* 15 (1987): 519–521. W. S. Tan, A. C. Wilbur, J. J. Jafar, et al., "Brain Death: Use of Dynamic CT and Intravenous Digital Subtraction Angiography," *American Journal of Neuroradiology* 8 (1987): 123–125.

29. *Rashi*'s commentary on Yoma 85a, s.v. *ad hechan.*

30. *Shulchan Aruch, Yoreh Deah* 370.

31. Commentary *Omar Haboneh* in Jacob Habib's *Eyn Yaakov,* Yoma 85a.

32. Arachin 7:1.

33. *Shulchan Aruch, Orach Chayim* 330:5.

34. *Ramo, Shulchan Aruch, Orach Chayim* 330:5.

35. Responsa *Shevut Yaakov,* vol. 1, no. 13.

36. N. Rabinowitz, "What Is the *Halakhah* for Organ Transplants," *Tradition* 9 (1968): 20–27.

37. *Mishnah Commentary,* Oholot 1:6.

38. *Mishneh Torah, Hilchot Rotze'ach* 2:8.

39. N. E. Rabinowitz, "Sign of Life: A Single Organism," *Techumin* 8 (1987 solidus 5747): 442–443.

40. *Mishneh Torah, Hilchot Tumat Met* 1:15.

41. A. Soloveichik, "Jewish Law and Time of Death," *Journal of the American Medical Association* 240 (1978): 109. See M. D. Tendler, "Jewish Law and Time of Death," ibid., which offers a response to the objections of Rav Soloveichik.

21

Organ Transplantation

Although corneal and kidney transplants have been successfully accomplished for several decades, the first heart transplant was performed in 1967 in Capetown.[1] By 1984, over seven hundred human heart transplants had been performed in the United States, with 80 percent of the recipients living at least one year after the surgery.[2] Single lung transplants began in 1963, and liver transplants much earlier. Combined heart-lung transplants have also been successfully done.[3] The first combined heart-liver transplant was performed in 1984 in Pittsburgh. Bone marrow transplants are standard therapy for some medical conditions and experimental for others.[4] An artificial heart was implanted into Barney Clark in 1982 in Salt Lake City, Utah.

These operations have raised many moral, ethical, theological, social, legal, political, and philosophical problems. This chapter addresses some of these problems, with emphasis on the Jewish view of organ transplants as derived from classical, biblical, talmudic, and more recent rabbinic sources.

Let us first briefly examine some of the questions other than those of Jewish law which are involved in organ transplants. From the theological standpoint, one can ask whether or not one is interfering with the will of God by "artificially" prolonging a person's life by giving him a new organ. If God had ordained a life span of forty years for a man with terminal renal failure, who are we to change destiny and give this man a new kidney and additional years of life? Does not only God give and take life? Are we interfering with a patient's desire (or right?) to die in dignity without heroic efforts to extend the duration of his life? Is an organ transplant heroic?

Moral and ethical problems in the use of artificial and human organs are discussed elsewhere in general and also from the Jewish standpoint.[5] Is the publicity surrounding liver and lung and combined organ transplants inappropriate and excessive in the light of what is dictated by medical ethical standards? Is artificial heart implantation ethical? Is it premature? Is such experimentation justifiable? Has it reached therapeutic application?

Social problems regarding organ transplantation are also self-evident. Who shall pay for the enormous expense of the procedure and the pre- and post-operative care? The patient? Society? Are only the rich entitled to benefit from this medical advance? Who should select the recipients? Since there are many more potential recipients than donors available, who should decide "who should live and who shall die"? The physician? A group of physicians? Society? The enormous costs of organ transplants are being actively discussed in Britain and the United States as both governments wrestle with the problem of limited resources for transplantation.[6] Other political and societal issues related to organ transplants, such as the problems in the identification of potential organ donors,[7] the procurement of organs,[8] the regulation of institutions where transplants may be performed, the establishment of a national or international registry of donors and recipients, the support of medical research related to organ transplants, and the prohibition of buying and selling organs for transplantation are beyond the scope of this chapter.

Philosophical questions can also be asked. If one considers the heart to be the seat of the soul, is one removing the patient's soul when one removes the diseased heart before implanting the new heart? René Descartes once said, "Je pense, donc je suis" (I think, therefore I am). This famous expression now takes on new meaning for the cardiac transplant recipient. Who is he? Whose soul does he have, his own or that of the donor?

Legal problems in organ transplantation are also of concern. The legal issues of organ procurement and organ donation are dealt with differently in different states and in different countries. A Uniform Anatomical Gift Act reforming the legal structure relating to donation of organs and tissues for transplantation was formulated and endorsed by the American Bar Association shortly after the first heart transplant was performed in 1967.[9] Another early legal problem concerned a donor heart derived from a sailor who had been fatally beaten. Once the heart had been removed from his body, it was no longer possible to corroborate forensic evidence obtained during his autopsy if challenged by the defense counsel, and as a result the coroner feared that the district attorney would not be able to properly prosecute the case.

Medical and ethical guidelines for organ transplantation have been established by many hospitals, states, medical societies, and national organizations, such as the American Medical Association and the National Academy of Sciences.[10] The United States Congress is presently addressing the political, social, and financial issues, and theologians are discussing the religious and spiritual aspects of organ transplantation. The remainder of this chapter discusses Jewish legal and moral considerations in organ transplants.

Jewish Legal Issues in Organ Transplantation

The halachic (Jewish legal) issues concerning the transplantation of a human organ can be conveniently subdivided into those which pertain to the recipient, those that involve the physician or medical team, and those that primarily affect the donor.

In regard to the recipient, what is the status of the transplanted organ? Does it become a permanent part of the recipient, or must it be returned to the donor upon the eventual death of the recipient? The donor may long since have been buried, and his identity and/or burial site may not be known. Furthermore, where a diseased organ such as a heart, liver, or lung is removed before implantation of a new organ, what does one do with the "old" or diseased organ? Can one just discard it? Must it be buried? Can one incinerate it or place it in formalin for preservation? Must it be treated with respect as part of a human being who was created in the image of God? This problem is not unique to organ transplantation but applies to any organ or part removed from a living human being. Thus, the rabbis discuss whether or not a gallbladder, stomach, uterus, appendix, foot, leg, or other diseased organ or limb removed at surgery or traumatically avulsed requires burial. An entire chapter in Rabbi Joseph Karo's *Code of Jewish Law* is devoted to this question.[11]

Another halachic question is whether or not the recipient is allowed to subject himself to the danger of the operative procedure. In Judaism, it is not proper to intentionally wound oneself for no valid medical reason.[12] Does this rule apply to surgery in general and to an organ transplant in particular? Furthermore, does the recipient transgress the biblical commandments *Take heed to thyself and keep thy soul diligently* and *Take ye therefore good heed unto yourselves,*[13] which both the Talmud and Maimonides interpret to mean the removal (i.e., avoidance) of all danger to one's physical well-being?[14]

Another Jewish legal issue concerns a recipient who is a priest (*kohen*). The latter are commanded not to become ritually defiled by corpse contact.[15] Does this question of ritual defilement[16] apply to an organ from a dead donor which is now to be implanted into a priest?

Finally, what are the halachic priorities, if any, for choosing a recipient in view of the shortage of organ donors? In Jewish law, a woman takes precedence over a man when both desperately need food[17] because it is less dignified and more shameful for a woman to go begging than a man.[18] A woman is ransomed before a man if both are captives,[19] but a man takes precedence over a woman if both are drowning because he is subject to more commandments.[20] Additional priorities are enumerated in the Talmud.[21] Do any of these priorities apply to organ transplant recipients? Should medical criteria be used exclusively in the selection of recipients?

In regard to the physician or medical team performing the organ transplant there are two major halachic issues. Does an organ transplant constitute standard medical therapy or human experimentation but with therapeutic intent? Corneal and kidney transplants can be considered standard medical therapy, whereas heart, lung, and liver transplants should still be viewed as experimental. Physicians are obliged to heal the sick using all standard therapies available.[22] Human experimentation is permissible in Jewish law under specific restricted conditions.[23] The more difficult issue is the establishment of criteria for determining whether a prospective donor is dead, for if the donor is still alive when the physician performing an organ transplantation removed one or more of his organs, the physician would be guilty of murder. The definition of death in Jewish law is discussed in detail in chapter 18 of this book. In relation to heart transplantation, the question of "killing" the recipient is also raised by several rabbis. When the recipient's diseased heart is removed prior to the implantation of a new heart, the patient is without a heart. Is the patient halachically dead? If so, are the physicians guilty of murder? Obviously not!

There are numerous Jewish legal questions concerning the organ donor. I have already mentioned the most important of all; namely, the establishment of the death of the donor before any organ is removed for transplantation. In addition, there is a biblical prohibition of desecrating or mutilating the dead.[24] How can one remove an organ for transplantation without desecrating the body? There is also a biblical prohibition of deriving benefit from the dead.[25] The recipient of an organ from a deceased person certainly derives benefit from the dead! Furthermore, there is a biblical prohibition of delaying the burial of the dead[26] and the positive commandment of burying the dead.[27] Another halachic consideration is that of ritual defilement for priests in the same room with either the donor or only the donor's organ or organs.[28] Do such organs transmit ritual defilement? Finally, in Jewish law is permission necessary either from the deceased prior to his demise or from the next of kin? Is one "robbing the dead" if one fails to obtain consent? Does the deceased have total rights over his body, or does it belong to God, who gave it to him on loan for the duration of his life?

Corneal Transplants

The rabbinic literature on eye (i.e., corneal) transplantation is extensive and includes numerous responsa written and published over the past several decades. The basic halachic principles governing corneal transplants apply to all organ transplants. Kidney and heart transplants involve several additional unique questions which are discussed separately below.

One of the classic responsa on eye transplants is that of Rabbi Issar Yehuda Unterman, who states that the prohibitions of deriving benefit from the dead, desecrating the dead, and delaying the burial of the dead are all set aside because of the consideration of saving a life (*piku'ach nefesh*).[29] These prohibitions would remain if there were no threat to life. For example, there is no *piku'ach nefesh* involved in a nasal bone transplant. The question then arises: Is an eye transplant in the category of *piku'ach nefesh?* In answering this question, Rabbi Unterman cites the Talmud: "If one's eye gets out of order, it is permissible to paint it on the Sabbath because the eyesight is connected with the perception of the heart."[30] Thus, eye illness does seem to constitute *piku'ach nefesh*, since one may desecrate the Sabbath to save an eye. Rabbi Unterman argues, however, that this case deals with preventing blindness, whereas in eye transplantation one attempts to restore vision, a totally different matter.

On the other hand, Unterman agrees that total blindness is considered a life-threatening situation, since the person so afflicted may fall down a flight of stairs or into a ditch and be killed. Thus, since blindness constitutes a true *piku'ach nefesh*, the problems of desecrating and benefiting from and delaying the burial of the dead are put aside.

What of a person blind in one eye? The concept of *piku'ach nefesh* does not apply, and thus on what grounds would corneal transplants be permitted? To answer this question, Rabbi Unterman provides us with an enlightening and original pronouncement. Once the eye is implanted into the recipient, it is not considered dead but a living organ. Thus, the prohibitions of deriving benefit from the dead and delaying the burial of the dead are not applicable, since no dead organ is involved. Furthermore, the problem of ritual defilement (*tum'ah*) is nonexistent, since *tum'ah* relates only to a dead organ or a dead body. Confirmation of this point is found in the Talmud, where it states: "The men of Alexandria asked Rabbi Joshua . . . was the [dead] son of the Shunammite woman [revived by Elijah the Prophet] unclean? He replied: A corpse is unclean, but a living person is not."[31] Thus, when the boy came back to life, the problem of *tum'ah* was eliminated.

One problem remains, however, in Rabbi Unterman's dissertation, and that is the prohibition of desecrating the dead to obtain the eye for a person with unilateral blindness. One still has to make an incision into the donor, and one does not have the concept of *piku'ach nefesh* to set aside the question of desecration. Unterman answers that since the eyes of a deceased person are closed for burial, removing one or both beforehand would not constitute a desecration. Only an incision into the body with an externally visible scar represents a true desecration, and this would be permitted for a real *piku'ach nefesh* such as blindness in both eyes.

Rabbi Jekuthiel Judah Greenwald states that the prohibition of deriving benefit from the dead applies only to flesh (*basar*) or organs but not to skin (*or*).[32] The cornea of the eye, according to Greenwald, is considered skin and not flesh, based on a passage in the Talmud and the commentary of *Tosafot* (s.v. *shema ya'aseh shetikhin*) thereon.[33] Rabbi Unterman and many others, however, reject this difference between skin and flesh.

Another point by Rabbi Greenwald is that the engrafted or transplanted cornea becomes an integral part of the recipient. An analogous situation is described in the Talmud, where it states: "If he grafted a young shoot on an old stem, the young shoot is annulled by the old stem and the law of *orlah* does not apply to it."[34] Similarly, when a cornea is transplanted, it does not retain its original status but becomes annulled on the recipient.

Rabbi Yitzchok Glickman adds that one must obtain permission from the deceased donor or the next of kin prior to performing a corneal transplant for two reasons.[35] Firstly, permission is necessary lest the physicians and perhaps the recipient be considered guilty of "stealing" the organ from the deceased, violating the biblical admonition *thou shalt not steal.*[36] The second reason for obtaining permission relates to the Judaic principle that when a deceased person is buried, he receives atonement for all sins committed during life. The shame of being buried in the ground and having earth thrown on one's coffin is sufficient to provide the deceased with atonement, provided the body is buried intact. An organ donor is hindered from achieving atonement *(kapparah)* for his sins through his death, since one or more of his organs remain alive. If he gave permission, however, he has voiced his acquiescence to delaying his atonement until his organ is later buried following the eventual death of the recipient. In the meantime, he has performed a charitable act in restoring the vision or saving the life of the recipient. Most other rabbinic responsa agree with the need for permission from the donor or his family. There are dissenting opinions, however.[37]

Rabbi Meyer Steinberg raises the problem of eye banks.[38] Is the permissibility for corneal transplantation only applicable to an immediate transfer of the cornea from donor to recipient, or may one place an eye in an eye bank for later use? Since the permissibility of organ transplantation rests primarily on the overriding consideration of *piku'ach nefesh,* it would seem that the recipient would have to be at hand (*lefaneinu,* lit. "before us"). Rabbi Steinberg answers that since the number of blind people is so large, it is as if there were always a recipient at hand. Rabbi Immanuel Jakobovits also permits "organs or blood to be donated for deposit in banks provided there is a reasonable certainty that they will be eventually used in life-saving operations [including the restoration or preservation of eyesight]."[39] Rabbi Unterman had already stated at the end of his remarks on eye transplants that blood donations to blood banks are permissible for the same reason.[40]

Rabbi Moshe Feinstein, in a lengthy responsum devoted exclusively to the prohibition of deriving benefit from the dead, raises the problem of a gentile donor for an eye transplant.[41] Rabbi Feinstein's conclusion is that it is permissible. Rabbi Eliezer Waldenberg only allows non-Jewish donors.[42]

Rabbi Jacob Weinberg takes exception to nearly all of Rabbi Unterman's arguments cited above but concludes that since rabbinic authorities who preceded him permitted eye transplants, he would be in accord with this ruling, providing, however, that the recipient is blind in both eyes.[43] Most other rabbinic responsa agree with Rabbi Unterman's ruling.[44] One outstanding exception is Rabbi Shmuel Huebner, who admits that most rabbis permit eye transplants but does not himself consider a blind or deaf person to be in the category of a dangerously ill person.[45] Therefore, the concept of *piku'ach nefesh* cannot be invoked, and thus, states Rabbi Huebner, the prohibitions of desecrating, deriving benefit from, and delaying the burial of the dead cannot be set aside.

A final question relating to eye transplants is whether or not the remainder of the donor's eye after the cornea has been transplanted into the recipient can be used for medical research. Most rabbis answer negatively because of the prohibition of deriving benefit from the dead, cited above. This prohibition does not apply, however, to organs removed at surgery from a live person. Such organs may be used for medical research provided one buries or burns or otherwise destroys the remnants thereof at the conclusion of the experiment, without allowing the organ to be treated with disrespect.[46]

Kidney Transplants

All the halachic principles discussed above relating to eye transplants are equally applicable to kidney transplants. In fact, many of the responsa deal with both eye and kidney transplants. A kidney transplant is only undertaken when both kidneys of the recipient are so diseased that life cannot continue without the removal of the body's waste products that accumulate in the blood. Elimination of such wastes can be accomplished by the intermittent use of an artificial kidney or its equivalent, or by the definitive implantation of a healthy human kidney to replace the patient's own nonfunctioning kidneys. All rabbinic authorities would agree that such a case constitutes *piku'ach nefesh*, or danger to life, and, therefore, the prohibitions revolving around the dead donor would all be set aside for the overriding consideration of saving a life.

In addition to cadaver kidneys, physicians also employ kidneys from live donors for transplantation. Here, new halachic questions arise. Is the donor allowed to subject himself to the danger, however small, of the operative procedure to remove one of his kidneys in order to save the life of another? Does the donor transgress the commandment of *Take heed to thyself and keep thy soul diligently* or *Take ye therefore good heed unto yourself?*[47]. We have already mentioned that the Talmud and Maimonides interpret these verses to refer to the removal of all danger to one's physical well-being.[48] We have also already stated that it is not permitted to intentionally wound oneself.[49] We also know that one may not set aside one person's life for that of another.[50] The question then remains: May one endanger one's own life by donating a kidney in order to save another's life?

The answer is found in commentaries on Maimonides and on Karo and later codes in nearly identical language:[51]

> The Jerusalem Talmud concludes that one is obligated to place oneself even into a possibly dangerous situation [to save another's life]. It seems logical that the reason is that the one's [death without intervention, i.e., the kidney recipient] is a certainty, whereas [the donor's] is only a possibility.

Some authorities claim that since many of the codes, including those of Maimonides, Isaac Alfasi, Jacob ben Asher, known as *Tur*, and Asher ben Yechiel, known as *Rosh*, omit this passage from the Jerusalem Talmud, the final ruling is not in accord therewith. However, based upon this passage, Rabbi Jakobovits states that a donor may endanger his own life or health to supply a "spare" organ to a recipient whose life would thereby be saved if the probability of saving the recipient's life is substantially greater than the risk to the donor's life or health.[52] This principle is applicable to all organ transplantation where live donors are used as a source of the organ in question. Rabbi Ovadiah Yosef also rules that it is at least permissible and perhaps even obligatory for a person to subject himself to a small risk to save the life of another.[53] Hence, one is certainly allowed to give a kidney to save the life of another person. Rabbi Jacob Joseph Weiss also agrees that one may accept a small risk (i.e., anesthesia, surgery, remaining with only one kidney) to save the life of another.[54]

Rabbi Eliezer Yehuda Waldenberg discusses at length the question of whether a healthy person must or may donate one of his organs for transplantation into a desperately ill individual in order to save the latter from certain death.[55] Waldenberg concludes that kidney transplants from a live donor are only permissible if a group of trustworthy physicians testify that there is no danger to life to the donor and if the donor is not coerced into consenting to the procedure. Rabbi Moshe Meiselman discusses the risk-benefit ratio involved in kidney transplantation from live donors, and concludes that one performs a meritorious act *(chesed)* by giving a kidney to save a life.[56] Meiselman also states that one is obligated to give blood and/or skin to save another because the risk to the donor is extremely small. Rabbi Moshe Hershler allows a person to accept a small risk to give a kidney to save someone's life but not to just alleviate the latter's suffering.[57] Hershler also discusses the use of a kidney from a mentally incompetent donor, stating that if the latter were of normal intelligence and knew that his kidney could save the life of his brother, he would certainly consent. May we, therefore, presume that consent is given, or must the guardian not allow any surgical procedure on a mentally incompetent person that is not for his direct benefit? No answer is given.

The majority of rabbinic responsa thus allow but do not require a live donor to subject himself to a small risk to save the life of a patient dying of kidney failure. A minority of rabbis even require such a donation to save a life. Rabbi David ben Zimra considers one who believes this requirement to be a religious obligation as a "pious fool."[58] Nevertheless, a person who donates an organ to save the life of another has clearly performed an act of loving-kindness of the highest order.[59]

Heart Transplants

In the transplantation of a human heart from a dead donor, the prohibitions dealing with desecrating the dead, delaying the burial of the dead, and ritual defilement are all set aside by the overriding consideration of *piku'ach nefesh*, saving a life. The major Jewish legal problem remaining is the establishment of the death of the donor. Prior to death, the donor is in the category of a *goses* (hopelessly ill patient), and one is prohibited from touching him or moving him or doing anything that might hasten his death.[60]

There are several types of death: intellectual death, when a person's intellect ceases to function; social death, when a person can no longer function in society; spiritual death, when the soul leaves the body; and physiological or medical death. We are concerned with the halachic, or Jewish legal, definition of death, which is discussed elsewhere in this book, based upon talmudic and rabbinic sources (see chap. 18). Cessation of respiration and absence of a heartbeat for a short time period represents the classical halachic interpretation of death. Today, an additional required criterion is the impossibility of resuscitation.

On the assumption that the donor is absolutely and positively dead, many rabbinic authorities permit heart transplants. Rabbi Jakobovits states:

> An organ may never be removed for transplantation from a donor until death has been definitely established. The prohibition of *nivul ha-met* [desecration of the dead] would then be suspended by the overriding consideration of *Piku'ach Nefesh*. Hence, in principle, I can see no objection in Jewish law to the heart operations recently carried out, provided the donors were definitely deceased at the time the organ was removed from them.[61]

Rabbi Isaac Arieli is quoted as having said that heart transplants are permissible if the donor is definitely dead, but only with the family's consent.[62] A similar view was expressed by Rabbi David Lifshitz.[63]

In August 1968, then Israeli Chief Rabbi Issar Yehuda Unterman delivered a lengthy discourse on heart transplants to the Congress of Oral Law meeting in Jerusalem. His remarks have since been published.[64] Unterman begins by stating that consent from the family of the donor must be obtained. Otherwise, the doctors and the recipient would transgress the prohibition of *Thou shalt not steal*. Unterman then reviews the halachic definition of death and states that under ordinary circumstances, death occurs when spontaneous respiration ceases. However, sudden unexplained death in young, otherwise healthy individuals must be followed by resuscitative measures. A *goses* need not be resuscitated when spontaneous respiration ceases. Unterman then briefly mentions the problem of organ banks and asserts that freezing organs for later use is allowed provided there is a good chance they will be used to save a life. Then the situation would be comparable to having the recipient at hand (*lefaneinu*).

A novel pronouncement by Rabbi Unterman is that heart transplants in general may not be halachically sanctioned until such time that the chances for survival from the procedure are greater than those for failure. That is, we invoke the requirement that the probability of success of the surgery shall be greater than the risk of the recipient. This ruling seems to be contrary to the pronouncements of earlier rabbis who allow a sick person to submit to dangerous surgery or dangerous medication if there is a small chance for cure, even if the risk of the operation or the treatment is much greater than the chance for cure.[65]

Unterman explains that the recipient of a new heart is in a different situation from all other desperately ill (but not necessarily dying) people. After his diseased heart is removed and before the new heart is implanted, the recipient has lost his *chezkat chayyim* ("hold on life," or the presumption of being alive). Once he loses his *chezkat chayyim*, the heart transplant recipient is no longer permitted to risk his life if the chances for success are not greater than the chances of failure. A person dying of cancer, on the other hand, never loses his *chezkat chayyim* and, therefore, may subject himself to any risk, however great, if there is a small chance for cure. The definition of *chezkat chayyim* is exemplified in the talmudic passage which states that if a messenger brings a bill of divorce from a distant place and the husband was an old man or sick at the time the messenger left, he should still deliver it to the wife on the presumption that the husband is still alive.[66] Unless we have positive information to the contrary, a person retains his *chezkat chayyim* until he is pronounced dead.

That the heart is the seat of life and that its removal causes one to lose one's *chezkat chayyim* is exemplified by the well-known case of a chicken that was slaughtered in accordance with Jewish law and was found to have no heart. Two rabbis gave diametrically opposing rulings regarding this chicken. Rabbi Tzvi ben Jacob Ashkenazi decreed that the chicken was kosher because without a heart there is no life, and since the chicken walked and ate in a normal manner, the heart must have been present.[67] After the chicken was opened, reasoned Rabbi Ashkenazi, a cat must have snatched the heart away and eaten it. Ashkenazi also cites the book of Jewish mysticism known as *Zohar* in which it is written that without a heart life cannot exist for even a moment. Furthermore, says Ashkenazi, Rabbi Joseph Karo, in his *Kesef Mishneh* commentary on Maimonides' *Mishneh Torah*, points out that Maimonides omits absence of the heart from his list of animals with defects which cannot be slaughtered for food (*terefot*) because such an animal would not be viable. Finally, rules Ashkenazi, even if witnesses were to come forward and say that they saw the chicken at all times and nothing had been removed from it, they are not believed, since that is impossible and against nature. The opposing viewpoint is that of Rabbi Jonathan Eyebeschuetz, who ruled that the chicken was not kosher and the witnesses were believed.[68] He also claims that physicians in Prague assured him that the heart might have been located outside its usual site, and without a normal heart in the normal location the chicken was nonkosher.

In either event, we see from both rabbis involved in this case that the heart is essential to life, and life is impossible without it. Therefore, concludes Rabbi Unterman, who cited this unusual controversy, in the case of a human heart transplant recipient, removing the patient's old heart removes from him his *chezkat chayyim*, or presumption of being alive, and thus the removal of the recipient's heart can be sanctioned only if the risk of death resulting from the surgery is estimated to be smaller than the prospect of lasting success. On the other hand, one must desecrate the Sabbath to rescue someone from under a collapsed building,[69] even if the person may be already dead, because he retains his *chezkat chayyim* until proven otherwise. Similarly, a patient dying of an incurable illness may subject himself to a dangerous medication or operation on the small chance that cure might be achieved, because this patient never lost his *chezkat chayyim*.

This original concept of Rabbi Unterman regarding the loss of the *chezkat chayyim* by the heart transplant recipient after his diseased heart is removed raises numerous questions. What is the status of this "lifeless" patient until the new heart is implanted? Is he legally dead? Is his wife considered a widow? Can she remarry? Are his children considered orphans, and how do the inheritance laws apply here, if at all? After he receives his new heart, he is certainly alive again. Does he have to remarry his wife? All these questions have already been answered negatively by Rabbi Azriel Rosenfeld.[70] Rosenfeld discusses the case of a person who has just died of an incurable disease and whose body is stored at a very low temperature for eventual thawing out and revival when the cure for the disease is found. If the answer to all the above questions is no, as Rosenfeld proves for a refrigerated person who "is certainly dead—by any ordinary definition—once he has been frozen," then certainly a heart transplant patient who has only lost his *chezkat chayyim* temporarily should be considered not to have lost his status as husband and father. He might be considered lifeless during this interim period between heart exchanges but certainly not legally dead.

Rabbi Chaim David Regensberg claims that if the heart transplant recipient were legally dead when the diseased heart is removed before the new heart is implanted, all open heart surgery would be prohibited.[71] In the latter, the patient's heart is not physically removed but temporarily disconnected from his circulatory system while the patient is attached to a heart-lung machine known as cardiopulmonary bypass. The patient is medically alive throughout, continues Regensberg. Otherwise, in implanting the new heart, physicians would be "resurrecting the dead," an act of which only Almighty God is capable. Therefore, concludes Regensberg, if the heart donor is totally dead, "one might allow heart transplants if one is dealing with trustworthy doctors." The transplanted heart also becomes an integral part of the recipient and is buried with him when he eventually dies.

The trustworthiness of the doctors involved in cardiac transplantation is a major issue discussed by several rabbis who object to this procedure because they believe that the donor's heart is removed before he is halachically dead. Rabbi Yaakov Yitzchok Weiss, answering an extensive inquiry from Britain's Chief Rabbi Jakobovits following the first heart transplant in South Africa, strongly condemns this procedure as an act of murder.[72] Weiss's responsum is entitled "whether it is permissible to transplant the heart of a sick person about to die into another ill person as treatment [for the latter]." Jakobovits had written to Weiss that a transplant operation may require artificial extension of the donor's "life" by the use of a respirator until the recipient can be prepared to receive the new heart. As a result, the following halachic question arises: Is it lawful to artificially prolong the "life" of the donor solely to preserve his heart long enough to effect the transplant, and having done so, is it lawful to then shut off the respirator, thus, in effect, manipulating the life and death of the donor at will? This question, which Rabbi Jakobovits believes is highly relevant to the whole problem,[73] was answered negatively by Rabbi Weiss.

Another early responsum dealing with transplantation is that of Rabbi Chaim Dov Gulewski.[74] Gulewski discusses the question of whether a person can renounce his desire to live in order to give his heart to another and, if this is permissible, whether the potential recipient is allowed to accept this heart and whether the surgeon is guilty of murder if he performs the transplantation. Rabbi Gulewski further offers legal definitions for a person who is considered a *terefah* (suffering from a serious organic disease and who cannot live more than twelve months) and a dying individual (*goses*). The law differs depending on whether this person is dying by Divine decree (*goses bi-yedei shamayim*), such as from incurable cancer or old age, or by human intervention (*goses bi-yedei adam*), such as a car accident or homicide.

Rabbi Aryeh Leib Grossnass writes that a person is alive in Jewish law if his breathing is maintained either spontaneously or artificially, even if all cerebral function has ceased.[75] Such an individual is classified as a *terefah* upon whom one may not operate save to heal him but not to use his heart, even with his permission, to save another. Once a person reaches the status of a *nevelah* (corpse), as defined in the Talmud,[76] one may remove his heart and transplant it into another. Grossnass also discusses the status of the recipient after his diseased heart is removed and before his "new heart" is implanted. Although halachically dead, if the operation is successful, it becomes clear that the patient was never really dead at all. A long discussion follows in Grossnass's responsum dealing with the question as to whether one is required or allowed to donate an organ, such as a kidney, to save another if there is a risk involved to the donor. The answer is as described above; namely, one is permitted but not obligated to do so.

Rabbi Moshe Feinstein, in a brief statement, added his voice to those condemning heart transplants in that he considers this procedure to involve double murder: murder of the recipient, whose diseased heart is removed and cannot legally be alive without a heart, and murder of the donor, whose heart is removed for transplantation before he is halachically dead.[77] However, careful reading of Feinstein's lengthy responsum on this subject discloses the following clarification of his position.[78] If the donor is absolutely and positively dead by all medical and Jewish legal criteria, no murder of the donor would be involved, and the removal of his heart or other organ to save another human life would be permitted. He reiterates this view at the end of his responsum defining death.[79] Concerning the recipient, when cardiac transplantation becomes an accepted therapeutic procedure with reasonably good chances for success, murder of the recipient would no longer be a consideration. Additional animal experimentation, continues Feinstein, is essential to overcome major obstacles, such as organ rejection, tissue compatibility typing, and immunosuppressive therapy, before heart transplantation in man can be condoned. In the present state of medical knowledge, however, where chances for success are minuscule and the recipient's life is probably shortened rather than lengthened by this procedure, heart transplantation must still be considered murder of the recipient. This opinion of Feinstein was written shortly after the first heart transplant was performed. Today, most of these obstacles have been overcome, and therefore Rabbi Feinstein would probably sanction cardiac transplantation provided the donor is definitely deceased at the time his heart is removed.

Rabbi Eliezer Yehuda Waldenberg also originally prohibited heart transplants because "the donor is not dead and the recipient has little chance for survival from the transplant surgery and would live longer with his own heart."[80] However, continues Waldenberg, if the chances for success are fifty-fifty, the procedure can be sanctioned provided the donor is dead. Other rabbinic responsa on heart transplantation all express the concern about the possible removal of the donor's heart before the establishment of his death.[81] Rabbi Shlomo Goren seems to summarize rabbinic opinion when he states that if the donor is dead and the recipient is dangerously ill and cannot live except for a very short time, "it would be hard to prohibit heart transplants provided there is a reasonable chance of success with the surgery."[82] Goren also discusses the spiritual and physical functions of the heart, the biologic and organismal role of the heart, the heart as the seat of human temperaments, and the definition of death in Jewish law.

Artificial Heart Implantation

The implantation of an artificial heart into Dr. Barney Clark raised many ethical and religious issues in regard to life and death and the "artificial" prolongation of life. A basic tenet of Judaism is the supreme value of human life. This principle is based in part on the belief that man was created in the image of God. Jewish law requires the physician to do everything in his power to prolong life, but prohibits the use of measures that prolong the act of dying. To save a life all Jewish religious laws are automatically suspended, the only exceptions being idolatry, incest, and murder.

As discussed above, Judaism considers organ transplantation to be a praiseworthy activity in that it provides prolongation of life for most patients undergoing this procedure. Hence, corneal, renal, and cardiac transplantation are sanctioned by most rabbis and even mandated by some, but with permission of the deceased or next of kin. For kidney transplants, live donors may be used. When cadaver organs are to be used, the organ may not be removed for transplantation until the donor has been pronounced dead.

The use of a totally artificial heart for implantation into a patient dying of heart disease avoids many of the ethical and religious issues involving the donor. Thus, the problems of deriving benefit from the dead, desecrating the dead, delaying the burial of the dead, and/or establishing the time of death of the donor do not exist with the use of an artificial heart. A recent review on organ transplants and Jewish law discusses the use of an artificial heart transplant.[83] Since in Judaism the concern for the patient's physical and mental welfare remains supreme to the end, and everything must be done to preserve both, the implantation of an artificial heart is consonant with the basic axioms of Judaism relating to the sanctity and infinite value of human life. This sanctioning of such a complex and controversial experimental treatment in Judaism is also predicated on the fulfillment of Jewish principles governing human experimentation, such as the lack of availability of a standard therapy, the expertise of the experimental team, the testing of such experimental procedures in animal models, and the reasonable expectation of therapeutic efficacy weighed against the potential risks.

Other Organ Transplants

The principles cited above regarding kidney and heart transplants are equally applicable to liver, lung, pancreas, colon, or other organ transplants. Where a patient's life is at stake, such organ transplantation is permissible, but consent from the donor or the next of kin should be obtained prior to the transplantation. The biblical injunctions regarding the donor proscribing desecration of the dead, deriving benefit from the dead, and delaying the burial of the dead are suspended for the greater consideration of saving the recipient's life. The donor must be dead according to Jewish legal criteria before any organ may be removed for transplantation. Live donors are acceptable if the risk to them is small compared to the certainty of death for the recipient without transplantation.[84]

Sex organ transplants are discussed elsewhere in this book in the chapter on *in vitro* fertilization and surrogate motherhood. Brain transplants, although not medically possible, are discussed from the Jewish legal viewpoint by Rabbi Azriel Rosenfeld.[85]

Epilogue

As a motto to our survey of Jewish legal attitudes toward heart and other organ transplantation, we might cite the prophecy of Ezekiel, as promised by Almighty God: *And a new heart will I give you, and a new spirit will I put within you, and I will take away the stone heart out of your flesh, and I will give you a heart of flesh.*[86] Although this scriptural reference is obviously meant in a figurative and spiritual sense, it seems to vividly depict the present epoch of cardiac and other organ transplantation.

Notes

1. C. N. Barnard, "A Human Cardiac Transplant: An Interim Report of a Successful Operation Performed at Groote Schuur Hospital, Capetown," *South African Medical Journal* 41 (1967): 1271–1274.

2. P. Gunby, "Organ Transplant Improvements, Demands Draw Increasing Attention," *Journal of the American Medical Association* 251 (1984): 1521–1527.

3. B. A. Reitz, "Heart Lung Transplantation: A Review," *Heart Transplantation* 1 (1982): 291–298.

4. R. Storb, "Human Bone Marrow Transplantation," *Transplantation Proceedings* 15 (1983): 1379–1384.

5. J. Hamburger and J. Grosnier, "Moral and Ethical Problems in Transplantation" in *Human Transplantation*, ed. F. T. Rapaport and J. Dausset (New York): Grune & Stratton, 1968), pp. 37–44; J. R. Elkinton, "Moral Problems in the Use of Borrowed Organs, Artificial and Transplanted," *Annals of Internal Medicine* 60 (1964): 309–313; M. D. Tendler, "Medical Ethics and Torah Morality," *Tradition* 9 (1968): 5–13.

6. R. Deitch, "The Government's Present Line on Cardiac Transplantation," *Lancet* 1 (1984): 407–408; J. K. Inglehart, "The Politics of Transplantation," *New England Journal of Medicine* 310 (1984): 864–868; J. K. Inglehart, "Transplantation: The Problem of Limited Resources," ibid. 309 (1983): 123–128.

7. T. D. Overcast, R. W. Evans, L. E. Brewen, M. M. Hoe and C. L. Livak, "Problems in the Identification of Potential Organ Donors," *Journal of the Americal Medical Association* 251 (1984): 1559–1562.

8. C. E. Koop, "Promoting Organs for Transplantation," ibid. (1984): 1591–1592.

9. A. M. Sadler, B. L. Sadler and E. B. Stason, "The Uniform Anatomical Gift Act: A Model for Reform," *Journal of the American Medical Association* 206 (1968): 2501–2506.

10. Judicial Council, "Ethical Guidelines for Organ Transplantation," *Journal of the American Medical Association* 205 (1968): 341–342; "Cardiac Transplantation in Man. Statement Prepared by the Board on Medicine of the National Academy of Sciences," ibid. 204 (1968): 805–806.

11. J. Karo, *Shulchan Aruch, Yoreh Deah*, no. 374.

12. Maimonides, *Mishneh Torah, Hilchot Shevu'ot* 5:17 and *Hilchot Chovel Umazik* 5:1, based on Baba Kamma 91b.

13. Deuteronomy 4:9 and 4:15.

14. Berachot 32b; Maimonides, *Mishneh Torah, Hilchot Rotze'ach* 11:4.

15. Leviticus 21:1–3.

16. Karo, *Shulchan Aruch, Yoreh Deah* nos. 369:1 and 374:2.

17. Ibid., no. 251:8, based on Horayot 3:7.

18. S. HaKohen, Commentary known as *Shach (Sifsei Kohen)* on Karo's *Shulchan Aruch, Yoreh Deah*, no. 251:8.

19. Karo, *Shulchan Aruch, Yoreh Deah* 252:8.
20. D. HaLevi, Commentary known as *Taz (Turei Zahav)* on Karo's *Shulchan Aruch, Yoreh Deah*, no. 252:8.
21. Horayot 13a, 13b, and 14a.
22. See above, chap. 1.
23. F. Rosner and J. D. Bleich, Editors. *Jewish Bioethics* (New York: Hebrew Publishing Co., 1979), pp. 377–397.
24. Arachin 7a, Chullin 11b, and Baba Batra 154b.
25. Karo, *Shulchan Aruch, Yoreh Deah*, no. 349:1–2, and Maimonides, *Mishneh Torah, Hilchot Avel* 14:21, based on Avodah Zarah 29b.
26. Karo, *Shulchan Aruch, Yoreh Deah*, no. 357:1, based on *his body shall not remain all night upon the tree* (Deut. 21:23). See also Sanhedrin 46b.
27. Maimonides, *Mishneh Torah, Hilchot Avel* 12:1, based on *but thou shalt surely bury him on that day* (Deut. 21:23). See also Sanhedrin 46b and Jerusalem Talmud, Nazir 7:1.
28. Maimonides, *Mishneh Torah, Hilchot Tumat Met* 3:1, and Karo, *Shulchan Aruch, Yoreh Deah*, no. 369:1.
29. Unterman, *Shevet mi-Yehudah* (Jerusalem, 1955), pp. 313–322.
30. Avodah Zarah 28b.
31. Niddah 70b.
32. J. J. Greenwald, *Kol Bo al Avelut* (New York, 1947), vol. 1, pp. 45–48.
33. Niddah 55a.
34. Sotah 43b. *Orlah* is the prohibition of using fruit during the first three years after planting a tree. See Leviticus 19:23.
35. Y. Glickman, "Regarding the Law of Grafting Organs from the Dead onto the Living," *Noam* 4 (1961): 206–217.
36. Exodus 20:13, Leviticus 19:11 and 13, Deuteronomy 5:17.
37. B. Z. Pirer, "Grafting an Organ from the Dead to a Living Person," *Noam* 4 (1961): 200–205.
38. M. Steinberg, "Grafting an Eye from the Dead to a Blind Person," *Noam* 3 (1960): 87–96.
39. I. Jakobovits, personal communication, Aug. 1, 1968.
40. Unterman, loc. cit.
41. M. Feinstein, Responsa *Iggrot Moshe, Yoreh Deah*, no. 229.
42. E. Y. Waldenberg, Responsa *Tzitz Eliezer*, vol. 14, no. 84.
43. J. Weinberg, Responsa *Seridei Esh, Yoreh Deah*, pt. 2, no. 120.
44. O. Yosef, Responsa *Yabiya Omer*, pt. 3, no. 22; Z. P. Frank, Responsa *Har Tzvi, Yoreh Deah*, no. 277 and others.
45. S. Huebner, in *Hadarom* 13 (1961): 54–64.
46. Feinstein, Responsa *Iggrot Moshe, Yoreh Deah*, no. 232; Waldenberg, Responsa *Tzitz Eliezer*, vol. 10, no. 25:8.
47. Deuteronomy 4:9 and 4:15.
48. Berachot 32b; Maimonides, *Mishneh Torah, Hilchot Rozte'ach* 11:4.
49. See ibid., *Hilchot Shevu'ot* 5:17 and *Hilchot Chovel Umazik* 5:1.

50. Oholot 7:6; Maimonides, *Mishneh Torah, Hilchot Rotze'ach* 1:9; Karo, *Shulchan Aruch, Yoreh Deah*, no. 425:2.

51. Joseph Karo's commentary known as *Kesef Mishneh* on Maimonides' *Mishneh Torah, Hilchot Rotze'ach* 1:14; Joshua Falk's commentary known as *Me'irat Einayim* on Karo's *Shulchan Aruch, Choshen Mishpat*, no. 426:1; Y. M. Epstein, *Aruch Hashulchan, Choshen Mishpat*, no. 426:4.

52. Jakobovits, personal communication, Aug. 1, 1968.

53. O. Yosef, "The Law of Kidney Transplantation," *Halachah Urefuah* 3 (1983): 61–63.

54. J. J. Weiss, Responsa *Minchat Yitzchok*, pt. 6, no. 103:2.

55. Waldenberg, Responsa *Tzitz Eliezer*, vol. 10, no. 25:7.

56. M. Meiselman, "Halachic Questions in Kidney Transplants," *Halachah Urefuah* 2 (1981): 114–121.

57. M. Hershler, "Kidney Transplants from Mentally Incompetent Donors," *Halachah Urefuah* 2 (1981): 122–127.

58. David ben Zimra, Responsa *Radvaz*, pt. 3, no. 625.

59. J. D. Bleich, "Organ Transplants," in *Judaism and Healing* (New York: Ktav, 1981), pp. 129–133.

60. Semachot 1:2 and Shabbat 151b; Maimonides, *Mishneh Torah, Hilchot Avel* 4:5; Karo, *Shulchan Aruch, Yoreh Deah*, no. 339.

61. Jakobovits, personal communication, Jan. 8, 1968.

62. I. Arieli, cited by Abraham ben Melech in *Panim el Panim*, no. 458, March 1, 1968, p. 16.

63. D. Lifshitz, personal communication, Feb. 16, 1968.

64. I. Y. Unterman, "Points of Halachah in Heart Transplantation," *Noam* 13 (1970): 1–9.

65. J. Reischer, Responsa *Shevut Yaakov*, pt. 3, no. 75, and Ch. O. Grodzinski, Responsa *Achiezer, Yoreh Deah*, no. 16.

66. Gittin 28a.

67. Tzvi ben Yaakov Ashkenazi, Responsa *Chachim Tzvi*, no. 74.

68. Y. Eyebeschuetz, Responsa *Kereti Upeleti*, no. 40:4.

69. Yoma 85a; Maimonides, *Mishneh Torah, Hilchot Shabbat* 2:19; Karo, *Shulchan Aruch, Orach Chayim*, no. 329.4

70. A. Rosenfeld, "Refrigeration, Resuscitation and Resurrection," *Tradition* 9 (1967): 82–94.

71. Ch. D. Regensberg, "Heart Transplantation in Halachah," *Halachah Urefuah* 2 (1981): 3–8.

72. Y. Y. Weiss, Responsa *Minchat Yitzchok*, pt. 5, nos. 7 and 8; also in *Hamsar* 20, no. 178 (1968): 3–9.

73. I. Jakobovits, personal communication, Dec. 18, 1968.

74. Ch. D. Gulewski, in *Hamaor* 20, no. 179 (1968): 3–16.

75. A. L. Grossnass, Responsa *Lev Aryeh*, pt. 2.

76. Chullin 88a.

77. M. Feinstein, "Final Legal Judgment in Heart Transplantation," *Ha-Pardes* 43 (1969): 4.

78. M. Feinstein, Responsa *Iggrot Moshe, Yoreh Deah*, pt. 2, no. 174.

79. Ibid., no. 146.

80. Waldenberg, Responsa *Tzitz Eliezer*, vol. 10, no. 25:5.

81. Y. Gershuni, "Heart Transplantation in the Light of Jewish Law," *Or Hamizrach* 18 (1969): 133–137; J. Levi, "Transplanting Organs from the Dead,' *Noam* 12 (1969): 289–313; M. M. Kasher, "The Problem of Heart Transplantation," *Noam* 13 (1970): 10–20; see also Kasher's *Divrei Menachem*, no. 27; N. Z. Friedman, "Heart Transplants in Halachah," *Assia* 1 (1976): 200–201; Ch. D. Levy, "Organ Transplants from the Living and from the Deceased in Halachah," *Assia* 4 (1983): 251–259.

82. S. Goren, "Heart Transplants as Viewed in Halachah," *Machanayim*, no. 132, (1970), pp. 7–17.

83. I. Ralbag, "Organ Transplants," in *Harefuah Le'or Hahalachah* (Jerusalem, 1983), vol. 2, pt. 2, pp. 87–124.

84. D. M. Feldman and F. Rosner. *Compendium on Medical Ethics* (New York: Federation of Jewish Philanthropies, 1984), p. 71.

85. A. Rosenfeld, "The Heart, the Head and the Halachah," *New York State Journal of Medicine* 70 (1970): 2615–2619.

86. Ezekiel 11:19 and 36:26.

22

Skin Grafting and Skin Banks

In the first volume of a compendium of halachah entitled *Techumin* published in Israel in 1980, Rabbi Shaul Yisraeli wrote an article entitled "The Treatment of Burns by Skin Transplantation from the Dead."[1] The question posed to Rabbi Yisraeli was whether or not it is permissible to prepare human skin from deceased people and store it in skin banks so that it is available for grafting or transplantation to burn victims in times of emergency, such as wars or fires. Most if not all rabbis accept the ruling of Rabbi Ezekiel Landau that biblical and rabbinic laws are suspended when danger to life is involved only if the patient whose life is to be saved is present and identified (*lefaneinu*).[2] The question regarding skin banks is that the potential recipients are not presently identified. Yet in times of emergency, the skin must be immediately available. Furthermore, skin grafting after burns is also performed for cosmetic and functional reasons without there being any danger to the life of the patient if the graft is not performed. Is such skin grafting permissible?

Rabbi Yisraeli divides his presentation into three parts: (1) the prohibition of deriving benefit from the skin of the deceased and whether or not permission for its use by the deceased prior to his death is acceptable in Jewish law; (2) whether or not it is permissible to derive benefit from the skin in a manner different than its normal usage; (3) whether or not there is an obligation to bury skin and not to leave it unburied overnight.

The talmudic commentary *Tosafot* is of the opinion that the skin of the dead is not biblically forbidden.[3] The prohibition of deriving any benefit from the dead is derived from the heifer whose neck was to be broken (*eglah arufah*).[4] The prohibition of deriving benefit from the *eglah arufah* is in turn derived from the word "forgive" (*kaper*) which is mentioned in regard to the *eglah arufah*,[5] just as it is mentioned in regard to sacrifices (*kapara*) from which no secular benefit may be derived. However, the skin of sacrifices is permitted. Therefore, the skin of the *eglah arufah* is permitted, and so, too, the skin of the dead is permitted. This is the reasoning of *Tosafot*.

The talmudic commentary of Rabbi Samuel Adels, known as *Maharsha*, cites Maimonides,[6] from whom Adels deduces that hides of sacrifices offered to idols are only prohibited if the hides are offered to the idols.[7] Since the prohibition of deriving benefit from a sacrifice is derived from the *eglah arufah*, and the skin of the *eglah arufah* is not prohibited, as stated by *Tosafot* above, it follows that Maimonides is also of the opinion that the skin of the dead is not biblically forbidden.

On the other hand, the opinion of Rabbenu Tam is that the skin of the dead is biblically proscribed because skin is no worse than shrouds specifically prepared for the dead, deriving benefit from which is prohibited.[8] This opinion is shared by *Ritva*[9] and by Rabbi Solomon ben Adret, known as *Rashba*,[10] who cite the Talmud to prove that even hair from a dead human being is prohibited because death renders the body prohibited for any use.[11] *Rashi* states that natural human hair never "lived" and is, therefore, not affected by death.[12] For this reason, Maimonides rules that one is permitted to derive benefit from the hair of a deceased person.[13] This reasoning, however, is only applicable to hair, since skin "lived" and should therefore be prohibited according to all opinions, thus posing a difficulty according to the view of *Tosafot* cited above that the skin of the dead is permissible.

Rabbi Yisraeli attempts to reconcile the apparently opposing views of *Tosafot* and Rabbenu Tam. He explains that the prohibition of deriving benefit from shrouds prepared for the dead relates to the honor of the dead, and the deceased, while still alive, can instruct that his honor be waived just as he can instruct that no eulogy be recited in his honor. Rabbenu Tam proscribes the use of skin from a deceased only if he did not specifically instruct that one forgo honors on his behalf after he dies. But if he did so instruct, there is no prohibition at all against using the skin for burn victims, not because of the need to save their lives but because there is no biblical prohibition to forbid it.

Another consideration relating to the use of human skin from the deceased for transplantation to burn victims is whether or not the prohibition of deriving benefit from the dead also extends and includes the prohibition of deriving benefit from something in a manner other than its normal usage. The Talmud states that with regard to all the prohibited articles in the Torah, we do not flagellate on their account except when they are eaten or used in the normal manner of their consumption or usage, respectively.[14] For example, if one eats raw forbidden meat, he is exempt. *Tosafot* points out that in regard to sacred things, including sacrifices, the only prohibition is on their use in the normal manner of their usage.[15] Since the prohibition of deriving benefit from the dead is derived from the heifer whose neck was broken (*eglah arufah*), and the latter prohibition is derived from an analogy to sacrifices,[16] it follows that the *eglah arufah* is only forbidden in the normal manner of its usage. This is the reason why Maimonides excludes *eglah arufah* from the list of things which are prohibited even in a manner different than their normal usage.[17] It also seems logical, therefore, that deriving benefit from the dead is only prohibited in the normal manner of its usage.

Rabbi Yisraeli cites other opinions which posit that the prohibitions of deriving benefit from sacrifices, from *eglah arufah*, and from the dead extend even to the manner other than their normal usage. He attempts to reconcile these opinions with those expressed by the Talmud, by *Tosafot*, and by Maimonides as cited above. Rabbi Yisraeli concludes that without the deceased's permission while he was still alive, there is a biblical prohibition against using his skin after his death, according to Rabbenu Tam. This prohibition extends even to its use in a manner different than its normal usage, such as storage in a skin bank for transplantation to a living human being. Such transplantation would only be permissible if the patient requiring the skin transplant is clearly identified and the procedure is needed because of danger to his life. For actual or potential danger to life, all biblical and rabbinic commandments except the cardinal three (idolatry, murder, and forbidden sexual relations) are suspended.

However, if the deceased gave permission for the use of his skin after his death, even Rabbenu Tam would agree that it is only prohibited if used in the manner of its normal usage. But if it is used in a manner diferent than its normal usage, there is no biblical prohibition involved. There is a difference of opinion discussed by *Tosafot* as to whether or not there remains a rabbinic prohibition.[18] In either event, it is permissible, according to all opinions, to transplant skin from a deceased person to a living patient even in whom there is no danger to life, since the skin is considered as being used in a manner different than its normal usage. An analogy is cited in the Talmud about Rabina, who was rubbing his daughter with undeveloped olvies of *orlah*[19] as a remedy.[20] He was permitted to do so either because his daughter was in danger from an inflammatory fever or because he was using the olives in a manner different than their normal usage.

The final part of Rabbi Yisraeli's article deals with the questions of whether or not there is an obligation to bury human skin, and whether or not there is a prohibition of "leaving part of the dead unburied until the morrow."[21] After citing and discussing various sources and opinions, Rabbi Yisraeli concludes that there is no commandment to bury skin and there is no prohibition of leaving it unburied. The issue of the shame or disgrace of not burying the skin of the dead is not applicable if one uses it for the healing of a patient or for sparing the patient pain and suffering and perhaps even saving his life. Furthermore, as mentioned before, if the deceased gave permission during his lifetime for his skin to be used for healing purposes, there is no prohibition involved in its use. Even according to the opinions of those who state that it is forbidden to derive benefit from human skin, it is permitted to do so for transplant purposes because that is considered to be using it in a manner different than its normal usage and hence permitted even for a patient in whom there is no immediate danger to life. Finally, Rabbi Yisraeli states that it is even permissible to prepare human skin for this purpose (i.e., skin banks) even before the patient who needs a skin graft has been identified, since, prior to its use, there is no question of deriving benefit therefrom. When a burn victim or other needy patient presents, then it is certainly permissible because of the medical indication.

The Israeli incursion into Lebanon in 1982 resulted in numerous casualties, including seriously burned soldiers who required skin grafting. The Rabbinic Council of the Israeli Chief Rabbinate was instructed by the country's two Chief Rabbis to research the topic of skin transplantation from deceased human beings to patients burned in war or in other situations. The deliberations and conclusions of the Council were summarized by Rabbi Shalom Meshash, Chief Rabbi of Jerusalem, in 1986 in an article entitled "Skin Banks for the Treatment of Burns."[22] Rabbi Meshash takes issue with many of the points made by Rabbi Yisraeli in his 1980 article. Rabbi Meshash's article was followed by another article written by Rabbi

Yisraeli entitled "Skin Transplants from the Dead" in which the latter refutes all the criticisms of Rabbi Meshash.[23] There then followed an exchange of letters between these two prominent rabbis.[24]

Rabbi Meshash begins his article by citing the mandate to the Rabbinic Council by the Chief Rabbis to investigate the topic of transplanting skin from the deceased onto patients who were seriously burned or wounded in war. There is no question but that it is permissible to do so if a burn victim is at hand and his life is actually or potentially at stake, because danger to life sets aside all biblical prohibitions. The question is whether or not it is permissible to prepare skin in advance from the deceased and to store it in a skin bank for later use when the need arises. Rabbi Meshash points out that each member of the Council had before him the 1980 article and opinion of Rabbi Yisraeli, which, in answer to the question, ruled in the affirmative.

Rabbi Yisraeli had cited the opinion of Maimonides that the hair and skin of the deceased are not biblically prohibited. However, asserts Rabbi Meshash, Rabbi Yisraeli omitted several citations from Maimonides in which the latter clearly prohibits the use of skin but not hair from the deceased.[25] Rabbi Meshash also states that there is even a difference of opinion, based on a talmudic argument between Rav and Rabbi Nachman bar Yitzchak,[26] about the permissibility of using the hair of the deceased. However, the majority of rabbinic decisors, including *Tur, Ritva, Ramban,* and *Rashba,* rule with Rabbenu Tam that the skin of the dead is certainly prohibited.[27] Rabbi Meshash takes issue with Rabbi Yisraeli's interpretation of Rabbenu Tam that the use of skin from the deceased is permissible if the latter specifically instructed that one may forgo honors on his behalf after he dies. Rabbi Meshash is of the opinion that a person does not have the right to forgo such honors. Rabbi Ben Zion Uziel states that a person does not have title over his body.[28] Rabbi Moshe Schick[29] and his teacher Rabbi Moshe Schreiber[30] assert that a person cannot disgrace his own body nor forgo honors due him because his body and soul are not his but belong to Almighty God. Similarly, Maimonides states that the life of a murdered person is not the property of the avenger of blood but the property of God.[31]

On the other hand, Rabbi Yisraeli is of the opinion that all these rulings apply to a person's body but not his skin, since skin is compared to shrouds, and therefore a person is allowed to renounce honors due him in regard to the use of his skin just as he can forgo honors due him in regard to the shrouds in which he is to be buried.

Rabbi Meshash also puts forth the thesis that the prohibition of deriving benefit from the dead is not derived from the laws pertaining to sacrifices but only from the heifer whose neck was to be broken (*eglah arufah*). Furthermore, the prohibition of the *eglah arufah* after its neck was broken is not derived from the laws of sacrifices. He also cites many sources that the prohibition of deriving benefit from the dead applies even if the skin is used in a manner different than its normal usage. Rabbi Meshash rejects Rabbi Yisraeli's conclusion that the skin of a deceased human being does not require burial. On the contrary, states Rabbi Meshash, he who fails to bury the skin of the deceased violates the biblical prohibition of leaving a body unburied overnight.[32] He cites evidence in favor of this viewpoint from the talmudic commentary of *Tosafot* and from the novellae of Rabbi Nissim Girondi, known as *Ran*.[33]

Following his lengthy remarks, Rabbi Meshash concludes it is not possible to permit the removal of human skin from the deceased to store it for later use except for a situation of danger to life where the patient whose life is to be saved is before us here and now (*lefaneinu*) according to the classic ruling of Rabbi Ezekiel Landau.[34] However, in our times, when there are wars in the world, and specifically in the land of Israel, which is surrounded by enemies, there is hardly a day that passes without someone getting killed, and certainly during actual times of war. Therefore, says Rabbi Meshash, "I searched and found" two possible grounds to perhaps permit skin transplantation using human skin from the deceased. The first reason is to counter the requirement of Rabbi Ezekiel Landau and Rabbi Moshe Schreiber that the dangerously ill patient must be at hand (*lefaneinu*) in order to allow the suspension of all biblical prohibitions in order to save his life.[35] If the patient is not at hand, even rabbinic prohibitions may not be waived. However, in our era, says Rabbi Meshash, quoting Rabbi Isaiah Karelitz, known as *Chazon Ish*,[36] there is no difference whether the patient is at hand or not, if the disease or dangerous medical condition is very common, for then it is as if the patient is at hand, and one may suspend biblical prohibitions such as desecrating the dead and take skin from the deceased and store it in a skin bank, because it will likely be used very soon for a burn victim. The situation is analogous to enemies besieging an Israeli city near the border as described in the Talmud.[37]

Rabbi Shlomo Goren[38] also quotes *Chazon Ish* and provides support for his viewpoint from the talmudic commentary of *Tosafot*,[39] which implies that if a dangerous medical condition is common, it is permissible to perform certain otherwise prohibited acts on the Sabbath even if the patient is not yet at hand. Therefore, continues Rabbi Meshash, since we are concerned about all the dangerously ill people throughout the land, common illnesses involving danger to life (such as cancer) are considered to constitute an equivalency to the dangerously ill patient being at hand (*lefaneinu*). Furthermore, since we in Israel are constantly in a state of war, one can certainly allow the storing of human skin in skin banks for later use. Rabbi Meshash also cites Rabbi Ben Zion Uziel,[40] who comments on Rabbi Landau's requirement of *lefaneinu* as follows:

> . . . to be sure, there are always many extant patients who are ill with that disease. And if we do not know of any at this precise moment, tomorrow or even today we will be apprised thereof. The situation is not at all comparable to the preparation of medications (*sechikat samamanim*) which can be compounded at any time or prepared from yesterday [i.e., before the Sabbath]. But in this situation [of autopsy to determine the cause of death], if the autopsy is not performed on this body because of the prohibition [of desecrating the dead], it will never be performed . . . and [the lack of vital information to be gained from the autopsy] may be responsible for the death of many people.

Rabbi Moshe Feinstein[41] rules that autopsy is permitted where a patient died after he received experimental chemotherapy for cancer, or received an experimental antibiotic or an unproven vaccine for the treatment or prevention of an infectious disease, or underwent an operation in which a new or experimental surgical technique was employed. In each of these situations, it is imperative to ascertain whether or not the drug or vaccine or surgical technique contributed to the patient's death and/or benefited the patient. Such information is critical for the physician in his decision regarding the possible use of the same drug, vaccine, or operation for other extant patients. Thus, Rabbi Feinstein also defines *lefaneinu* to include patients with common life-threatening diseases even though a specific patient whose life is to be saved has not yet been identified.

The same reasoning is used to allow the donation of corneas to eye banks and blood to blood banks without an immediate transfer from donor to recipient. Since the permissibility of organ transplantation rests primarily on the overriding consideration of *piku'ach nefesh* (danger to life), it would seem that the recipient would have to be at hand (*lefaneinu*). Rabbi Meyer Steinberg, however, rules that since the number of blind people is large, it is as if there is always a recipient at hand.[42] Rabbi Isser Yehuda Unterman, in his remarks on eye transplants,[44] also permits blood donations to blood banks for the same reason.

The reason offered by Rabbi Meshash to allow the use of human skin for transplantation from the deceased onto burn victims is the thesis cited by Rabbi Unterman whereby an organ that functions when transplanted from a cadaver into a live recipient does not involve the prohibition of deriving benefit from the dead.[45] If part of the deceased is "alive" and functioning in another person, the prohibition does not exist, because the Torah prohibited deriving benefit from the "dead" but not from the "alive." So, too, the dry bones (i.e., human skeletons) which Ezekiel brought back to life were fully alive, did not convey ritual uncleanliness, and it was permitted to derive benefit from them.

Rabbi Meshash's final statement in his essay "Skin Banks for the Treatment of Burns"[46] is the following:

> For the above-cited reasons, many rabbinic decisors permit the taking of skin from the deceased for the use of extant patients who may present at a later time, and one can rely on this ruling in actual practice. However, the Rabbinic Council of the Chief Rabbinate was correct in limiting this procedure to the banking of only fifty skins and no more. Had it not been so, we would again be faced with the concerns of the *Noda Biyehudah* [Rabbi Ezekiel Landau] that we might come to perform anatomical dissection on all dead people. The procedure should also be performed in great privacy in a manner that does not constitute a desecration of the dead.

In his 1986 article on skin transplantation from the dead,[47] Rabbi Yisraeli reiterates the opinion of *Tosafot* and Maimonides that it is permissible to derive benefit from the skin of the deceased. Even Rabbenu Tam allows such benefit—if the deceased asked that one forgo any honors due him—since the prohibition of deriving benefit from skin of a dead person relates to a violation of his honor and if he wishes he can forgo that honor. Yisraeli admits that a person can only forgo such honors in regard to his skin and his shrouds but not his body. Yisraeli reviews and rebuts all the arguments against the contents of his 1980 article made by Rabbi Meshash in his above-described essay. Rabbi Yisraeli concludes that there are three opinions in regard to the prohibition of deriving benefit from the dead.

1. The view of *Tosafot* (Niddah 55a and Zevachim 71b) that there is no prohibition in regard to the skin of the dead.
2. The view of Rabbenu Tam (Sanhedrin 40a) that there is a prohibition of deriving benefit from his shrouds. However, if the deceased while alive specifically instructed that one use the skin after he dies, there is no prohibition because he is allowed to issue such instructions and they are valid.
3. The view of Nachmanides and others that the skin of the deceased is prohibited from being used just like the rest of the body. The source of the prohibition is derived from sacrifices, and, therefore, the prohibition applies only if the skin is used in the normal manner of its usage. However, since the use of skin for transplantation and other medical usages is in a manner other than its normal usage, there is no prohibition involved.

The two 1986 essays by Rabbis Meshash and Yisraeli are followed by an exchange of letters between the two rabbis in which they reiterate and amplify their respective viewpoints regarding the permissibility of deriving benefit from the skin of deceased human beings.[48]

They both conclude, however, that the use of human skin from the deceased for transplantation to burn victims or others who have immediate need thereof is entirely permissible because of the overriding consideration of *piku'ach nefesh* (actual or potential danger to life). The two rabbis also sanction the storage of human skin in skin banks in Israel for later use because it is very probable that it will be needed in view of the frequent occurrence of burns both during war and even in peacetime. This fact makes Jewish law consider the situation as if the potential recipient is already identified, thus satisfying the requirement of Rabbi Ezekiel Landau that the patient whose life is to be saved is at hand (*lefaneinu*). Rabbi Meshash, however, limits skin banking to the needs of fifty patients and insists that the skin-removal procedure be performed in great privacy, with preservation, as much as possible, of the dignity and honor of the deceased skin donors.

Notes

1. S. Yisraeli, "Ripuy Keviyot al Yedei Hashtolat Or Min Hamet," *Techumin* (Winter 5740/1980): 237–247.
2. E. Landau, Responsa *Noda Biyehudah, Madura Tanina, Yoreh Deah*, no. 210.
3. Niddah 55a, s.v. *sheyma*.
4. Deuteronomy 21:1–9 and Avodah Zarah 29b.
5. Deuteronomy 21:8.
6. M. Maimonides, *Mishneh Torah, Hilchot Avodah Zarah* 7:3.
7. S. Adels, *Gilyon Maharsha* on Avodah Zarah 29b, s.v. *ve'orot levuvim*.
8. Commentary of Rabbenu Tam, in *Tosafot* Sanhedrin 48a, s.v. *meshamshin*.
9. *Novellae Ritva* on Niddah 55a.
10. S. Adret, Responsa *Rashba*, pt. 1, no. 365.
11. Arachin 7b.
12. Commentary of *Rashi* on Arachin 7b.
13. Maimonides, *Mishneh Torah, Hilchot Avel* 14:21.
14. Pesachim 24b.
15. Pesachim 26a, s.v. *shayni*.
16. Avodah Zarah 29b.
17. Maimonides, *Mishneh Torah, Hilchot Yesodei Hatorah* 5:8.
18. Avodah Zarah 12b, s.v. *elah*.
19. Newly planted trees whose fruits are forbidden for the first three years. Leviticus 19:23 ff.
20. Pesachim 25b.
21. Deuteronomy 21:23.
22. S. Meshash, "Bank Or Letsorech Ripuy Keviyot," *Techumin* 7 (1986 solidus 5746): 193–205.
23. S. Yisraeli, "Hashtalat Or Mayhamet," *Techumin* 7 (1986 solidus 5746): 206–213.
24. S. Meshash and S. Yisraeli, "Or Hamet (Chalifat Michtavim)," *Techumin* 7 (1986/5746): 214–218.
25. Maimonides, *Mishneh Torah, Hilchot Tumat Met* 3:11, *Hilchot Ma'achalot Assurot* 4:21, and *Hilchot Avel* 14:21.
26. Arachin 7b.
27. Commentary of Rabbenu Tam in *Tosafot*, Sanhedrin 48a, s.v. *meshamshin*.
28. B. Z. Uziel, Responsa *Mishpetei Uziel, Yoreh Deah*, no. 28; p. 212a.
29. M. Schick, Responsa *Maharam Schick, Yoreh Deah*, no. 344.
30. M. Schreiber, Responsa *Chatam Sofer, Yoreh Deah*, no. 336.
31. Maimonides, *Mishneh Torah, Hilchot Rotse'ach* 1:4.
32. Deuteronomy 21:23.
33. N. Girondi, *Chiddushei Haran* on Chullin 122a.

34. E. Landau, Responsa *Noda Biyehudah, Madura Tanina, Yoreh Deah*, no. 210.
35. See above, n. 30.
36. I. Karelitz, *Chazon Ish, Hilchot Avelut*, no. 208:7.
37. Eruvin 45a and Taanit 21b.
38. S. Goren, *Me'orot*, pt. 2.
39. Pesachim 46b, s.v. *rabbah.*
40. See above, n. 28.
41. F. Rosner and M. D. Tendler, *Practical Medical Halachah*, 2nd ed. (New York: Association of Orthodox Jewish Scientists and Feldheim Publishers, 1980), pp. 67–69.
42. M. Steinberg, *Noam* 3 (1960): 87–96.
44. I. Y. Unterman, *Shevet Yehudah* (Jerusalem, 1955), pp. 313–322.
45. I. Y. Unterman, *Hatorah Vehamedinah*, vols. 5–6, p. 210.
46. See above, n. 22.
47. See above, n. 23.
48. See above, n. 24.

23

Autopsy

The purpose of postmortem examination—autopsy—is to modify, elaborate, confirm, or reject antemortem diagnoses, thus aiding the medical profession in understanding human illness. It is performed to correlate the clinical aspects of disease for diagnostic and therapeutic evaluations, to determine the cause of death, to evaluate incompletely known disorders or discover new diseases, to serve an educational function through demonstration of tissue alterations as they relate to pathogenesis and to the therapeutically altered or natural courses of disease, and to collect data for statistical analysis of disease incidence.

There is little doubt that autopsies sometimes are a revelation to the physician, sometimes of the expected, at other times of unanticipated disease. Cases where autopsy disclosed unexpected findings are well documented in the medical literature. There is also no dispute concerning the value of autopsy as an essential component of medical education. These and other reasons for the performing of autopsies, however, still leave many questions unanswered. How many autopsies are "needed"? How should they be done? Who should do them? It is incorrect to assume that since autopsies are good, we must have more of them. It is also fallacious to presume that the more autopsies we perform, the better-quality medicine we have. A senior editor of the *Journal of the American Medical Association* refutes this assumption when he states:

> It is a pernicious misconception that the mere performance of postmortem dissection leads to progress in medical science, or the discovery of new diseases, or the advancement of medical

> frontiers. We lose sight of the fact that progress depends not on the autopsy, but on the person who is examining the material. Those who believe that the more autopsies we perform, the more medical science will advance, are actually pleading not for more autopsies but for persons who can profitably utilize the data of autopsies, persons who have imagination, originality, persistence, mental acuity, sound education and background, the indispensably prepared mind without which observations are quite sterile. It is a grave disservice to confuse the performance of autopsies with the spark of insight which the autopsy may trigger. We want the insight; and autopsies alone, no matter how numerous, are not the equivalent. We must not confuse the performance of postmortem dissection with the autoptic attitude. They may indeed coincide, but they need not.[1]

Current medical diagnostic techniques have decreased the value of the "routine" autopsy. Greater stress should be placed on the postmortem examination in selected cases rather than in a fixed percentage of deaths. From the Jewish religious viewpoint, however, even where an autopsy is sanctioned or even mandated, different answers must be provided, particularly to the question of how an autopsy is to be done. In most religions, including Judaism, the physical remains of a deceased person must be treated with honor and respect. Judaism requires not only that the dead be treated with utmost dignity and honor but that no desecration of the dead be performed except where such an act may immediately save a life. Even in such a situation, all organs examined and/or removed must be returned to the body prior to burial. Burial must not be delayed. No benefit may be derived from the dead except where a life is at stake.

Early attempts at presenting the Jewish view on autopsies in the English medical literature have been woefully inadequate.[2] This chapter discusses the Jewish attitude toward anatomical dissection and postmortem examinations as developed in biblical, talmudic, and rabbinic literatures. There is a need for Jewish physicians to obtain answers to the following questions: When, if ever, does Jewish law sanction or even mandate an autopsy? When is it permissible for a Jewish physician to request permission for an autopsy from the next of kin? Does Jewish law require permission in a case where autopsy is allowed? From whom must permission be sought—the bereaved family or the deceased prior to his demise? What if the deceased specifically asked that his body be dissected after his death? What constitutes desecration of the dead? Can one use cadaver organs for transplantation? How should a postmortem examination be performed when it is allowed or required in Jewish law?

The earliest responsum on autopsy was authored in the eighteenth century by Rabbi Ezekiel Landau.[3] It is this responsum upon which all subsequent rabbinic and Jewish legal decisions are based. Landau was asked by rabbinical authorities in London concerning a patient with a bladder calculus (probably urinary bladder, but possibly gallbladder) who had died following an unsuccessful operation. The question posed was whether it was permissible to make an incision into the body of the deceased at the site of the previous surgery, and to directly observe the root of the illness (and the cause of death). The purpose was to learn what the proper therapy should be in future cases and to avoid unnecessary surgery. Rabbi Landau answered that autopsy constitutes a desecration of the dead, and is only permissible to save the life of another patient who is immediately at hand *(lefaneinu)*. In the case before him, however, the life of no specific living patient was under consideration, and the autopsy was solely to learn therefrom for a future patient with a similar affliction. This possibility was too remote to permit an autopsy. Furthermore, concluded Landau, "if we would be lenient in this matter, heaven forbid, they would dissect all dead people in order to learn the arrangement of the internal organs and their functions, so as to know what therapy to give to the living."

The only other eighteenth-century rabbinic responsum dealing with autopsy is that of Rabbi Jacob Emden, who was asked by a medical student whether he could participate in the dissection of dogs on the Sabbath as a part of his anatomy training.[4] Rabbi Emden replied that numerous prohibitions relating to the Sabbath are involved. Dissection of human bodies, he continued, is prohibited because one is not permitted to derive any benefit from the deceased.

In the nineteenth century, there were five recorded responsa dealing with autopsy, by Rabbis Schreiber, Ettlinger, Schick, Auerbach, and Bamberger.[5] All take an essentially negative view toward the performance of autopsy except if the lives of other existing (not future) patients might thereby be saved. Rabbi Ettlinger also allows autopsy if the deceased had willed his body for that purpose during his lifetime.

Twentieth-century rabbinic responsa on the Jewish attitude toward autopsy and anatomical dissection of the dead are quite numerous.[6] The various principles upon which the Jewish legal rules governing the performance of postmortem examinations are cited in all the responsa and are detailed by Rabbi Isaac Arieli, who discusses whether or not autopsies are permitted for the following: (a) the sake of studying anatomy; (b) as a general procedure to gain knowledge; (c) to determine the cause of death; (d) to save an existing seriously ill patient; (e) to save future patients who may present a similar disease; (f) in the case of a common disease; (g) in the case of a rare disease; (h) in the case of a genetic disorder; (i) on a person who asked that this procedure be performed after his death; (j) transplantation of an organ from a dead person to a living individual; and (k) on a stillbirth.[7]

The prohibition of desecrating or disgracing the dead is based upon the biblical passage *And if a man has committed a sin worthy of death, and he be put to death, and thou hang him on a tree, his body shall not remain all night upon the tree but thou shalt surely bury him the same day.*[8] The Talmud interprets this phrase to mean that just as hanging all night is a disgrace to the human body, so too any action which constitutes a disgrace to the deceased is prohibited.[9] If the Torah was concerned for the body of a convicted criminal, then certainly, *a fortiori*, the body of a law-abiding citizen should be treated with the proper respect, and be interred without being subjected to shame or disgrace.

Two talmudic passages dealing with autopsy are relevant, although neither deals directly with dissection of the dead for purely medical purposes. One case deals with criminal law, the other with civil law. The first case deals with a murderer for whom the Divine Law prescribes death. The Talmud asks:

> Why do we not fear that the victim may have been afflicted with a fatal organic disease, for whose killing a person is not punishable as a murderer? Is it not because we follow the majority, and most victims of murderers are not so afflicted? And should you say that we can examine the body—this is not allowed because it would thereby be mutilated. And should you say that since a man's life is at stake, we should mutilate the body, then one could answer that there is always the possibility that the murderer may have killed the victim by striking him in a place where he was suffering from a fatal wound, thus removing all traces of the wound. In such a case, it is clear that no amount of postmortem examination would show that the victim was afflicted with a fatal disease.[10]

Therefore, it is proved, concludes the Talmud, that we follow the majority and do not perform an autopsy. In this case, the findings of an autopsy, even if it were permitted, would have been irrelevant to the conviction of the murderer, and insufficient to acquit him.

The second case is the story told in Bene-Berak that a person once sold his father's estate and died.[11] The members of the family protested that he was a minor at the time of his death and, therefore, not eligible to sell any of his father's estate. Hence, the property he sold should belong to the surviving members of the family. They came to Rabbi Akiva and asked whether the body might be exhumed and examined, so as to ascertain the age of the deceased by performing a postmortem examination. Rabbi Akiva replied that one is not permitted to dishonor the dead; and furthermore, the signs of maturity usually undergo a change after death. Hence, the examination would not produce reliable evidence of his age.

Neither talmudic case deals with autopsy for medical purposes, but both illustrate the objection to this procedure on the grounds that it would constitute a desecration of the dead, a biblically prohibited act.

The next major objection in Jewish law against routine autopsy is the multifaceted problem of burial of the dead. Firstly, the biblical phrase *Thou shalt surely bury him*[12] tells us that it is a positive commandment to bury the dead.[13] Secondly, whoever keeps his dead unburied overnight transgresses a negative commandment. This rule is deduced from the earlier part of the same biblical phrase: *His body shall not remain all night.* If one performs an autopsy, one may be transgressing the prohibition of delaying burial of the dead. Thirdly, the body must be interred whole, for if one leaves out even a small portion, it is as if no burial at all took place.[14] According to Maimonides, the infinitive *Thou shalt surely bury him* indicates that the command regarding burial concerns all dead, not only those executed by the court.[15] A fourth facet of the burial problem is the question as to whether burial, in addition to averting disgrace (by later putrefaction of the body), also represents atonement for the sins committed during life.[16] Judaism posits the thesis that the shame of being buried in the ground and having earth thrown upon one's coffin is sufficient to atone for all one's sins. Thus the sages of the Talmud tell us that, "all Israelites have a portion in the world-to-come."[17] Such atonement at the time of burial only takes effect if the entire body is buried. If one fails to return all removed organs to the body for burial, one also prevents atonement, since such a burial is incomplete.

Another serious objection to autopsy in Jewish law is the prohibition of deriving any benefit from the dead, as deduced in the Talmud.[18] The question of whether observation alone constitutes a benefit, or whether parts of the deceased must be used, such as for organ transplantation, in order to be considered deriving benefit from the dead, is a legal technicality, as is the question of whether the prohibition is biblical or rabbinic in origin.

Other halachic questions are also raised concerning autopsies. For example, can a priest ritually defile himself for the burial of a first-degree relative if the deceased has had an autopsy, particularly if organs are removed? Or can mourning begin if burial is effected but parts of the body have not been buried? Do the prohibitions regarding autopsy apply to a stillbirth? According to the Jewish concept of the soul being bound to the body, does not the soul suffer pain and/or disgrace if the body is dissected? Is permission for autopsy required to avoid the question of stealing, particularly in regard to organ transplants? Who may give such consent? The deceased in his lifetime? The family? Society?

The Jewish legal view toward autopsies, as discussed by most rabbinic authorities is summarized by Rabbi Arieli as follows:

a. A postmortem examination is a desecration and disgrace to the dead and biblically forbidden.
b. There is suffering to the soul which is bound to the body when the latter is desecrated.
c. The body of a Jew is holy.
d. If one leaves any part of the deceased unburied, one transgresses the positive commandment of burying the dead, and the negative commandments of delaying the burial of the dead and defiling the land. There is no rest for the deceased until his entire body returns to the earth.
e. If the relatives are able to effect burial of the entire body, then the laws of *aninut* (time prior to the onset of mourning) apply until they have done so.
f. If any part of the body is missing, priestly relatives may not actually defile themselves for the deceased.
g. Autopsy on a stillbirth is prohibited.
h. In addition to the reasons mentioned above, dissection for medical studies is prohibited because one would be deriving benefit from the dead, which some but not all rabbis also state is not allowed.
i. Dissection of the dead to save another person's life is permitted, provided such a patient is available, and there is a reason-

able prospect that the autopsy will directly save that life. But to save the life of some patient at a future time, autopsy is prohibited.

j. Autopsy to establish the cause of death is adjudicated like the case of a patient who may be present in the future (i.e., prohibited).
k. Autopsies are permitted in cases of hereditary diseases, just as if a patient whose life could be directly saved is at hand.
l. If the deceased in his lifetime freely consented to an autopsy, many authorities allow it, and it is permitted.
m. Corneal grafts from the dead to the living are permitted, but the transplantation of other organs requires further investigation.
n. The family, while not empowered to permit autopsies, may prevent them. In some cases, anyone can prevent an autopsy.[19]

These conclusions are based primarily on the classic responsum of Rabbi Ezekiel Landau (see above), who allows autopsies only if they would save the life of a patient immediately at hand *(lefaneinu)*. Britain's Chief Rabbi Immanuel Jakobovits comments:

> Rabbi Arieli is prepared to extend this principle even to patients who are not locally at hand, but who—through modern means of communication—may benefit from the findings of autopsies elsewhere, provided the ailment concerned is widespread enough to warrant the assumption that some other sufferer at the same time may be cured through these findings. But in fact, adds Rabbi Arieli, while the disease may be widespread, the likelihood of a cure being discovered as a result of any particular autopsy is very remote indeed. In these circumstances, therefore, one would not be justified in setting aside the ban on disfiguring the dead for the [almost hypothetical] sake of saving life. . . . Equally restrictive is Rabbi Arieli's rejection of autopsies to establish the cause of death, since he regards the link between such operations and the saving of life once again too tenuous. . . . he is inclined [however] to permit autopsies on bodies or persons who gave their consent in their lifetime.[20]

The consensus of rabbinic opinion today seems to permit autopsy only in the spirit of the famous responsum of Rabbi Ezekiel Landau, i.e., if it may directly contribute to the saving of a life of another patient at hand. In the case of hereditary diseases, the family or future offspring of the deceased are considered to represent patients at hand, and thus autopsies are allowed. However, as pointed out by Rabbi Jakobovits, in applying the eighteenth-century ruling of Rabbi Landau, one must take into account the following new circumstances:

a. With the speed of present-day communications, such patients are in fact at hand all over the world, and the findings of an autopsy in one place may aid a sufferer in another immediately.
b. Without autopsies, some of the worst scourges still afflicting mankind cannot be conquered.
c. Autopsies now bear a relationship to the saving of life not only in the hope they hold out for finding new cures for obscure diseases, but also in testing the effects and safety of new medications.
d. On the other hand, the very frequency of autopsies increases the danger that they will become a sheer routine, without any regard for their urgency, and without proper safeguards for the respect due to the dead.
e. With some patients in Israel refusing to be admitted to hospitals for fear of autopsies, the consideration of the saving of life now also operates in reverse.

Rabbi Chayim David Regensberg concludes that autopsy is permissible "if the pathologist honestly and firmly believes that he will thereby help other patients and a new therapy may be revealed thereby and become immediately known throughout the world."[21] Rabbi Immanuel Jakobovits recommends:

> While no general sanction can be given for the indiscriminate surrender of all bodies to postmortem examinations, the area of sanction should be broadened to include tests on new drugs and cases of reasonable suspicion that the diagnosis was mistaken; for autopsies under such conditions, too, may directly result in the saving of life. . . .
>
> Any permission for an autopsy is to be given only on condition that operation is reduced to a minimum, carried out with the greatest dispatch in the presence of a Rabbi or religious supervisor if requested by the family, and performed with the utmost reverence and with the assurance that all parts of the body are returned for burial.
>
> Just as it is the duty of Rabbis to urge relatives not to consent to an autopsy where the law does not justify it, they are religiously obliged to insure that permission is granted in cases

where human lives may thereby be saved, in the same way as the violation of the Sabbath laws in the face of danger to life is not merely optional but mandatory.

The most detailed exposition of autopsy in Jewish law is the recent essay by Rabbi Yitzchok Ralbag,[22] who begins by stating that the Talmud compares a deceased human being to a Scroll of the Law *(Sefer Torah)*[23] and says that a dead body must be treated with dignity and respect.[24] He who treats a dead body with disrespect transgresses a biblical commandment.[25] The deceased must be buried promptly, including all organs or parts that might have been removed for whatever reason. Cremation is not permitted in Judaism. Desecrating the dead, deriving benefit from the dead, and delaying or not burying the dead are all biblical prohibitions. The prohibition of deriving benefit from the dead, according to Ralbag and others, does not include a cardiac pacemaker, which may be removed from the deceased for use in another patient. Many rabbis also permit observation on dead bodies for the sake of studying anatomy but not the anatomical dissection itself. Observation alone is not considered to constitute deriving benefit from the dead. Ralbag cites at least two rabbinic respondents who state that if a man wills or sells his body to medical science, anatomical dissection is still prohibited because a human being is not master over his body, which is given to him by his Creator to use and not to abuse or desecrate.[26] At least one rabbi, however, asserts that a person has enough rights over his body to allow him to will his body to science, since he can forgive the desecration of his body.[27] His remains, however, must be buried.

Summary of Rabbinic Opinion on Autopsy

The Medical Ethics Committee of the Federation of Jewish Philanthropies of New York has succinctly summarized the biblical, talmudic, and rabbinic views concerning autopsies.[28]

Since Judaism teaches that man is created in the image of God, every dignity must be extended to the human body in death as in life. It is for this reason that the body must be regarded as inviolate. It is well known that, except in certain very limited circumstances, Jewish law does not sanction the performance of autopsies. It is, however, the consensus of rabbinic opinion that postmortem examinations may be performed for the purpose of gaining specific information of benefit in the treatment of other patients already afflicted by a life-threatening disease. A case in point would be a person with cancer who has died after receiving an experimental drug or drug combination which had been administered to a group of patients. Postmortem examination to ascertain possible toxicity, foreboding potential harm to other patients on the same course of treatment, or for purposes of obtaining information concerning the therapeutic efficacy of the drug or drug combination, would be warranted according to *Halachah* when such information is deemed to be essential in the treatment of other patients already suffering from the same illness.

Another instance where autopsy is not only allowed but probably mandated is the situation of life-threatening infectious disease, such as Legionnaire's disease. At a convention in Philadelphia in 1976, several hundred Legionnaires were afflicted with a pneumonia-like illness and many died. Jewish law would probably dictate autopsy on those who died in order to discover the offending organism (now known) and treatment (now available) in order to save the lives of the other patients afflicted, many of whom were dying of the same illness.

The dominant consideration in permitting an autopsy is the immediacy of the constructive application of the findings. This "here and now" principle, once limited to the medical needs of a local community, can now be extended, through the excellence of communications and scientific reporting, to the whole medical world. Results of autopsies in New York can be available in London in a matter of minutes. However, a routine autopsy cannot be sanctioned, although great benefit may accrue at some distant future time.

Another area where autopsy is permissible in Jewish law is genetic disease. A postmortem examination may be performed on a child who dies of a fatal genetic disease in order to obtain information that might save the lives of future children in the same family who may be afflicted with the same disease. Although the baby whose life is to be saved has not yet been born or even conceived, the "here and now" (*lefaneinu*) principle is rabbinically satisfied in the case of lethal genetic diseases.

The autopsy should be done as a surgical procedure with the same dignity, respect, and consideration that would be accorded a living patient undergoing an operation. It should be performed in dignified surroundings. The deceased should be draped and only the area of incision exposed. Proper decorum should be observed; and the behavior of the surgical-pathological staff should be appropriate to the situation. The usual autopsy involves an incision extending over the entire length of the abdominal and thoracic cavities, and examination of all internal organs, including the brain. These procedures cannot be countenanced when—as is usually the case—all pertinent potentially life-saving information may be acquired by means of a much more limited incision and examination of only those organs or areas crucial for obtaining this information. Organs may not be removed if they can be examined *in situ*. All organs and body fluids must be returned for burial.

A special autopsy consent form has been prepared in consultation with a number of physicians and legal scholars.[29] It is designed to provide for detailed specification of the nature and scope of the postmortem examination for which permission is sought. This consent form requires the physician to state in precise clinical terms the information he seeks, and to specify the area to be incised and the organs to be examined in obtaining such information. The authorization signed by the next of kin limits the extent of the postmortem procedure to that which is absolutely necessary in order to secure pertinent, potentially life-saving information of immediate applicability. Use of the consent form morally and legally obligates the pathologist to respect the directives of the next of kin. It specifies the limitations placed upon the autopsy procedure and, in addition, ensures that all organs, tissues, and fluids will be returned for burial as required by Jewish law.

The Israeli Autopsy Controversy

Nowhere has the controversy over autopsies been more intense and bitter than in the State of Israel, where we have often seen Jew pitted against Jew, rabbi against physician, and friend against friend. The issue was first raised prior to Israel's establishment when the Hadassah Hospital in Jerusalem asked the Chief Rabbinate whether it was permitted to perform anatomical dissections for medical-student teaching. The answer was that no objection exists for such anatomical dissections in cases where the deceased had freely willed his body for such purposes prior to his death.[30] Regarding autopsy or the dissection of bodies to discover pathologic anatomy, the agreement reached between Chief Rabbis Herzog and Frank, and Dr. Yasski, the then director of the Hadassah Hospital, stated that the Chief Rabbinate would not oppose autopsy in the following situations:

a. if the autopsy is required by law,

b. if the cause of death cannot be established without an autopsy; and where three physicians attest to this fact,
c. to save a life; and
d. in cases of genetic or inherited disease where the family may be guided or counselled concerning future children. . . .

The deceased must be buried in accordance with Jewish law and all organs removed for examination must be returned for burial.

On August 26, 1953, the Israeli Parliament (*Knesset*) passed the Anatomy and Pathology Law. One of the major provisions of this law is that if a person agreed, in writing, that his body could be used for science, it is permitted to dissect that body for medical instruction and research. A second major provision of the law states that a physician may perform an autopsy to establish the cause of death, or in order to use one or more of the organs of the deceased for transplantation to a critically ill recipient. The Ministry of Health was empowered to make amendments and decrees to implement and interpret the law.

The law was unclear as to who had the final word over whether an autopsy should be performed or not, the family of the deceased or the medical authorities. Some clarification emerged from the "Collected Amendments" (*Kovetz ha-Takkanot*, 10 Shevat 5714), in which section 2 of the Anatomy and Pathology Law is explained as follows: If a person dies without leaving written consent for autopsy, his next of kin may request that the body not be disturbed, and no autopsy should then be performed. Next of kin is specifically defined. Furthermore, if the deceased had no family, the burial society (*Chevra Kaddisha*) may also object to autopsy, in which case it is not to be done. If the body is unclaimed, the medical school can utilize the body for teaching and research purposes. However, a panel of three physicians was still empowered to order an autopsy if the cause of death could not be established without such a procedure.

Physicians were accused of taking advantage of this ambiguity in the law, in many instances overruling the wishes of families against performing autopsies. It was alleged that blank autopsy forms were signed by two physicians even prior to the death of the patient, so that only one physician would need to sign the order for an autopsy once the patient died, a practice contrary to the spirit of the law, and against the wishes of the family. Physicians were accused of desecration of the dead, because they removed internal organs and filled the body cavities with rags.

When Yitzchok Raphael became Deputy Minister of Health late in 1961, the Israeli Parliament charged him with the formation of a committee to consider the law concerning autopsies, and to present its conclusions and recommendations to the government for action. The desires of the family of the deceased were to be considered in the committee's deliberations. In 1962 a committee was appointed by Dr. Raphael

> to make a thorough study of the *de facto* and *de jure* situations, including all the relevant ordinances and operational directives and to present to the Ministry of Health conclusions to guide the Ministry's future actions in the matter. The committee is to take into consideration the needs of medical practice and research, the sensibilities of the public in the matter, the law of the land and Jewish legal [halachic] law.

The full committee met seventeen times, and its subcommittees held additional meetings. It took testimony from fourteen experts. All the members of the committee made a sincere effort to work in a spirit of mutual understanding, despite differences of opinion among some of them. They found a common language, and it transpired that for the needs of real life a solution could be found in halachic literature that provides for all contingencies. The detailed report submitted by the committee said in part:

> Having carefully weighed the data put before us, the testimony we have heard, and the pamphlets and articles we have read, we have come to the conclusion that, despite the great gap that appears to exist between the two points of view expressed before us, there is a way of satisfying at least part of the demands of both sides.

The following recommendations were accepted unanimously:

A. The 1953 law should be amended to include halachic principles.
   1. An autopsy should be performed only when, by thus establishing the exact cause of death, it will provide information which will make it possible to save lives, and
   2. in order to perform a transplant to treat a patient who has been specifically marked for this particular transplant.

B. An autopsy shall not be performed if the deceased had, in his lifetime, expressed opposition to it, or if, after his death, certain specified next of kin express opposition, except

1. if there are grounds to suspect that not establishing the cause of death might constitute a danger to the public or to the family, or
2. if there are grounds to suspect that death was caused by medical error which, if it is not ascertained, might lead to deaths.

C. The next of kin shall be given enough time to express their opposition.
D. The section of the law concerning penalties should be extended to apply also to false autopsy certificates.
E. A control committee should be set up consisting of a doctor, a rabbi, and a Christian clergyman.

These very restrictive amendments to the 1953 Anatomy and Pathology Law also required that in a case where physicians invoke item B above (danger to society or a medical error), the matter should come for adjudication before a rabbi or Christian clergyman. An appeals board was also to be established by the Ministry of Health. Deputy Minister of Health Yitzchok Raphael stated that he was certain that the Knesset would not adopt such a restrictive law where the family has the final word.[31] The rate of autopsy would drop to near zero, and the nonreligious elements in the government would defeat any such proposal. After much deliberation and discussion with various members of the cabinet, Dr. Raphael presented to the Knesset on December 25, 1964, the following compromise bill:

a. The concept of objection to autopsy by the burial society or a relative to the deceased is added to the 1953 law.
b. Autopsy is permitted to establish the cause of death if this will make possible the saving of lives.
c. An organ from a deceased may be used for transplant purposes for a patient who has been specifically designated for that transplant.
d. Autopsy will not be performed if the deceased had, in his lifetime, expressed opposition to autopsy after his death.
e. Autopsy will not be performed if there is opposition to autopsy from the person whose name appears in the hospital chart, and who is to be called in case of emergency, or from certain specified relatives, or a specified burial society.
f. Items d and e above are overruled if there are grounds to suspect that not establishing the cause of death might constitute a danger to the public, or to the family, or if there is a suspicion that death was caused by a medical error which, if

not ascertained, might lead to further danger to life. Such a suspicion must be certified in writing by a panel of three physicians.

g. Autopsy is not to be performed until at least five hours have elapsed from the time of notification of death to the responsible family member or burial society, as in item e. Sabbaths and Jewish holy days are not included in the five-hour waiting period.
h. The Minister of Health will appoint a control commission to supervise the implementation of the law. Among the members of this commission should be a physician, rabbi, and Christian clergyman.
i. Penalties are to be imposed upon a physician who falsely certifies to the need for an autopsy, punishment to consist of three years imprisonment.

This new proposal was much more restrictive than the 1953 law but more moderate than the earlier proposal in that it did not require each case to be presented for rabbinic judgment. In spite of strong objections from many sides, particularly the medical profession and the nonreligious elements in the government, the proposal was presented to the Israeli Parliament as the "Anatomy and Pathology Law. Revised 1965." Renewed controversy among the various factions in the government brought the debate to fever pitch. Some demanded that the earlier version of the bill, as originally proposed by the special Wahl Commission, be brought to the floor for a vote. Yet others had intermediate or compromise suggestions, but none were adopted because the parliamentary debate took place shortly before election time, and members of the Knesset felt that votes might be influenced by that consideration. The whole matter was referred back to the special commission and to a committee made up of members of the coalition parties. As a result of these new deliberations, the following modification of the earlier proposal was made:

a. To delete the concept of the burial society objecting to an autopsy, except as it was defined in the 1953 law.
b. To allow autopsy in exceptional cases, even if this means overruling the expressed wishes of the deceased before his death or the objections of the next of kin.

   The exceptional cases are where three physicians certify in writing that there exists the possibility that death was due to an unusual unknown cause or due to an accident, and without establishing the cause of death there may result danger to life; or where there is suspicion that a danger to society or to an individual exists which may be overcome by establishing the precise cause of death, or where a need exists to use an organ from the deceased for transplantation purposes. Corneas may be preserved in an eye bank.

c. To delete completely the paragraph dealing with a control commission to supervise implementation of the law.
d. To broaden the matter of transplantation.

This new "revision of the revision," which was now acceptable to the medical community but not to the religious elements in the government, was presented to the Fifth Knesset at the end of the session in 1965. In the haste of adjourning, the bill was referred back to a parliamentary committee. The Sixth Knesset failed to act on the bill. In the meantime, autopsies continued to be performed in the major hospitals of Israel over the opposition of families of the deceased, burial societies, and the rabbinate. Polarization between the medical and religious communities reached a climax with an incident in the Kaplan Hospital in Petach Tikvah. An autopsy had been performed and the family of the deceased stormed the hospital, wreaked havoc causing extensive property damage, and physically assaulted members of the medical staff of the hospital. As a result of this incident, the Ministry of Health issued a circular to all hospitals in Israel directing that patients who stipulate that their bodies not be dissected if they die should not be admitted to the hospital.

This directive outraged both the religious and nonreligious public. Demonstrations were held in Israel and throughout the world demanding that indiscriminate autopsies cease at once. Many violent incidents ensued in the various confrontations. The Chief Rabbinate of Israel published a statement on October 15, 1966, which asserted:

> In view of the great calamity in the matter of autopsy, we express our opinion that autopsy in any form whatsoever is prohibited by the law of the Torah. And there is no way to allow it except in a manner of immediate danger to life, and then only with the approval in each instance of a brilliant rabbi who is authorized to do so.

The statement was signed by Chief Rabbis Issar Yehuda Unterman and Isaac Nissim, Rabbi Yechezkel Abramsky, and 356 rabbis from the entire State of Israel. The fourteen pages of signatures end with the following pronouncement: "This judgment is a warning against the passage of any law which would negate it."

Needless to say, this extreme viewpoint of the Chief Rabbinate generated more protest, more controversy, more violence. Accusations, counteraccusations, and denials flew between the Hadassah Medical Center in Jerusalem and ad hoc organizations such as the Committee for Safeguarding Human Dignity. The Association of Orthodox Jewish Scientists, headquartered in New York, sent a letter to Prime Minister Levi Eshkol on May 5, 1967, part of which follows:

> We would like to emphasize that in spite of our appreciation of the contributions of postmortem examination to modern medicine, we are firm in our conviction that the primary rights of disposition of the remains of a deceased individual—not merely the right to object to an autopsy—must be granted to the next of kin. This practice is almost universal in scientifically advanced countries. We are certain that non-coercive means can be found to assure adequate numbers of postmortem examinations to preserve Israel's position in the medical world.
>
> We urge you to act immediately to achieve passage of legislation, vesting permission for autopsy in the hands of the family of the deceased. Until such legislation is passed, we urge you to prevail upon the medical community to declare a voluntary moratorium on autopsies, except when specific consent is obtained from the family of the deceased.
>
> With the prevailing climate of distrust and controversy, your personal intervention is urgently needed to terminate this destructive internecine war within the Jewish community. We urge you to act now.

The controversy did not abate, however. Stories were published in the Israeli lay and medical press[32] as well as in American lay and medical publications.[33] Acts of incitement and provocation, slanders, derogations, disturbances, and personal threats and abuse against physicians continued. On the other hand, autopsies continued to be performed at major Israeli hospitals in spite of the objections of next of kin. People were afraid to be admitted to an Israeli hospital for fear their body might be dissected if they should die.

Ten years later (i.e., in 1977), the Israeli autopsy situation was as follows:

a. There was no change in the law.
b. There seemed to have been a change in the practice in many hospitals in that far fewer autopsies were being done in oppo-

sition to the wishes of the family. In general, people were still not formally asked, but expressed opposition was much more frequently honored.

c. There seemed to be some Ministry of Health internal administrative guidelines which instructed hospitals not to do autopsies against family wishes. The existence of such a guide was confirmed by the head of the ministry, but a copy thereof could not be obtained.

Thus, there was a *de facto* change in practice as a result of the realities of pressures and conflict but no change of Israeli law.

Any new Israeli law concerning autopsy necessarily must take into account the religious and social sensitivities of the population, as well as the needs of the medical community in its dedication to provide the best possible medical care for the sick. In those circumstances where Jewish law does permit an autopsy, the procedure must be performed according to all halachic principles, including the return of all removed organs to the body for burial. Only in an atmosphere of mutual trust can the rabbinate and medical profession arrive at a solution which will satisfy the requirements of both.

It is hoped that more rabbis will speak out in the near future concerning the areas of disease (i.e., genetic and infectious diseases, experimental drug therapy, and others) where autopsy may be permitted or is mandated and how it should be conducted. Physicians, on their part, particularly pathologists, must make arrangements to perform limited autopsies without undue delay. They must return all organs to the body for burial, removing only minute pieces for microscopic examination. Photographs of the gross pathology can be taken for later use rather than saving whole organs. Only with a recognition of the problems of medicine and Jewish law by both sides—that is, physician and rabbi—can progress be made toward a mutually acceptable solution. This is true not only in the United States, but also in Israel, because in the matter of autopsy, medicine and Judaism do, in fact, strive toward a common goal, the eradication of disease.

Notes

1. L. S. King, "Of Autopsies" (editorial), *Journal of the American Medical Association* 191 (1965): 1078–1079.

2. C. D. Spivak, "Postmortem Examination among Jews," *New York Medical Journal* 99 (1914): 1185; J. L. Belford, "Religious Views of Autopsies," *Long Island Medical Journal* 9 (1915): 484; J. Gottlieb, "A Review of Jewish Opinions Regarding Postmortem Examinations," *Boston Medical and Surgical Journal* 196 (1929): 726–728; E. P. Joslin, "Autopsies upon Jews and Gentiles," ibid., pp. 728–729; M. Plotz, "The Jewish Attitude toward Autopsies," *Modern Hospital* 45 (1935): 67–68; H. L. Gordon, "Autopsies According to the Jewish Religious Laws," *Harofé Haivri* 1 (1937): 201–203 (Engl.) and 130–141 (Heb.); O. Saphir, "Religious Aspects of the Autopsy," *Hospitals* 12 (1938): 50–55; B. J. Abeshouse, "The Problem of Autopsies on Orthodox Jewish Patients," *Sinai Hospital Journal* (Baltimore) 6 (1957): 76–98; A. Kottler, "The Jewish Attitude on Autopsy," *New York State Journal of Medicine* 57 (1957): 1649–1650; H. Ribner, "Jewish Law, Social Prejudice and Autopsy," *Bulletin of the Maryland University School of Medicine* 44 (1959): 21–25.

3. E. Landau, Responsa *Noda Biyehuda*, pt. 2, *Yoreh Deah*, no. 210.

4. J. Emden, Responsa *She'elatz Yavetz*, pt. 1 no. 41.

5. M. Schreiber, Responsa *Chatam Sofer, Yoreh Deah*, no. 336; J. Ettlinger, Responsa *Binyan Zion*, nos. 170–171; M. Schick, Responsa *Maharam Schick, Yoreh Deah*, no. 347; B. Z. Auerbach, *Nachal Eshkol*, pt. 2, no. 117; S. Bamberger, Responsa *Zecher Simchah*, no. 158.

6. M. Winkler, Responsa *Levushei Mordechai, Orach Chayim*, pt. 2, no. 29; S. Sofer, Responsa *Ketav Sofer, Yoreh Deah*, no. 174; E. H. Shapira, Responsa *Minchat Eliezer*, pt. 4, no. 25; E. Y. Waldenberg, Responsa *Tzitz Eliezer* vol. 4, no. 14; Y. M. Shapiro, Responsa *Ohr HaMeir*, pt. 1, no. 74; M. T. Halevy, Responsa *Divrei Malkiel*, pt. 2, no. 92; D. Hoffman, Responsa *Melamed Leho 'il, Yoreh Deah*, no. 109; Y. Zweig, Responsa *Porat Yosef*, no. 17; M. Y. Zweig, Responsa *Ohel Moshe*, pt. 1, no. 4; B. Z. Uziel, Responsa *Mishpetei Uziel, Yoreh Deah*, pt. 1, nos. 218–29 and pt. 2, no. 110; A. D. Kook, *Da' at Kohen*, no. 199; D. M. Manesh, *Chavatzelet Hasharon, Yoreh Deah*, no. 95; S. T. Rubenstein, *Torah she-be-al Peh*, (1964), pp. 67–74; V. Silberstein, ibid. pp. 82–86; M. D. Wilner, in *Hatorah Vehamedinah* 5–6 (1953–54): 202–212; S. Yisroeli, ibid., pp. 213–226; O. Hadaya ibid., pp. 191–201; Y. H. Levin, in ibid. 7–8 (1955–57): 222–227; Ch. Hirshenson, *Malki Bakodesh* (Hoboken, N.J., 1923), pt. 3, pp. 6–9 and 137–152; Y. Raphael, in *Or Hamizrach* 16 (1966): 5–13; N. S. Schechter, in *Noam* 5 (1962): 159–164; S. Sharashefsky, in ibid. 7 (1964): 387–392; M. Feinstein, in ibid. 8 (1965): 9–16; O. Hedaya, in ibid., pp. 68–74; H. Z. Grossberg, in ibid., 10 (1967): 204–207; S. Y. Levine, in *Hapardes* 1951, pp. 138–141; J. J. Greenwald, in *Kol Bo Al Avelut* (New York 1947), vol. 1, pp. 33–63; J. M. Tukazinsky, *Gesher Hachayim* (Jerusalem, 1960), vol. 1,

pp. 70–74; D. Margalit, *Korot* 4 (1966): 41–64; E. L. Globus, in *Harefuah* 60 (1961): 196–200; Y. Silberstein, in *Machanayim*, 123 (1970): 108–113; G. Felder, in *Assia* 1 (1976): 216–220.

7. I. Arieli, in *Noam* 6 (1963): 82–103 and *Torah she-be-al Peh*, 1964 pp. 40–60.

8. Deuteronomy 21:22–23.

9. Sanhedrin 47a.

10. Chullin 11b.

11. Baba Batra 154a.

12. Deuteronomy 21:23.

13. Sanhedrin 46b.

14. Jerusalem Talmud, Nazir 7:1.

15. Maimonides, *Mishneh Torah, Hilchot Sanhedrin* 15:8.

16. Sanhedrin 46b.

17. Sanhedrin 10:1.

18. Avodah Zarah 29b and Nedarim 48a.

19. Arieli, loc. cit.

20. I. Jakobovits, *Torah she-be-al Peh*, 1964, pp. 61–66. See also the following by Rabbi Jakobovits: *Harofe Haivri* 2 (1961): 233–238; ibid. 1 (1960): 210–222 and 2 (1961): 212–221; *Tradition* 1 (1958): 77–103; *Jewish Medical Ethics* (New York: Bloch 1959), pp. 132–152; *Jewish Law Faces Modern Problems* (New York: Yeshiva University Press 1965), pp. 81–87; *Journal of a Rabbi* (New York: Living Books, 1966), pp. 173–193; *Machanayim*, 123 (1970): 114–119.

21. Ch. D. Regensberg, "Autopsies in Jewish Law," *Halachah Urefuah* 2 (1981): 9–14.

22. Y. Ralbag, "Dissection of the Dead," in *Harefuah Le'or Hahalachah* (Jerusalem, 1983), vol. 3, pt. 1, pp. 1–86.

23. Shabbat 105b and Moed Katan 25a.

24. Berachot 18a.

25. Sanhedrin 46b.

26. M. Schick, Responsa *Maharam Schick, Yoreh Deah*, nos. 344, 347, and 349; M. Sofer, Responsa *Chatam Sofer, Yoreh Deah*, nos. 144 and 336.

27. Y. Y. Ettlinger, Responsa *Binyan Zion*, nos. 170 and 171.

28. D. M. Feldman and F. Rosner, ed., *Compendium on Medical Ethics*, 6th ed. (New York: Federation of Jewish Philanthropies, 1984), pp. 120–125.

29. Ibid., pp. 126–128.

30. Chief Rabbi Isaac Herzog's responsum on this subject was publicized in the Hebrew periodical *Kol Torah*, vol. 1 (1947).

31. Minister Raphael's comments were published in the Hebrew periodical *Gevilin*, vol. 25.

32. P. Gillon, "Autopsies," *Jerusalem Post*, Mar. 24, 1967. Y. Rosenthal, "Nettichat Geviyot Raq be-Hetar Rav," *Ha-Aretz*, Dec. 4, 1966; V. Resnekov, Editorial on Autopsies, *Quarterly Review of the Israel Medical Association* 23 (1967): 3–11.

33. M. M. Greenberg, "The Autopsy Crisis in Israel," *Jewish Observer*, September 1966, pp. 5–9; M. N. Chalef and J. Goldberg, "Are Autopsies Really Prohibited?" *Jewish Press*, Sept. 2, 1966, pp. 20–21; M. Birnbaum, "Eye Witness to Autopsy Mill Tells of Experiences in Israel," ibid., Oct. 7, 1966; P. Robbins, "Unauthorized Autopsy on Israel Hero Performed," *Guardian* 3, 2 (1967): 1; D. M. Maeir, "An Examination of the Autopsy Problem," *Yeshiva University Alumni Review* 7, 4 (1967): 2 and 8; D. Sohn, "Israel Autopsy Debate," *New York State Journal of Medicine* 68 (1968): 398–401; "Autopsy Dispute Brings Israeli M.D.'s Under Fire," *Medical World News*, June 9, 1967, p. 45.

24

Embalming and Cremation

Introduction

Balm is defined in Webster's dictionary as an aromatic preparation or any of various aromatic plants or odors, or a balsamic resin especially from small tropical evergreen trees. Embalming of a body, therefore, is the filling of that body with sweet aromatic odors to perfume it. Another definition of embalming is the injection of preservatives into a body to prevent or delay its putrefaction. Mummification is the embalming of a body or its treatment for burial with preservatives in the manner of the ancient Egyptians.

The reason for this ancient Egyptian practice is probably related to their profound belief in immortality. Not only was the soul immortal but it was believed that at some later time it would return to the body to continue the earthly life. It was, therefore, desirable to preserve the body and the dead person's possessions.[1] The natural drying out of the body by solar heat (mummification) is the oldest method of preserving a corpse. The ancient Egyptians may have simply tried to dry corpses in the hot desert sands or, as in one of the chambers found at Thebes, in rooms which were artifically heated.[2] In the rainless desert, the corpses often remained well preserved for thousands of years.

The method of embalming as practiced by the ancient Egyptians in the fifth century B.C.E. is described by the Greek historian Herodotus as follows:

> The brain was drawn out with a hook in fragments through the nose. Then an incision was made in the left flank, and certain organs were removed. The heart was left untouched. The body

> cavity was now filled with spices and the whole body was next placed in a solution of salts for about two months. Then it was dried, covered with special paste, and wrapped in linen bandages. The organs removed were preserved in special jars.[3]

A slightly expanded account of Herodotus' description of ancient Egyptian embalming is provided by Garrison, who claims that the Egyptians already knew the antiseptic virtues of extreme dryness and of certain chemicals like nitre and common salt.

> The brain was first drawn out through the nostrils by an iron hook and the skull cleared of the rest by rinsing with drugs; the abdomen was then incised with a sharp flint knife, eviscerated, cleansed with wine and aromatics, filled with myrrh, cassia and spices and the wound sewed up. The body was then steeped for seventy days in sodium chloride or bicarbonate [natron] and afterward washed and enveloped completely in linen bandages smeared together with gum. The relatives put it in a wooden coffin, shaped like a man, which was deposited in the burial chamber along with four Canopic jars containing the viscera. . . . the departed spirit was furnished with food, drink and other appointments and conveniences.[4]

The Egyptian embalming procedure was carried out not by physicians but by technicians known as "paraschistes," who were "held in such aversion that they were driven away with curses, pelted with stones, and otherwise roughly handled, if caught."[5] Embalming was also known to the ancient Persians and Assyrians.[6]

The Embalming of Jacob

The Hebrew word *chanitah* or *chanatah* refers not only to embalming but also to blossoming or ripening. The term designates a certain stage in the development of fruit trees[7] when the obligation of giving tithe from the fruit occurs. Quoting the Jerusalemic Talmud, Rabbi Samson Raphael Hirsch states that this stage is

> the time when the fruit is so ripe that it or its seed or pip, if sound, would grow, accordingly when the essential materials are collected together in it to the essential degree of formation, accordingly when it is already penetrated by the aromatic essences which give the fruit its characteristic taste. Now em-

balming is nothing else but filling out and penetrating the arteries and veins and soft tissues of the body which have been emptied out, with aromatic materials, so perhaps therein lies the connection between the two uses of the word *chanatah*.[8]

The Bible describes embalmers or physicians[9] and mentions embalming only with reference to Jacob and Joseph, who both died in Egypt.[10] The key scriptural passage, *And Joseph commanded his servants the physicians to embalm his father and the physicians embalmed Israel*,[11] is explained differently by many of the classic biblical commentators. Rabbi Shlomo ben Yitzchak, popularly known as *Rashi*, states that embalming is a matter of using aromatic spices. Rabbi Jonathan ben Uziel's Aramaic translation of the Bible asserts that Joseph commanded the physicians "to spice his father." Rabbi Abraham Ibn Ezra uses the expression "like a powder." Rabbi Joseph H. Hertz comments that the embalming of Jacob was not in imitation of the custom of the Egyptians, who took care to preserve the body after death and keep it ready for occupation by the soul. Joseph's purpose was merely to preserve it from dissolution before it reached the Cave of Machpelah.[12] Julius Preuss also asserts that the embalming of Jacob was needed specifically because of the necessity to preserve the body during its long transport from Egypt to Canaan.[13] However, contrary to Hertz, Preuss is of the opinion that Joseph had his father's body embalmed according to Egyptian practice, not according to the rules of his own people.

The embalming of Jacob is vividly described in the book of Jewish mysticism known as the *Zohar* as follows:

> Apparently, this embalming was like that of any other person. It cannot have been on account of the journey to Canaan, because Joseph also was embalmed and yet he was not taken out of the country. The real reason was that it was the custom to embalm kings in order to preserve their bodies. They were embalmed with very special oil mixed with spices. This was rubbed on them day after day for forty days. After that, the body could last for a very long time. For the air of the land of Canaan and of the land of Egypt corrupts the body [251a] more rapidly than that of any other country. Hence they do this to preserve the body, embalming it within and without. They place the oil on the navel, and it enters into the body and draws out the inside, and thus preserves it inside and outside. It was fitting that Jacob's body should be so preserved, since he was the body of the

> patriarchs. Similarly Joseph, who was an emblem of the body, was preserved both in body and soul—in body, as it says, *and they embalmed him*, in soul, as it is written, *and he was put in a coffin in Egypt.*[14]

Rabbi Yitzchak Ralbag cites the commentary of Rabbi Moshe Hagiz in his book *Leket Hakemach*, which explains the words of the *Zohar* as follows: It is impossible that the sons of Jacob would allow him to be embalmed like ordinary people who are disemboweled and whose heads are opened and brains removed. Rather, the Egyptian physicians injected balm oil into his navel.[15]

On the other hand, the talmudic commentary of Rabbi Yom Tov Lippman Heller, popularly known as *Tosafot Yom Tov*, in relation to King Hezekiah, who dragged the bones of his wicked father Manasseh on a bed of ropes in order to atone for the latter's sins, states as follows:

> . . . it was their custom to first bury the dead. After the body decomposed they would gather the bones and bury them. . . . But for kings it was not the custom to first bury them and then gather their bones. Rather, before they were buried they were embalmed, which consisted of the removal of all their internal organs and their replacement with spices and the anointing of the body both on the inside and on the outside. The embalming prevented the decay and putrefaction of the body. And the skin and the flesh would slowly dissolve until only the bones remained. And so do we find by Saul: *and they took the body of Saul and the bodies of his sons . . . and they burnt them there; and they took their bones and buried them.*[16] Thus embalming is called burning. . . . there is great benefit in this type of embalming in that the body does not decay nor putrefy and no worms develop in it.[17]

The definition of embalming as cited by *Tosafot Yom Tov* is also found in other Jewish sources. Rabbi Shlomo ben Adret, known as *Rashba*, permits calcium to be spread over bodies already in the grave in order to hasten the decomposition of the flesh and then adds: "embalmers open the abdomen and remove the intestines."[18] Rabbi Moshe Schreiber, known as *Chatam Sofer*, also defines embalming as does *Tosafot Yom Tov* but asserts that the embalming of Jacob was without any physical contact with the body because the purpose of disembowelment as part of embalming is to prevent decay and putrefaction because of the dirt in the bowels.[19] However, continues *Chatam Sofer*, since Jacob was spiritually pure and physically clean, he did not require removal of his internal organs and he was therefore embalmed by having oil poured into his navel.

The biblical commentary of Rabbi Bachya ben Asher states that embalming means that they used to perfume the body with spices, as it is written concerning King Asa, *And they laid him in the bed which was filled with sweet odors and divers kinds [of spices] prepared by the perfumer's art*,[20] and this was after the washing.[21] Bachya also states that the expression *and they embalmed him* means that the physicians were commanded to do so because they were experts in the natural sciences, but they did not touch the body of Jacob. Joseph apparently asked the physicians to tell him the secrets of the embalming procedure, but they did the embalming of Jacob themselves.

Hirsch points out the sharp contrast in Egyptian and Jewish ideas:

> To the Egyptian the *body* was embalmed so that its individuality should persist. But the soul did not remain in its personal individuality, but wandered from body to body—even to animal bodies—in manifold metamorphosis. To the Jew the soul persists, the body wanders, once the soul has gone home to the circle where it belongs, the body has nothing more to do with the individual. But rather, it is a commandment, as soon as possible to bring it in as close contact as possible to the dissolving earth. It becomes earth again, and can then go through all the possible changes and vicissitudes of earthly matter. The Egyptian believes in the wandering of the soul, and tries to protect the body from all possible wandering or change. The Jew believes in an eternal personal existence of the soul, and hands the body over to material earthly change. Perhaps it was just the lack of belief in Egypt of the permanent individuality of the soul, as well as the embalming of corpses which resulted in the colossal building of pyramids designed for dwellings for the dead. As one believed the soul to be wandering, one wanted at least to keep the body. Embalming was accordingly not Jewish, and Joseph here might only have made a concession to the Egyptian customs as they would have considered an omission as showing a great lack of piety. Perhaps also the reason for Jacob making Joseph swear not to bury him in Egypt was, as our Sages remark, to avoid the Egyptian making an idol out of

> his body, for at bottom, the preserving of mummies in Egypt usually resulted in making it into a god and praying to it. The physicians embalmed "Israel," in accordance with his status.[22]

According to the biblical commentary of Rabbi Meir Leib ben Yechiel Michael, popularly known as *Malbim*, the practice of embalming as practiced in Egypt is known to us from mummies, which are embalmed bodies which are preserved and have not decayed over several thousand years. Even if the Egyptians practiced embalming because of their beliefs, it is astonishing to consider how Joseph could do so with the body of his holy father. *Malbim* then distinguishes between the Divine soul (Heb. *neshamah*) of a human being, which leaves the body immediately at death and returns to its source, and the animalistic soul (Heb. *ruach*) or spirit, which does not. Burial is necessary so that the body decays and allows the animalistic soul to separate from it. In righteous people such as Jacob, both the Divine and the animalistic soul depart immediately at death and, therefore, burial in the ground to allow decay of the body is unnecessary. That is why the Egyptians embalmed him to preserve his pure body.

In his collection of biblical commentaries known as *Yalkut Me'am Lo'ez*, Rabbi Yaakov Koli describes the two methods of embalming.[23] One method is where fragrant spices are mixed in the best aromatic oils and this mixture is poured on and rubbed over the entire body, so that some of the mixture is absorbed into the body. The other method is the ancient Egyptian practice of removing the internal organs, including the brain, and the instillation of aromatic substances into the body to dry it and preserve it. Both methods were meant to delay or prevent decay of the body. He does not say which method was used for Jacob.

Rabbi Yitzchak Ralbag states that the sages and the biblical commentaries imply that the embalming of Jacob did not involve any desecration of his body,[24] an act strictly forbidden in Judaism.[25] Ralbag supports his statement with the scriptural phrase *And Jacob came whole.*[26] Ralbag also cites the biblical commentary known as *Da'at Zekenim*, which interprets the embalming of Jacob as follows: "they sweetened his body after they injected the aromatic substances to cleanse the dirt in his intestines; and so that the body not putrefy they then injected into it sweet substances to give it a good odor."

According to Herodotus, the Egyptian process of embalming required seventy days, which is at variance with the biblical statement that it required only forty days, the period that the Bible assigns to the Egyptians' mourning for Jacob: *And forty days were fulfilled for him, for so are fulfilled the days of embalming; and the Egyptians wept for him three score and ten days.*[27] *Rashi* states that they completed the embalming in forty days but they wept for him for seventy days: forty days during the period of embalming and thirty more days for mourning. They wept so long for him because a blessing had come to them on Jacob's arrival in Egypt, for the famine then ceased and the waters of the Nile again increased. Bachya explains the *three score and ten days* as forty days for the embalming and thirty days of mourning. *Malbim* asserts that embalming to the Egyptians was like the reconstruction of the body for eternal life when the soul returns to it after three thousand years; hence, forty days is comparable to the formation of a human embryo and thirty days of mourning. In his biblical commentary, Rabbi Ovadiah Seforno states that the Egyptians mourned for Jacob not only because of Joseph and at the latter's command but because Jacob was also worthy of leadership and royal honor.

The Embalming of Joseph

At the end of the Book of Genesis, the embalming of Joseph is cited: *So Joseph died, being one hundred and ten years old: and they embalmed him, and he was put in a coffin in Egypt.*[28] Ibn Ezra states that the word *they* refers to the physicians, whereas others interpret *they* to refer to Joseph's brothers.[29] Seforno claims that Joseph's bones were placed in the same coffin, that he was embalmed, and that he was not buried in the ground. According to the Talmud, the Egyptians made a bronze coffin for Joseph and placed it in the Nile so that the river's waters would be blessed.[30] Bachya's biblical commentary adds that the Egyptians wanted to hide Joseph's coffin so that the Jews would not find it and be unable to leave Egypt without the bones of Joseph.

Herod's "Embalming" of His Beloved in Honey

The Talmud relates that Herod the Great was a slave of the Hasmonean house and had set his eyes on a certain maiden of that house.[31] One day he heard a voice from heaven say, "Every slave that rebels now will succeed." So he rose and killed all the members of his master's household, but spared the maiden. When she saw that he wanted to marry her, she went up onto a roof and cried out,

"Whoever comes and says, I am from the Hasmonean house, is a slave, since I alone am left of it, and I am throwing myself down from this roof." He preserved her body in honey for seven years. Some say that he had intercourse with her, others that he did not. According to those who say that he had intercourse with her, his reason for embalming her was to gratify his desires. According to those who say that he did not have intercourse with her, his reason was that people might say that he had married a king's daughter.

According to Preuss, honey was also used as a preservative substance in Mycenae and Babylon.[32] Preuss also cites Democritos, who said that if one preserves bodies in honey, they come back to life again, a statement ridiculed by Pliny. Josephus points out that the body of the poisoned Aristobulus lay preserved in honey for a long time, until Antonius sent it to the Jews for burial.[33] The method of preserving bodies in honey is not described, but nowhere is the suggestion made that evisceration, as practiced by the ancient Egyptian embalmers, is part of the procedure.

Cremation and "Burnings for Kings"

Several scriptural passages are cited to prove that burial is a religious obligation in Judaism,[34] and that nonburial is regarded as a punishment to the wicked.[35] The Talmud derives the obligation of burial from the biblical phrase *his body shall not remain all night upon the tree, but thou shalt surely bury him the same day.*[36] This rule is codified by Moses Maimonides and Joseph Karo in their famous codes of Jewish law.[37] Hence, disposal of a dead body by cremation is contrary to Jewish teaching. In fact, the Talmud considers the burning of a corpse to be an idolatrous practice.[38]

The accounts of cremation in Jewish antiquity are mostly based on the erroneous interpretation of the word "burning" in relation to death.[39] Burning is one of the four types of captial punishment[40] but does not mean cremation. The manner in which burning was effectuated for someone convicted of a capital offense is described in detail in the Talmud.[41] The main biblical passages which are cited in relation to cremation refer to the deaths of King Asa, King Zedekiah, and Saul and his sons. King Asa was laid in a bed which was filled with herbs and spices prepared according to the apothecary's art. The exact scriptural quotation follows:

> *And Asa slept with his fathers and died in the forty-first year of his reign. And they buried him in his own sepulchres which he*

> *had hewn out for himself in the city of David; and they laid him in the bed which was filled with sweet odors and divers kind [of spices] prepared by the perfumer's art; and they made a very great burning for him.*[42]

Rashi states that the great burning refers to fragrant spices which were burned to a powder and then sprinkled on Asa. An alternative explanation offered by *Rashi* is that the burning refers to the customary funeral pyre of the bed and other personal articles of the deceased king, which were burned as a sign of honor to him. Such burnings in honor of deceased kings, according to the Talmud, are not considered idolatrous practices and, therefore, not prohibited.[43] Rabbi David Altshul, in his biblical commentary known as *Metzudat David*, also interprets the burning to refer to King Asa's bed and utensils, "as was customary for kings." Rabbi David Kimchi, known as *Radak*, states that "they burned spices and perfumes, and the sages explained that it was customary to burn flax and personal possessions of kings after their death." The same honor was paid to the patriarchs, and the greater the value of the things burned, the greater the honor.[44] Spices worth seventy talents were also burned when the talmudic sage Rabban Gamliel the Elder died.[45]

It was prophesied for King Zedekiah: *thou shalt die in peace, and with the burning of thy fathers, the former kings that were before thee, so shall they make a burning for thee.*[46] *Rashi* again states that it was the custom to burn the bed and personal articles of deceased kings in their honor. The same interpretation is given by *Metzudat David* and *Radak*. For King Jehoram, however, *his people made no burning for him like the burning of his fathers.*[47]

After the death of Saul and his sons, the Bible states:

> *And all the valiant men arose, and went all night, and took the body of Saul and the bodies of his sons from the wall of Beth-Shan; and they came to Jabesh, and burnt them there. . . . And they took their bones and buried them.* [48]

Rashi explains that they burned for them as one burns for kings. *Metzudat David* and *Radak* offer three explanations of this burning. First, their beds and utensils were burned, as was the custom to honor a deceased king. Second, they burned fragrant spices, as they did to embalm Jacob and Joseph. Third, perhaps the bodies were so badly decomposed that it would have been an affront to the dead to bury them in that state, and therefore they burned the flesh and buried the bones.

These burnings for deceased kings but not for ordinary citizens are specifically permitted by Maimonides and Karo in their codes.[49] Preuss asserts that the aforementioned burnings were for the kings but not the king himself.[50] An apparent biblical case of cremation is recorded in the prophet's statement that God will punish Moab because they were so vindictive against their enemies that they would not allow the slain body of the king of Edom to be honorably buried but burned it to ashes to be used as lime.[51] This case, however, dealt with a non-Jewish king. Another exceptional biblical case is the burning by King Josiah of the bones of idolatrous priests[52] to fulfill the prophecy of *the man of God out of Judah.*[53]

Preuss points out several indirect references to cremation in the Talmud.[54] Thus, ritual defilement is discussed in relation to "the ashes of burned corpses."[55] An inheritance dispute is described in a case where the testator made the specific request "burn me."[56] The Sadducees literally interpreted the biblical command of burning for capital offenses to mean cremation and once burned a priest's adulterous daughter.[57] A curse on the wicked states that even their bones should be burned[58] or pulverized.[59] The Talmud also presumes that the Romans practiced cremation when it quotes Titus as having said, "Burn me and strew my ashes over the sea."[60]

Recent Rabbinic Opinions on Embalming and Cremation

Rabbi Jekuthiel Judah Greenwald describes modern embalming to consist of the insertion of a tube into the abdomen of the deceased to remove the bad odor and dirty liquids from the deceased and the removal of his blood through the blood vessels in his extremities.[61] Then balm is instilled into his heart through a tube so that his flesh will become hard and not decay. In some places, continues Greenwald, only the blood is removed through the extremities and embalming fluid injected, and no more. This, in fact, is the most widely practiced method of embalming today, in which no incisions are made in the body and no organs are removed. Embalming fluid is injected into major veins or arteries of the deceased, displacing the blood which flows out. The injection is continued until the fluid emanating from the vessels is clear. Embalming fluid may also be injected into the abdominal cavity but without incisions or bowel removal.

Another method cited by Greenwald and discussed in greater detail by Rabbi Joshua Baumol[62] is called "freezing," in which nothing is done to the body of the deceased except that various spices are placed in his nose so that the body will not dry out rapidly. This type of "freezing" is permissible. However, two Jewish legal issues which are of concern where embalming is performed, as defined above by Greenwald, are the prohibition against desecrating the dead[63] and the prevention of the decay and hence atonement of the deceased.[64] Greenwald adds that according to Rabbi Moshe Schreiber, the embalming of Joseph was performed in the manner of embalming used today, but it was permitted because it was for his honor.[65] Rabbi Yitzchok Ralbag states that although the embalming of Jacob and Joseph may have been done for their honor, it is not permissible for any ordinary citizen to be embalmed if that involves desecration of the dead by the making of incisions and/or removal of organs or if it involves delaying the natural decay of the body, because the body must return to the earth and the soul to God, and the body decay precedes the soul's return to God.[66] Furthermore, states Ralbag, it is likely that the embalming of Jacob and Joseph only involved the perfuming and spicing of their body, but embalming as we know it today is prohibited.

Rabbi Yechiel Michael Tokazynsky expresses concern about the removal of the blood of the deceased as part of the embalming process as well as the effect of the embalming fluid in delaying the decay of the body.[67] Such decay is part of the goal of burial of bodies so that the soul can return to God. Tokazynsky recognizes the need during hot weather to transport bodies between cities and even between countries for burial and allows the injection of spices and aromatic fluids through the nose or navel to temporarily preserve the body from decay without emptying the body of blood. For travel over great distances, such as from the United States to Israel, embalming fluid may be injected into the blood vessels. However, the blood and other body fluids which are expressed as a result of the injection should be placed in a bottle and sent along with the body for burial. He also states that the embalming of Jacob and Joseph was done because their bodies had to be transported from Egypt to Israel.

Rabbi J. David Bleich states that the embalming process, wherein the blood of the deceased is replaced by an embalming fluid, is strictly forbidden by Jewish law as a gross desecration of the body.[68] Morticians who embalm the remains of a Jewish deceased person as a matter of course violate the religious sensibilities and rights of the deceased and the survivors. A rabbi should be consulted regarding procedures for the purpose of transportation.

In regard to cremation, Bleich states that cremation of the remains of a Jewish person is a gross desecration strictly forbidden by Jewish law.[69] It is an act that reflects a total negation of belief in the resurrection of the dead, which is a basic principle of faith. When a person mandates cremation of his remains, his ashes are not to be interred in a Jewish cemetery, and in many cases, the surviving family is not required to observe the usual mourning period. Bleich also adds that cosmetic treatment of the body of the deceased is forbidden. Public viewing of the body is considered an outrageous humiliation of the dead, in complete violation of the spirit and the letter of the *Halachah* (Jewish law). By the same token, relatives are forbidden to embrace the deceased or even touch him except when involved in preparation for interment.

Britain's Chief Rabbi Immanuel Jakobovits also states that cremation after death is a denial in the belief in a hereafter for body and soul.[70] The same opinion is expressed by Tokozynsky, who asserts that cremation is a denial of the belief in bodily resurrection and an affront to the dignity of the human body.[71]

Finally, Rabinowicz quotes Chief Rabbi Nathan Adler of Britain, who in 1887, though opposed to cremation, permitted the ashes of a person who had been cremated to be interred in a Jewish cemetery.[72] The decision was sustained in 1891 by his successor, Rabbi Herman Adler, who quoted the authority of Rabbi Isaac Elchanan Spector. So too, continues Rabinowicz, was the opinion of Chief Rabbi Zadok Kahn of France.

Epilogue

For a more detailed discussion of Jewish practices and procedures after death, including the washing and cleansing and ritual purification of the body, the use of coffins to effectuate burial, the different types of graves, such as vaults, sepulchres, caves, or the ground, the funeral, and the like, the reader is referred elsewhere.[73] The Medical Ethics Committee of the Federation of Jewish Philanthropies of New York, in its *Compendium on Medical Ethics*, summarizes the Jewish view of procedures after death.

> The inviolate right of a person to life, which differentiates mankind from all other animal species, extends an aura of

holiness over the body even after the Divine soul leaves it. The sanctity of an individual does not cease with death. The body, like the soul, is the property of the One who created it. It is therefore not permitted to injure or mutilate the body except when overriding consideration for the preservation of life and health make such action necessary. . . .

Reverent treatment of the body and speedy interment are biblically-ordained precepts. Cremation, freeze-storage of the body, and above-ground burial crypts, are all in violation of Jewish law and practice. The duty to bury in the ground applies to all parts of the body and is the obligation of the next of kin. Even where testamentary direction to be cremated has been given, Jewish law requires that it be ignored as an unwarranted desecration of the body.[74]

Notes

1. C. Singer and E. A. Underwood, *A Short History of Medicine*, 2d ed. (New York and Oxford: Oxford University Press, 1962), pp. 3–4.
2. H. Karplus, "Embalming," in *Encyclopaedia Judaica*, (1972) vol. 6, cols. 718–719.
3. Singer and Underwood, loc. cit.
4. F. H. Garrison, *An Introduction to the History of Medicine*, 3d ed. (Philadelphia: Saunders, 1924), pp. 50–52.
5. Ibid.
6. A. Goldstein and M. Schecter, *Otzar Harefuah Vehabriyut. Lexicon Refui.* (Tel Aviv: Dvir, 1955), p. 416.
7. Song of Songs 2:13.
8. S. R. Hirsch, *The Pentateuch*, trans. Isaac Levy, Vol. 1. Genesis, 2d ed. (London, 1963), p. 680.
9. Genesis 50:2.
10. Ibid. 50:2–3., Ibid. 50:26.
11. Ibid. 50:2.
12. J. H. Hertz, *The Pentateuch and Haftorahs*, 2d ed. (London: Soncino Press, 1962), p. 188.
13. J. Preuss, *Biblical and Talmudic Medicine*, trans. F. Rosner (New York: Hebrew Publishing Co., 1978), p. 512.
14. H. Sperling, and M. Simon, transl., *The Zohar* (London: Soncino Press, 1934), vol. 2, p. 392. The biblical quotation at the end is from Genesis 50:26.
15. Y. Ralbag, in *Harefuah Le'or Hahalachah*, (Jerusalem: Institute for Research in Medicine and Halachah, 1983), vol. 2, pp. 9–14.
16. I Samuel 31:12–13.
17. Heller, Commentary on Pesachim 4:9.
18. Responsa *Rashba*, pt. 1, no. 369.
19. *Chatam Sofer, Yoreh-Deah*, no. 336.
20. II Chronicles 16:14.
21. In Jewish law a dead person is washed and anointed. See the talmudic discussion in Shabbat 23:5.
22. Hirsch, loc. cit.
23. Y. Koli *Yalkut me'am Lo'ez: Sefer Bereshit* (Jerusalem: Mossad Yad Ezrah, 1968), p. 817.
24. Ralbag. loc. cit.
25. F. Rosner and J. D. Bleich, *Jewish Bioethics* (New York: Hebrew Publishing Co., 1979), pp, 331–348.
26. Genesis 33:18.
27. Ibid. 50:3.
28. Ibid. 50-26.
29. Koli, op. cit., p. 840.
30. Sotah 13a.

31. Baba Batra 3b. According to a footnote in the Soncino edition of the Talmud (Baba Batra, p. 10), the maiden was Marianne, daughter of Alexander, a son of Aristobulus II.
32. Preuss, op. cit., p. 513.
33. Josephus, *Antiquities*, bk. 14, chap. 7:4, and *The Jewish War*, bk. 1, chap. 9:1.
34. Genesis 3:19, I Kings 14:13, and elsewhere.
35. Jeremiah 16:4.
36. Sanhedrin 46b, based on Deuteronomy 21:23.
37. Maimonides, *Mishneh Torah, Hilchot Sanhedrin* 15:8, Karo, *Shulchan Aruch, Yoreh Deah* 362:1 ff.
38. Avodah Zarah 1:3.
39. E.g., Joshua 7:15 and 7:25.
40. Leviticus 20:14 and 21:9.
41. Sanhedrin 52a.
42. II Chronicles 16:13–14.
43. Sanhedrin 52b.
44. Avodah Zarah 11a.
45. Ibid.
46. Jeremiah 34:5.
47. II Chronicles 21:19.
48. I Samuel 31:12–13.
49. Maimonides, *Mishneh Torah, Hilchot Avel* 14:26; Karo, *Shulchan Aruch, Yoreh Deah* 345:1.
50. Preuss, op. cit., p. 521.
51. Amos 2:1.
52. II Kings 23:16.
53. I Kings 13:1–3.
54. Preuss, op. cit., p. 523.
55. Oholot 2:2.
56. Jerusalem Talmud, Ketubot 11:34b.
57. Sanhedrin 52b.
58. Jerusalem Talmud Shebiit 8:38b.
59. Genesis Rabbah 28:3.
60. Gittin 56b.
61. J. J. Greenwald, *Kol Bo Al Avelut* (Jerusalem: Feldheim, 1972), chap. 1, sec. 3, p. 51.
62. J. Baumol, *Emek Halachah*, nos. 48 and 49.
63. Rosner and Bleich, loc. cit.
64. Sanhedrin 47b.
65. Schreiber, loc. cit.
66. Ralbag, loc. cit.
67. Y. M. Tokazynsky, *Gesher Hachayim*, 2d ed. (Jerusalem, 1960), pt. 1, chap. 5, pp. 73–74.
68. J. D. Bleich, *Judaism and Healing*, (New York: Ktav, 1981), p. 179.
69. Ibid., pp. 175–183.

70. I. Jakobovits, *Journal of a Rabbi* (New York: Living Books, 1966), pp. 292–293.

71. Tokazynsky, loc. cit.

72. H. Rabinowicz, "Cremation," in *Encyclopaedia Judaica* (1972), vol. 5, cols. 1072–1073.

73. Preuss, op. cit., pp. 516–521; I. Jakobovits, *Jewish Medical Ethics* (New York: Bloch, 1975), pp. 216–152; Bleich, op. cit., pp. 175–183.

74. D. M. Feldman, and F. Rosner *Compendium on Medical Ethics*, 6th ed. (New York: Federation of Jewish Philanthropies, 1984), p. 109.

PART IV
General Issues

25

Animal Experimentation

Introduction and Background

Throughout history, animals have played an important role in man's understanding of himself and his environment. Veterinary medicine was already quite advanced in ancient India one thousand years before the common era.[1] The Greeks practiced dissection on pigs and other animals. Galen studied the anatomy and physiology of the Barbary ape because of its similarity to man. Over the years, a wide variety of animal "models" have made invaluable contributions to the understanding, treatment, and cure of human diseases. These models provide essential tools for studying a broad spectrum of infectious, neoplastic, hereditary, metabolic, and other human disorders. Much of our knowledge of our own bodies and many medical discoveries stem from experiments with laboratory animals. The discovery and identification of hormones and vitamins and the testing of most antibiotics and chemicals would have been impossible without such experiments.[2]

Humane considerations in the use of experimental animals have been discussed, often with considerable vigor, for more than a century. Medical research workers whose studies involve experiments on animals have been and continue to be criticized because they are said to needlessly repeat and duplicate experiments, subject animals to unnecessary pain and distress, use too many animals, and obtain insignificant information.[3] Scientific groups counter by asserting that experimental procedures may cause pain and distress to animals, that anesthesia is used whenever it will not interfere with the research, that although many experiments may not be significant, there is no way of determining this fact in advance, and that duplication and confirmation of experimental results are essential parts of the scientific process.

The place and importance of the experimental animal in medicine today is hotly disputed by the so-called antivivisectionists and the scientific community. One writer suggests that whenever we use animals for experiments we should ask ourselves whether the animal is the best system to investigate the problem, whether the animal must be conscious during the procedure, whether pain or discomfort to the animal could be lessened or eliminated, whether the number of animals to be used could be reduced, and whether the problem is worth solving anyway.[4] The abolition of experiments on animals is both impracticable and improbable, but the regulation of animal experimentation is both practical and possible.[5]

In Britain, concerns about animal experimentation began early in the nineteenth century with the establishment in 1824 of the Royal Society for the Prevention of Cruelty to Animals, whose main focus was and is to stop painful animal research. Partially in response to these concerns, and because antivivisection in England had become a raging controversy, the British Association for the Advancement of Science in 1870 developed guidelines for conducting physiological experiments, including steps to minimize suffering and to discourage experiments on animals which were not clearly legitimate. In 1875, Queen Victoria established a royal commission to investigate the use in Britain of live animals for experiments, to study the cruelty that might be involved, and to suggest possible ways to prevent it. The report of the commission resulted in the subsequent passage in 1876 of the now famous Cruelty to Animals Act. The main features of the act include the licensing of experimenters, the establishment of an inspectorate, and the Pain Rule. Pain to the animal had to be minimized, experiments had to have the goal of alleviating human suffering, and experiments on domestic animals, such as cats, dogs, and horses, required special certification.

The immediate impact of the Cruelty to Animals Act was to drastically reduce animal experimentation. In response, the medical and scientific communities in 1882 established the Association for the Advancement of Medicine by Research, whose goal was to promote research and to seek a just implementation of the 1876 Cruelty to Animals Act. The administrative approval of applications for licenses to experiment on living animals was transferred from the Home Secretary to this association, which issued licenses to large numbers of qualified scientists. Experimental science and medicine increased rapidly. The controversy in Britain did not abate, and many antivivisectionists and humane societies are to this day trying to abolish most if not all animal experimentation. Many scholarly works dealing with antivivisection have been published and are summarized by Lowe.[6] The 1876 Cruelty to Animals Act is still in effect today, although the House of Lords held new hearings in 1980 with the intent of making the first real modification of the venerable act in over a century. Two years earlier, the Council of Europe assembled an expert committee to draw up a convention to protect animals used in research and testing from unlicensed exploitation.[7] The draftsmen of the Home Office in London are awaiting final agreement on the European convention on animal experiments before recommending new legislation to replace and update the 1876 Cruelty to Animals Act.

In the United States, the American Society for the Prevention of Cruelty to Animals (ASPCA) was founded in 1866. The following year and again in 1880, antivivisection bills were presented to the New York State legislature. Both failed. In 1883, the first antivivisection society was founded in Philadelphia. It was not until the end of the nineteenth century, when scientific disciplines were found to be necessary for the education of physicians, that protests against the use of animals for experimentation became organized. Activities by American animal-protection groups have increased since that time and culminated in proposed federal legislation which, if passed, would not only restrict the use of animals for research but would also interfere with the kinds of research that could be conducted. Present laws relating to research animals, including the Federal Laboratory Welfare Act (1966), the Animal Welfare Act (1970), and its amendments (1976), cover only the transportation, procurement, and care of animals; they expressly exempt the treatment animals receive in research study. In the Ninety-sixth Congress in 1980, two major bills were introduced. The first, H. R. 4805, known as the Research Modernization Act, would have established a National Center of Alternative Research and required the diversion of 30 to 50 percent of all federal funds supporting research involving the use of animals to be spent for the development of alternative methods for such research. Included in this diversion would be all research funds of the National Institutes of Health, National Science Foundation, Food and Drug Administration, Department of Defense, Department of Agriculture, Department of the Interior, Environmental Protection Agency, Veterans Administration, and military medical centers. The second major bill, H.R. 6847, was intended to amend the existing Animal Welfare Act. Both bills failed. The former was reintroduced in the Ninety-seventh Congress as bill H.R. 556.

The National Institutes of Health (NIH) reauthorization bill, S. 540, the only legislation passed by the 98th Congress which dealt with animal research issues was vetoed by the President. All other bills and resolutions affecting the Animal Welfare Act and other animal research and testing issues—there were a dozen—died with adjournment. While the 98th Congress did halt the use of dogs and cats in the Department of Defense wound laboratories by amendment to the FY 84 appropriations bill, efforts to prohibit the use of all species of animals from wound research were not successful.

On February 19, 1985, Congressman Robert Torricelli of New Jersey filed H.R. 1145 in the U.S. House of Representatives, identical to H.R. 5098 which he introduced the previous year. The Torricelli bill would provide for a comprehensive, full-text literature search before the approval of federal funding for any proposed research involving animals because "overwhelming numbers of laboratory animals are used in duplicative research . . .". The bill would also establish a National Center for Research Accountability to review all research proposals involving animals approved by Federal agencies.

On a state level more than 100 bills were introduced in 1984 mostly dealing with the availability of pound animals for research and amendment of animal cruelty laws.

American scientists are facing three possibilities: mandatory regulation through legislation, self-regulation, or some combination of both. The Committee on Animal Research at the New York Academy of Sciences recommended a program to establish ethical standards and humane guidelines to reduce where possible the number of animals and to avoid unnecessary duplication of experiments. The position of the National Institutes of Health (NIH) is that there are valid scientific reasons as well as humane considerations for affording experimental animals good care and compassionate use. It is the responsibility of those who use animals to care for them. NIH policy requires that recipients of its awards assure NIH that they are carrying out this responsibility. NIH uses the National Academy of Sciences–National Research Council Guide for the Care and Use of Laboratory Animals to define acceptable animal-care standards and a set of twelve Principles for the Use of Animals to define humane animal use.[8]

Are there alternatives to animal experiments? A recent book

discussing alternatives such as cell cultures, *in vitro* assays, and vaccine production has aroused considerable debate.[9] Whether or not this book will make any difference in the attitudes of the confirmed antivivisectionists is uncertain, but it may help to convince those who are less committed that animal experimentation must remain a significant component of biological and medical research in the foreseeable future.[10] Some even consider the subject of alternatives to animal experimentation as a phony debate and a nonsubject.[11] Animal rights groups strongly support such alternatives. One such group has for the first time awarded a grant to a medical research institution to develop an *in vitro* alternative to the Draize irritation test, which uses skin or eye reactions of rabbits to indicate possible toxic effects of proposed formulations of cosmetics intended for beauty care.[12]

The scientific community marshaled its forces to counteract the activities of animal-protection groups and their powerful lobbying efforts on the legislative front. The American Registry of Certified Animal Scientists asserted that the time has come for animal scientists to assert their prerogatives, promote their expertise, and practice their talents. The time has come for the animal-science profession to lead the animal-welfare movement so far as domestic-animal production, research, and teaching are concerned.[13] Restricting research on animals would severely reduce the number of experiments that might shed light and provide knowledge to enable medical science to alleviate human suffering.[14]

Recently, the ethical and philosophical issues in experimenting on animals and especially higher animals have been topics of extensive discussion and debate.[15] Editorials and commentaries in the British and American medical literatures continue to speak out on this topic.[16] The last word has not yet been heard.

The views of the world's great religions on the use of animal experimentation for scientific purposes need to be brought to the attention of both scientists and animal-protection groups. The present essay presents the moral and religious tenets of Judaism as applied to animal experimentation.

Judaism's Prohibition of Cruelty to Animals

PROLOGUE

The All-Merciful One shows mercy over all His creatures, including animals, and provides food for their sustenance.[17] A righteous man has regard for his animal.[18] Rabbi Gamliel Beribbi said: *And he shall give thee mercy, and have compassion upon thee and multiply thee* means that he who is merciful to others, mercy is shown to him by heaven, while he who is not merciful to others, mercy is not shown to him by heaven.[19]

Jews are inherently a compassionate people, for it is written *And (He will) show thee mercy and have compassion upon thee,* teaching that whoever is merciful to his fellow beings is certainly of the children of our father Abraham, and whosoever is not merciful to his fellow beings is certainly not of the children of our father Abraham.[20]

BIBLICAL SOURCES

The Jewish attitude toward animals has always been governed by the consideration that they, too, are God's creatures,[21] and *His tender mercies are over all His works,*[22] including animals. Not only is cruelty to animals prohibited (see below), but humaneness, compassion, and mercy to animals are demanded of man by God. God *gives to the beast its food, causes the grass to spring up for the cattle, satisfies every living thing,* and *preserves man and beast.*[23] God's concern extends from the lion, king of the beasts, to the raven, one of the most despised of birds.[24] When Moses obtained water from the rock by Divine intervention, the water was to give drink to *the congregation and their cattle.*[25] One reason for the commandment to let the fields lie fallow in the Sabbatical year is that the food which grows naturally there during that year shall be *for thy cattle and for the beasts that are in thy land.*[26]

Animals must have their Sabbath rest the same as man, as it states: *but the seventh day is a Sabbath unto the Lord, in it thou shalt not do any manner of work, thou, nor thy son, nor thy daughter, nor thy man-servant, nor thy maid-servant, nor thy cattle,* and later Scripture commands: *six days shalt thou do thy work, but on the seventh day, thou shalt rest; that thine ox and thine ass may rest.*[27] We thus clearly see the humanitarian teaching of affording complete rest to one's domesticated animals on the Sabbath. In the repetition of the Decalogue in Deuteronomy, this teaching is reiterated.[28] The Chief Rabbi of Great Britain explained that care and kindness to animals are included in the Decalogue because this duty is of profound importance for the humanizing of man.[29]

Thoughtfulness for animals as a religious duty is demonstrated in numerous biblical narratives. Rebekah proved that she was the proper wife for Isaac, son of Abraham the Patriarch, by the fact that she brought water not only for Abraham's servant Eliezer but also for his camels.[30] The parable with which Nathan rebuked King David took for granted that a lamb can be a household pet to be treated kindly.[31] A righteous man is merciful and pays attention to the needs of his beast.[32] God Himself admonished Jonah saying: *and should not I have pity on Nineveh, that great city, wherein are more than six score thousand persons . . . and also much cattle?*[33]

Numerous biblical commandments have as one possible explanation or allusion the prohibition of cruelty to animals. These include the prohibitions against muzzling an ox as it threshes to deprive it of food while it is working, the slaughtering of an animal and its young on the same day, the eating of a limb cut off from a living animal, the plowing with an ox and an ass together, and the command to release the mother bird from the nest before taking the young.[34] The prohibition of not muzzling the ox when he treads corn applies to all animals employed in labor. In his biblical commentary, Rabbi Abraham Ibn Ezra suggests that the reason for not plowing with an ox and an ass together is that the ox, being the stronger, would pull harder and thus cause pain to the ass.[35] In his philosophical masterpiece, the *Guide for the Perplexed*, Moses Maimonides explains some of these laws as follows:[36]

> It is likewise forbidden to slaughter *it and its young on the same day*,[37] this being a precautionary measure in order to avoid slaughtering the young animal in front of its mother. For in these cases animals feel very great pain, there being no difference regarding this pain between man and the other animals. For the love and the tenderness of a mother for her child is not consequent upon reason, but upon the activity of the imaginative faculty, which is found in most animals just as it is found in man. This law applies in particular to ox and lamb, because these are the domestic animals that we are allowed to eat and that in most cases it is usual to eat. . . . This is also the reason for the commandment to *let [the mother] go from the nest.*[38] For in general, the eggs over which the bird has sat and the young that need their mother are not fit to be eaten. If then the mother is let go and escapes of her own accord, she will not be pained by seeing that the young are taken away.

The homiletical commentary on the Bible known as the *Midrash Rabbah* states that just as God shows mercy to man, so too has He shown mercy to cattle.[39] Whence this? For it is said, *Ye shall not kill it and its young both in one day.*[40] And in the same way that God had compassion upon the cattle, so too was God filled with mercy for the birds, as it is said, *If a bird's nest chance before thee . . . thou shalt not take the dam with the young.*[41]

Commenting on the scriptural verse *And whether it be cow or ewe, ye shall not kill it and its young both in one day,*[42] the Midrash asserts as follows:[43]

> Rabbi Berachiah said in the name of Rabbi Levi: It is written, *A righteous man regardeth the life of his beast.*[44] *Righteous man* applies to the Holy One, blessed be He, in whose Torah it is written, *Thou shalt not take the dam with the young.*[45]

Elsewhere the Midrash relates that a creeping thing ran past Rabbi Judah the Patriarch's daughter. She was about to kill it when he said to her: "My daughter, let it be, for it is written, *And His tender mercies are over all His works.*"[46] Even the regulation regarding the hired servant, *In the same day shalt thou give him his hire,* is homiletically applied to the beast.[47]

Moses and David were chosen as leaders because God noted their gentle and understanding treatment of their flocks.[48] Legend tells how Moses, while still Jethro's shepherd, sought out a stray lamb and tenderly carried the tired creature in his arms back to the fold. A voice from heaven cried out: "Thou art worthy to be My people's pastor."

When Balaam smote his ass, the angel rebuked him saying: *wherefore hast thou smitten thine ass these three times?*[49] This verse is a classical text for the preaching of humane treatment of animals. Castration or emasculation of animals is also prohibited, based on the verse *and that which is mauled or crushed or torn or cut you shall not offer unto the Lord; nor shall you do this in your land.*[50]

The major biblical source for the prohibition of cruelty to animals is the law that if one sees an animal staggering under a burden too heavy for it, one must stop and help unload it, even if the animal belongs to one's enemy.[51] This law shows the humanitarian motive toward the animal and the charitable motive toward the enemy. This law is codified by Maimonides in his famous *Mishneh Torah,* where he rules that a person is enjoined to unload the burden from an animal that is crouching under the weight of the burden, even if the owner is not present with the animal, and even if the animal belongs to a heathen.[52]

In his *Guide for the Perplexed*, Maimonides explains the prohibition of cruelty to animals as follows:[53]

> As for the dictum of the sages: [To avoid causing] suffering to animals is [an injunction to be found] in the Torah—in which they refer to its dictum *wherefore hast thou smitten thine ass*[54]—it is set down with a view to perfecting us so that we should not acquire moral habits of cruelty and should not inflict pain gratuitously without any utility, but that we should intend to be kind and merciful even with a chance animal individual, except in case of need—*Because thy soul desireth to eat flesh*,[55] for we must not kill out of cruelty or for sport.

Maimonides here clearly prohibits hunting for sport (see below). He also introduces the concept of meat consumption to satisfy one's appetite. Many Jewish sects were strictly vegetarian. In fact, prior to the Flood, meat consumption was not yet sanctioned. Adam and Eve were blessed by God, who told them: *Be fruitful and multiply, and replenish the earth and subdue it; and have dominion over the fish of the sea, and over the fowl of the air, and over every living thing that creepeth on the earth.*[56] To *have dominion over* means to use for work purposes,[57] but not to eat, since God also told Adam and Eve: *Behold, I have given you every herb yielding seed, which is upon the face of all the earth, and every tree. . . . to you shall it be for food; and to every beast of the earth, and to every fowl of the air and to every thing that creepeth upon the earth, wherein there is a living soul (I have given) every green herb for food.*[58] Thus, man and animals were originally vegetarians,[59] although the sacrificing of animals to God had been previously allowed.[60] After Noah and his family saved the animals from extinction, God made a concession to man by giving him the right to consume meat,[61] provided the animals are humanely slaughtered. It has been suggested that the Jewish method of ritual slaughter, particularly the laws that the knife be exceedingly sharp and without the slightest notch, are motivated by consideration for the animal because this method is the most painless.

Eating a limb cut off from a living animal is prohibited even to non-Jews.[62] In his *Guide for the Perplexed*, Maimonides explains the reason for this prohibition: because such an act would make one acquire the habit of cruelty.[63] Maimonides continues by asserting that

> the commandment concerning the slaughtering of animals is necessary. For the natural food of man consists only of the plants deriving from the seeds growing in the earth and of the flesh of animals, the most excellent kinds of meat being those that are permitted to us [i.e., kosher animals]. No physician is ignorant of this. Now since the necessity to have good food requires that animals be killed, the aim was to kill them in the easiest manner, and it was forbidden to torment them through killing them in a reprehensible manner by piercing the lower part of their throat or by cutting off one of their members, just as we have explained.

TALMUDIC SOURCES

The Talmud, both in its legal (halachic) and its homiletical (aggadic) portions, is replete with references relating to the mandate to be kind to animals and the prohibition of cruelty to animals. The Talmud states that small appliances were made for rams so that their tails would not knock against rocks.[64] Furthermore, straps were placed on the legs of fowl to prevent the legs from knocking each other. A jaw bar was placed around the neck of an ass with a bruise to prevent it from chafing it afresh and to allow it to heal.[65] After an ewe was sheared, a compress saturated in oil was placed on its forehead so that she would not catch cold. When an ewe kneeled for lambing, two oily compresses were made for her: one was placed on her forehead and the other on her womb, so that she would be warmed. A chip of wood was placed in the nostril of an ewe to make her sneeze, so that worms in her head would fall out. Hedgehog skins were placed over cows' udders to prevent hedgehogs from sucking the udders.[66]

The Talmud also asserts that one helps fledglings ascend into or descend from a hen coop by overturning a basket for them in front of the coop.[67] One may assist an animal in giving birth on the Sabbath, and the newborn calf or lamb or other baby animal is held, so that it does not fall on the ground. One also blows into the baby animal's nostrils to clear them of mucus and puts the teat into its mouth so that it can suck. If an animal falls into a canal filled with water on the Sabbath, one must relieve it of its suffering pending its rescue after the termination of the Sabbath. One must feed it and, if necessary, place pillows or mattresses underneath the animal to enable it to raise itself out of the water and escape from its suffering, even though one is normally prohibited on the Sabbath from handling articles not previously designated for that purpose.[68] Maimonides codifies this rule when he states that if an animal falls into a cistern or irrigation canal one may bring pillows and blankets to place under it because Sabbath laws are waived by the duty to alleviate the animal's suffering.[69]

Thus, one may desecrate the Sabbath and Jewish holidays to relieve the suffering of an animal, since cruelty to animals is a biblical prohibition which takes precedence over rabbinically enacted Sabbath laws. To save animals from suffering is regarded as a stronger reason for desecrating the Sabbath than to save oneself from personal loss.[70] Elsewhere in the Talmud there is debate as to whether the prohibition of cruelty to animals is biblical or rabbinic in nature.[71] Although most talmudic sages and codes of Jewish law consider it to be a biblical command to relieve the suffering of an animal, some sages, such as Rabbi Jose the Galilean[72] and Rabbi Gamliel,[73] consider it to be enjoined merely by rabbinic law.

A person should not buy an animal or a bird unless he can properly provide for it.[74] A man is forbidden to eat before he gives food to his beast,[75] since Scripture first says *And I will give grass in thy field for thy cattle* and then *thou shalt eat and be satisfied.*[76] Maimonides confirms that the sages of old would not partake of a meal before they fed their cattle.[77] The All-Merciful One shows pity to living creatures.[78] A man who confined his neighbor's animal in a place exposed to the sun, so that it died of sunstroke, was held liable.[79] When one rabbi wanted to hamstring some mules, he was told by another rabbi not to do so because he would be causing suffering to animals.[80] Only in very exceptional cases may cattle be disabled,[81] where the commandment forbidding cruelty to animals is waived.[82]

The story is told that a calf being taken to be slaughtered broke away and hid its head under the skirts of Rabbi Judah the Prince. He said to it: "Go, for this wast thou created." Thereupon they said in heaven: "Since he has no pity, let us bring suffering upon him." So Rabbi Judah suffered from a toothache for thirteen years; he was cured when he saved the lives of a litter of kittens.[83]

Although meat consumption was permitted to man after the Flood, the Talmud recommends that meat be eaten only when one has an overwhelming desire for it.[84] Although one may eat meat after ritual slaughter of an animal, one may not eat flesh cut from a living animal.[85]

THE CODES OF JEWISH LAW

The major codes of Jewish law, the *Mishneh Torah* of Moses Maimonides and the *Shulchan Aruch* of Joseph Karo, consider cruelty to animals to be a biblical offense. Many of the talmudic rules and regulations cited above in regard to kindness to animals and the alleviation of suffering of animals are codified by both Maimonides and Karo. Karo states that a person who meets his friend on the way and the latter's animal is crouching from its burden must help unload that animal, as it is written: *thou shalt surely release it with him.*[86]

One must help unload the animal even repeatedly and without recompense,[87] to which Moses Isserles, known as *Ramah,* in his gloss on Karo's code, adds: "because cruelty to animals is a biblical offense."[88] Maimonides' similar ruling on this matter has already been cited earlier in this chapter.

Maimonides also asserts that a person must dismount from his animal on the Sabbath to prevent it from suffering.[89] Similarly, if one returns from a journey on Friday night with a laden animal, one may unload its pack on the Sabbath for the same reason. Under no circumstances may one leave a laden animal unloaded until after the Sabbath, since one would cause it to suffer.[90]

Other religious laws are waived to save animals from distress or pain and to preserve their health. Karo rules that the prohibition of muzzling an ox or any other animal when it plows the field to restrain it from eating freely is set aside if the food on which the animal works is injurious to its bowels and would cause diarrhea.[91] Karo also rules that if an animal ate an overdose of horse beans on the Sabbath and is in distress, one may cause it to run around the yard until it becomes exhausted and thus cured.[92] If an animal is suffering from plethora, it may be placed in water on the Sabbath to cool it.[93]

Other relaxations of the Sabbath and Festival laws for the sake of sick animals are quoted by Jakobovits[94] and include permission to capture them, to anoint fresh and painful animal wounds with oil or salve, to bleed an animal if it suffers from a seizure of blood, to assist an animal in giving birth and care for its young, to remove flies irritating an animal, notwithstanding the small wound thus caused, to ask a non-Jew to milk an animal if the milk causes distress to the animal, and to anoint placental fluid on a newborn animal rejected by its mother to make its mother have compassion on her young.[95]

Although the carrying of objects through a public thoroughfare is ordinarily prohibited on the Sabbath, an animal is permitted to carry objects which are worn for its protection,[96] or for health reasons, or for the prevention of pain, such as a bandage around a wound or splints to protect a fracture.[97]

Animal Experimentation in Jewish Law

In his gloss to Karo's code, Isserles *(Ramah)* states that anything necessary for medical or other useful purposes is excluded from the prohibition of cruelty to animals.[98] Hence, he adds, "it is permissible to pluck feathers from living geese" in order to obtain quills for writing without considering the ban on causing pain to animals. Nevertheless, concludes Isserles, "one refrains from doing so because it is an act of cruelty." Jakobovits cites the fifteenth-century sources upon which Isserles based his ruling, none of which actually specifies any medical use to which living animals can be put.[99] Nevertheless, all subsequent permissive rabbinic rulings on animal experimentation for medical research are based on this statement by Isserles that for medical or other useful purposes, the prohibition of cruelty to animals does not apply. Isserles also states that the consideration of cruelty does not apply if the removal of some feathers from a bird's neck[100] or of some wool from a sheep's neck[101] is essential to prepare the animal for ritual slaughter. The digest of rabbinic responsa known as *Otzar Haposkim* offers two additional reasons for removing the goose feathers: it is good for them, and it makes them fatter.[102]There seems to be no known scientific rationale for this assertion.

In the eighteenth century, Jacob Reischer was asked whether or not a Jewish physician is permitted to test the effects of a new drug on an animal, such as a dog or cat, in order to discover whether it might prove injurious or even fatal before applying it to human beings. His strongly affirmative answer[103] was based in part on several earlier responsa[104] which rule, like Isserles, that anything required for a useful purpose for mankind, including medical uses, is excluded from the biblical prohibitions of wanton destruction[105] and cruelty to animals. Reischer asserts that if the Sabbath must be descrated to save a human life, the prohibition of cruelty to animals must also be set aside for the same reason. The reservation of Isserles about refraining from feather plucking from living geese because it is an act of cruelty, concludes Reischer, refers to someone who is plucking individual feathers one by one, thus causing pain. However, where the dog or cat is to be given a medicinal potion, no immediate pain or discomfort is inflicted. Hence, although the animal may later become ill or even die, for the sake of finding a cure for human illness, it is permitted.

In the nineteenth century, Jacob Ettlinger expressed the view that the permissive ruling of Isserles in Karo's code that the prohibition of cruelty to animals is waived for any medical or useful purpose is limited to medical needs but not for financial gain.[106]

Rabbinic opinions expressed during the present century are, on the whole, inclined to permit animal experimentation for medical research. In a lengthy responsum, Mordechai Jacob Breisch asserted that Isserles' concern of cruelty is primarily a moral but not a legal objection to animal experimentation.[107] Hence, continues Breisch, for reasons of piety *(midat chasidut)* one should avoid cruelty to animals. In the same volume and subsequently in his own responsa work,[108] Yechiel Weinberg answers Breisch by pointing out that animals were created only to serve man,[109] and that the prohibition of cruelty to animals applies only where no need at all is served thereby. Considerations of piety on the part of an individual, albeit ordinarily laudatory, cannot be sanctioned when the welfare of the general population might be affected. Further, "what right have you to assume that the pain of animals counts more than the pain of sick people who might be helped [by animal experimentation]?" Weinberg, therefore, concludes that it is permissible to conduct animal experimentation for medical research.

Not only is the prohibition of cruelty to animals inapplicable when the health of the general population is at stake but also when the honor of the public is involved. This principle was first cited by the twelfth- and thirteenth-century talmudic commentary of various Franco-German talmudists known collectively as *Tosafot.*[110] Excessive individual piety in regard to cruelty to animals in situations where human life may be at stake is thus inappropriate. It is, therefore, a commandment to kill all dangerous animals, such as snakes or insects which carry disease. It is also permissible to perform medical research by vivisection, provided that every effort is made to eliminate the animal's suffering as far as possible, since "it is known that thousands of persons have already been cured by discoveries made through anatomical research in this manner."[111]

Jakobovits quotes Wohlgemuth, who states that Judaism justifies vivisection of animals as long as this procedure may be conducive to the saving of human life.[112] However, in exercising this right, measures must be taken to protect the animals from all unnecessary suffering and to exclude any operation which has no bearing whatsoever on the advancement of human health.

Hunting for sport would thus be condemned in Judaism because no medical or other benefit to mankind is obtained thereby. In fact, rabbinic rulings have always forbidden hunting as a sport because cruelty for its own sake is abhorrent. Bleich cites the various rabbinic authorities who have addressed this issue and points out that the fundamental criterion in animal experimentation, establishing a line of demarcation between the permissible and the forbidden, is the relationship of the act to a legitimate human need.[113] "Pain may be inflicted upon the animal only to the degree absolutely necessary in order to obtain the required information. Otherwise, the pain does not serve to satisfy a legitimate need and is prohibited. . . . The benefits must be practical in nature and not simply the satisfaction of intellectual curiosity." Ezekiel Landau prohibits hunting for sport because it not only serves no purpose but may also endanger the hunter's life.[114] Landau also asserts that the prohibition of cruelty to animals only applies to the infliction of pain during life. Hence this prohibition does not apply to hunting and other situations where the animal is put to death.

Friedman explains the statement of Isserles that "one refrains [from plucking feathers from geese] because it is an act of cruelty" to refer only to animals whose primary purpose is to serve man as a beast of burden or to provide man with eggs, milk, wool, and the like.[115] It would be cruel to kill such an animal for food, says Friedman, before it has served its primary purpose. Chaphutta discusses at length whether the prohibition of cruelty to animals is biblical or rabbinic in origin.[116] He also differentiates between animals and birds, on the one hand, where, other than for human need, the prohibition applies, and reptiles and insects, on the other hand, where it does not apply at all. He also distinguishes between vivisection on a live animal, where cruelty may occur, and anatomical dissection on a dead animal, where no cruelty is involved. Chaphutta concludes, as do most other rabbis, that animal experimentation for medical research is permissible.

The distinction between animals and insects had already been enunciated earlier by Jacob Emden, who said that "the prohibition of cruelty to animals only applies to animals which can perform work for man's needs. However, in regard to flies and gnats and other insects and the like, there is no prohibition of cruelty to animals, and it is permissible to kill them."[117] The same thesis seems to be implied in the Talmud, which states that the Holy One, blessed be He, did not create anything in this world without purpose; He created the snail as a remedy for the scab, the fly as an antidote to the hornet's sting, the mosquito crushed for a serpent's bite, the serpent as a remedy for an eruption, and a crushed spider as a remedy for a scorpion's bite.[118]

The most recent writings on animal experimentation in Jewish law are those of Steinberg and Metzger.[119] These authors review in detail the classical biblical, talmudic, and other Judaic writings as well as the more recent rabbinic responsa concerning the Jewish sources for the prohibition of cruelty to animals; the debate as to whether this prohibition is biblical or rabbinic in origin; scientific animal experimentation for medical, financial, or other human needs; whether or not the killing of an animal, as in ritual slaughtering or hunting, involves the prohibition of cruelty to animals; and whether or not the law prohibiting cruelty to living creatures also includes the infliction of pain on humans.

Summary and Conclusion

Jewish law not only forbids cruelty to animals but requires that we be kind to them, have compassion for them, and treat them humanely. Thus, if one sees an animal collapsing under a heavy burden, one must unload it. One may not muzzle an animal to deprive it of food while it is working. In fact, one may not partake of any food until one has first assured the provision of food for one's animals. That animals may not work on the Sabbath is a rule enunciated among the Ten Commandments, indicating that care of and kindness to animals are of profound importance for the humanizing of man.

These and other biblical and rabbinic moral and legal rules concerning the treatment of animals are based on the principle that animals are part of God's creation for which man bears responsibility. Moses Maimonides offers an insight into these rules in that he states that the prohibition of causing suffering to animals was set down with a view to perfecting humans so that we do not acquire moral habits of cruelty. Rather we should not inflict pain gratuitously without any utility, but should be kind and merciful even with a chance or stray animal. The reason why man is forbidden to eat a limb cut off from a living animal is because this act would make him acquire the habit of cruelty. The same reason is given for the rule forbidding the slaughtering of an animal and its young on the same day and the commandment to release the mother bird before taking the young.

There are many additional rules which the rabbis enacted to guard animals against hunger, overwork, disease, distress, and suffering. Wanton hunting and killing of animals for sport is prohibited. It is forbidden to inflict a blemish on an animal. Numerous Sabbath laws relating to forbidden acts are waived when such acts are intended to relieve pain of an animal. A person is not permitted to buy animals unless he can properly care and provide for them.

On the other hand, Judaism also espouses the concept that everything that was created in this world by Almighty God was created to serve mankind. Animals may thus be used as beasts of burden and for food, providing they are humanely slaughtered. Scientific experiments upon laboratory animals during the course of medical research designed to yield information that might lead to cure of disease are sanctioned by Jewish law as legitimate utilization of animals for the benefit of mankind. However, wherever possible, pain or discomfort should be eliminated or minimized by analgesia, anesthesia, or other means. Otherwise the pain does not serve to satisfy a legitimate human need and its infliction is prohibited. In addition, animal experimentation is only permissible by Jewish law if its purpose is to obtain practical benefits to mankind and not simply the satisfaction of intellectual curiosity. Furthermore, if alternative means of obtaining the same information are available, such as tissue culture studies, animal experimentation might be considered to fall under the category of unnecessary cruelty to animals and be prohibited.

Notes

1. J. R. Held, "Animals for Medical Research and Testing," *Bulletin of the Pan American Health Organization* 15 (1981): 36–48.

2. T. H. Jukes, Editorial, "Animal Research is Vital to Human Health," *American Council on Science and Health News and Views* 3 (1982): 4.

3. J. A. Sechzer, "Historical Issues Concerning Animal Experimentation in the United States," *Social Science and Medicine* 15F (1981): 13–17.

4. W. Lane-Petter, "The Place and Importance of the Experimental Animal in Medicine Today," *Proceedings of the Royal Society of Medicine* 65 (1972): 343–344.

5. W. N. Scott, "Humane Considerations in the Use of Experimental Animals," *Journal of the South African Veterinary Association* 49 (1978): 159–160.

6. F. M. Loew, "Animal Experimentation: Book Reviews," *Bulletin of the History of Medicine* 56 (1982): 123–126.

7. Editorial "Legislation and Animal Research: Is Reform Due?" *British Medical Journal* 1 (1979): 1035–1036.

8. C. McPherson, "Regulation of Animal Care and Research? NIH's Opinion," *Journal of Animal Sciences* 51 (1981): 492–496.

9. D. H. Smyth, *Alternatives to Animal Experiments* (London: Scolar Press in association with the Research Defense Society, 1978).

10. J. P. Payne, Editorial, "Animal Experimentation," *British Journal of Anaesthesiology* 50 (1978): 871–872.

11. S. Shuster, "In Ignorance Arrayed," *British Medical Journal* 1 (1978): 1541–1542.

12. P. Gunby, "Animal Rights Group Awards Research Grant," *Journal of the American Medical Association* 245 (1981): 1803.

13. S. E. Curtis, "Who Should Regulate Animal Care and Research? ARCAS's Opinion," *Journal of Animal Sciences* 51 (1981): 479–482.

14. C. R. Gallistel, "Bell, Magendie and the Proposals to Restrict the Use of Animals in Neurobehavioral Research," *American Psychologist* 36 (1981): 357–360.

15. M. W. Ross, "The Ethics of Experiments on Higher Animals," *Social Science and Medicine* 15F (1981): 51–60; T. Regan, "Animal Rights and Animal Experimentation," *Progress in Clinical and Biological Research* 50 (1981): 69–83; B. J. Cohen, "Animal Rights and Animal Experimentation," ibid. 50 (1981): 85–92.

16. Editorial, "Animal Experiments," *British Medical Journal* 2 (1982): 368; Editorial, "Protection for Laboratory Animals?" *Nature* 293 (1981): 173–174; D. H. Smyth, Editorial, "Tissue Culture as an Alternative," *Journal of the Royal Society of Medicine* 73 (1980): 229–230; M. B. Visscher, Commentary, "Current Attempts to Prevent the Use of Animals in Medical Research," *Journal of the American Medical Association* 245 (1981): 1223–1224.

17. Psalms 145:9; 147:9.
18. Proverbs 12:10.
19. Shabbat 151b, citing Deuteronomy 13:18.
20. Betzah 32b, citing Deuteronomy 13:18.
21. H. Revel, "Protection of Animals," in *Universal Jewish Encyclopedia*, (1939), 1, pp. 330–331; C. Roth, "Cruelty to Animals," in *Encyclopaedia Judaica* (1972), vol. 3, cols. 5–7; M. L. Bamberger, "Tza'ar Ba'aley Chayim" [Cruelty to animals], in *Otzar Yisrael*, ed. J. D. Eisenstein (Berlin, 1924), vol. 9, pp. 49–51; I. Jakobovits, "The Medical Treatment of Animals in Jewish Law," *Journal of Jewish Studies* 7 (1956): 207–220.
22. Psalms 145:9.
23. Ibid. 147:9, 104:14, 145:16, 36:7.
24. Job 38:39–41.
25. Numbers 20:8.
26. Leviticus 25:7.
27. Exodus 20:10, 23:12.
28. Deuteronomy 5:14.
29. J. H. Hertz, *The Pentateuch and Haftorahs*, 2d ed. (London: Soncino Press, 1962), p. 767.
30. Genesis 24:14.
31. II Samuel 12:3.
32. Proverbs 12:10.
33. Jonah 4:11.
34. Deuteronomy 25:4, Leviticus 22:28, Genesis 9:4 and Deuteronomy 12:23, ibid. 22:10, ibid. 22:6–7.
35. Ibn Ezra, commentary on Deuteronomy 22:10.
36. Maimonides, *Guide for the Perplexed* 3:48.
37. Leviticus 22:28.
38. Deuteronomy 22:6–7.
39. Deuteronomy Rabbah 6:1.
40. Leviticus 22:28.
41. Deuteronomy 22:6.
42. Leviticus 22:28.
43. Leviticus Rabbah 27:11.
44. Proverbs 12:10.
45. Deuteronomy 22:6.
46. Genesis Rabbah 33:3, citing Psalms 145:9.
47. Exodus Rabbah 31:7, citing Deuteronomy 24:15.
48. Ibid. 2:2.
49. Numbers 22:32.
50. Leviticus 22:34.
51. Exodus 23:5.
52. Maimonides, *Mishneh Torah, Hilchot Rotze'ach* 13:1, 13:8, 13:9.
53. Maimonides, *Guide for the Perplexed* 3:17.
54. Numbers 22:32.
55. Deuteronomy 12:20.

56. Genesis 1:28.
57. Psalms 8:7–9.
58. Genesis 1:29–30.
59. Sanhedrin 59b.
60. Genesis 1:29 and 9:3.
61. Ibid. 9:3.
62. Ibid. 9:4; Deuteronomy 12:23; Sanhedrin 56a–57a and 59a–b, and Chullin 101b.
63. Maimonides *Guide for the Perplexed* 3:48.
64. Shabbat 54b.
65. Ibid.
66. Ibid.
67. Ibid. 128b.
68. Ibid.
69. Maimonides, *Mishneh Torah, Hilchot Shabbat* 25:26.
70. Shabbat 117b.
71. Baba Metzia 32a–b.
72. Ibid. 33a.
73. Ibid. 154b.
74. Jerusalem Talmud, Ketubot 4:8.
75. Berachot 40a and Gittin 62a.
76. Deuteronomy 11:15.
77. Maimonides, *Mishneh Torah, Hilchot Avadim* 9:8.
78. Sanhedrin 55a.
79. Ibid. 76b.
80. Chullin 7b.
81. Joshua 11:6.
82. Avodah Zarah 13a.
83. Baba Metzia 85a.
84. Chullin 84a.
85. Sanhedrin 54b.
86. Karo, *Shulchan Aruch, Choshen Mishpat* 272:1, citing Exodus 23:5.
87. Ibid. 272:4, 272:5.
88. Ibid. 272:9.
89. Maimonides, *Mishneh Torah, Hilchot Shabbat* 21:9.
90. Ibid. 21:10.
91. Karo, *Shulchan Aruch, Choshen Mishpat* 338:7, referring to Deuteronomy 25:4.
92. Ibid., *Orach Chayim* 332.3.
93. Ibid. 332:4.
94. I. Jakobovits, "The Medical Treatment of Animals in Jewish Law," *Journal of Jewish Studies* 7 (1956): 207–220.
95. Karo, *Shulchan Aruch, Orach Chayim* 316:2, 332:2, ibid., *Yoreh Deah* 313:1; ibid., *Orach Chayim* 523:3, 523:1, 305:20, 523:3.
96. Ibid. 305:1.
97. Ibid. 305:11.

98. Karo, *Shulchan Aruch, Even Ha'ezer* 5:14.
99. Jakobovits, op. cit.
100. Moses Isserles' commentary on *Yoreh Deah* 23:6.
101. Ibid. 24:8.
102. *Oztar Haposkim, Even Ha'ezer*, vol. 1 (1974), p. 255.
103. J. Reischer, Responsa *Shevut Yaakov*, p. 3, no. 71.
104. G. Ashkenazi, Responsa *Avodat Gershuni*, no. 13; Jacob ben Samuel, Responsa *Bet Yaakov*, no. 42.
105. Based on Deuteronomy 20:19.
106. J. Ettlinger, Responsa *Binyan Zion*, no. 108.
107. M. J. Breisch, Responsa *Chelkat Yaakov*, p. 1, no. 30.
108. Y. Weinberg, in Responsa *Chelkat Yaakov*, p. 1, no. 31, idem, Responsa *Seridei Esh*, p. 3, no. 7.
109. Kiddushin 82a–b.
110. Commentary of *Tosafot* on Avodah Zarah 11a, s.v. *Okarin*.
111. J. D. Eisenstein, (ed.) *Otzar Yisrael* (1907–13), vol. 9, p. 50.
112. Jakobovits, op. cit.
113. J. D. Bleich, *Judaism and Healing* (New York: Ktav, 1981), pp. 123–125.
114. E. Landau, Responsa *Noda Biyehudah*, p. 2, *Yoreh Deah*, no. 10.
115. N. Z. Friedman, "Nisuyim Mada'eyem al Gufot Ba'ale Chayim" [Scientific experiments on living creatures], *Noam* 5 (1962): 188–194.
116. A. Chaphutta, "Bedin Tzar Ba'ale Chayim Letzorchei Refuah" [On the law of cruelty to animals for medical needs], *Noam* 4 (1961): 218–225.
117. J. Emden, Responsa *She'elat Yaavetz*, p. 1, no. 110.
118. Shabbat 77b.
119. A. Steinberg, "Tzar Ba'ale Chayim Le'ohr Hahalachah" [Cruelty to animals in Jewish law], *Assia* 1 (1976): 263–269; Z. Metzger, "Nisuyim Refuyim BeBa'ale Chayim" [Medical experiments on living animals], in *Harefuah Le'Ohr Hahalachah* (Jerusalem, 1983), pp. 1–50.

26

The Allocation of Scarce Medical Resources

Introduction

This chapter attempts to illustrate some of the current ethical dilemmas in the allocation of limited medical resources and discusses some of the present practices used to cope with these dilemmas. The propriety and feasibility of legislative solutions to the problem of scarce medical resource allocation will not be discussed. The thrust of this essay is to focus on the ethical and moral issues with emphasis on the Jewish viewpoint.

Let me define the problem. A private or voluntary hospital has no duty to furnish its services to everyone. However, if it opens an emergency room, it obligates itself to provide emergency care to the community. A doctor is not required to provide resources not generally available. He must, however, provide a level of care consonant with standard medical practice of good quality. At present, hospitals and doctors make most of the decisions in the allocation of their resources, although often neither is totally happy with that responsibility. Limited funds may not allow the hospital to buy both additional respirators and additional dialysis machines or new defibrillators. The hospital must then decide what to buy or replace. A physician with a limited supply of a new drug must decide which patient will receive it and to which patient it will be denied. Should a group of laymen be given the decision-making power to relieve the hospital and doctors of the ethical problems? How would such a group of laymen decide? What criteria would they use? Should lawyers, legislators, and judges assume the role of allocating scarce medical resources and determine hierarchies of criteria for the distribution and allocation of such resources?

The Example of Hemodialysis

Let us examine hemodialysis to illustrate the ethical issues involved in a classic situation involving the allocation of scarce medical resources. In 1973, the United States Congress legislated that all patients with kidney failure who need hemodialysis or kidney transplantation should have access thereto and that Medicare would assure the cost for the entire End Stage Renal Program. Prior to 1973, allocation decisions were made in a two-step process. First, rules of exclusion were applied to narrow the number of potential treatment recipients. Second, rules of selection were applied to choose between the remaining applicants.[1] Some factors, such as age, may be invoked in both the exclusion and the selection process.

Factors of exclusion may include: (a) *patient desires*, such as inability or unwillingness to travel to a distant location for treatment or preference for a particular doctor or hospital; (b) *hospital function* and orientation, such as veterans' hospitals, which only service veterans and only for service-related disabilities; (c) *age*, such as exclusion of patients below ten or above sixty years of age; (d) *treatment requirements*, such as the need to come to the hospital several times a week for hemodialysis or the need for running water and electricity for home dialysis; (e) *psychosocial requirements*, such as psychological stability, intelligence, and cooperation of the patient and stability of the family; (f) *medical criteria*, such as the relative contraindication of hemodialysis for diabetics and patients with certain other disorders; (g) *maximum utilization requirements*, such as the exclusion from an acute hemodialysis program of patients requiring chronic hemodialysis; (h) *ability to pay;* (i) *social worth* of the patient, such as the exclusion of drug addicts, criminals, prostitutes, and the mentally retarded or psychotic; (j) *physician bias*.

All these rules of exclusion can be criticized to a greater or lesser degree. For example, there may be more justification for medical criteria and treatment requirements for exclusion than age, ability to pay, or social worth. Rules of exclusion are preferable and easier to apply than rules of final selection. Properly applied, exclusion criteria are "probably less subjective, less arbitrary, and more acceptable to patient and doctor than the rules of final selection."[2] Serious ethical and moral dilemmas in the face of limited resources are posed where either exclusion or selection rules or both are unavoidable, as in the pre-1973 hemodialysis situation.

The two basic approaches in the selection process of patients for the allocation of scarce medical resources are: (a) comparison of the *social worth* of the various patients remaining in the selection pool; and (b) selection based on chance, such as a *first come–first served* rule or selection by lot. Most physicians seem to prefer the selection of patients by a lot or on a first-come basis.[3] A waiting-list procedure is also probably more acceptable to the patient and his family than a social-worth evaluation. Ethical problems, however, would arise when exceptions need to be made in applying the first come–first served rule. Should the President of the United States or a brilliant scientist receive preference in the allocation of a scarce resource? Should a mother of little children or a young person be preferred over a single or older person? Does not such preference negate the first come–first served rule and apply the social-worth approach which is so objectionable to many people? Practical necessity and the public conscience may, however, require exceptions to be made.

Another approach is to combine the exclusion and the selection criteria into a single slightly different set of both medical and social factors, such as constituency (e.g., children's hospitals will not serve adults), progress of science, prospect of success, life expectancy, family role, potential future contributions, and past services rendered.[4] Each of these factors is not totally objective. Rescher, the author of this system of scarce-resource allocation, recognizes its imperfections and suggests that an element of chance or random selection should also be introduced, but "limited and circumscribed by other weightier considerations, along some such lines as those set forth above."

Another approach is advocated by Childress, who presents a methodology and ethical argumentation for randomness as the most equitable means of distributing scarce medical resources after medical selection has been made.[5] He strongly criticizes the social-worth criteria and condemns Rescher for failing to give attention to the moral values that random selection might preserve.

A variety of formulations for the allocation of scarce medical resources based on different concepts of social justice is provided by Outka.[6] These include: (a) to each according to his merit; (b) to each according to his societal contribution; (c) to each according to his contribution in satisfying whatever is freely desired by others in the open marketplace of supply and demand; (d) to each according to his needs; and (e) similar treatment for similar cases.

In 1973, when Congress passed the now famous End Stage Renal Program (PL 92-603), all ethical problems relating to hemodialysis were seemingly solved. Hemodialysis was no longer to be considered exotic or "extraordinary" care. This formerly scarce medical resource was to be made available to all who needed it and was to be paid for by Medicare. The number of patients being dialyzed increased from less than two thousand in 1968 to more than seventy thousand in 1981. Many patients previously not dialyzed, such as diabetics and old people, were entered into dialysis programs, but the total cost of the program became prohibitive. In 1982, major governmental reductions in budgetary allocations for many programs began to be implemented. The resources for hemodialysis are again becoming scarce and limited, as they were prior to the 1973 legislation. The ethical dilemmas described above are again with us, but now new dimensions have been added.

The critical issues are not only who the allocators should be, but what should be decided. Is it worthwhile to dialyze all patients with end-stage renal disease? Is it worthwhile to expend the time of medical personnel to search for a dialysis program for a social outcast? How can one square such a decision with the suffering and indifference to mothers with screaming babies in the emergency room of that same hospital.[7]

Between 1973 and 1982, when Medicare paid for most hemodialysis in the United States, criteria were relaxed, the number of eligible patients multiplied manyfold, and hemodialysis facilities were markedly expanded. Economic necessity now dictates new decisions and allocations. The magnitude of the problem may become masked again, as it was before 1973, since directors of renal units often do not admit to any shortfall in available places, claiming that medically suitable patients are not being rejected. In other words, a process of rationalization occurs in which medical indications are unconsciously determined by medical resources or by private financing.[8]

Societal Allocation of Resources

So far I have discussed priority decision-making in resource allocation on the part of the doctor, hospital, or institution. The foregoing brief history of governmental involvement in hemodialysis raises the issue of society's allocation of its enormous but finite resources. Should the government proceed with the development of a new bomber for the defense of this country, or should those financial resources be allocated to the health of its citizens? Should hemodialysis take priority over hypertension screening or the treatment of cancer? Political decisions for health may be based on considerations other than rational medical thinking. This governmental macro-allocation process differs in several respects from the micro-allocation decision of the doctor at the bedside. The macro-allocation process is far removed from the clinical setting, is impersonal and not emotionally charged, involves large numbers of patients on a nationwide scale, and is not subject to the urgency of acting swiftly in a life-or-death situation. Macro-allocation or governmental decisions, such as the distribution of funds for medical research, strongly influence the course and direction of this research and consequently, to a large extent, determine whether a mode of therapy will ever exist. Governmental decisions can reduce or even eliminate the problem of scarcity,[9] as exemplified by the 1973 hemodialysis legislation and funding.

The proper level for governmental regulation and funding of research, development, and operation in areas of scarcity is beyond the scope of this paper. A model for more effective governmental allocation of scarce medical resources is described elsewhere.[10] To argue that funds should be shifted from highway construction or military budgets to health care is really naive. Even with major shifts in priorities, problems of allocation of the health dollars will still exist. The various alternatives, such as allocation on the basis of ability to pay, or to have the right connections, or the patient's social worth, or on strict medical criteria, or by lot, or by taking turns or standing in line on a first come–first served basis, or any combination of criteria, will continue to be debated. Allocations will continue to be made by individual physicians, clinics, hospitals, institutions, and governmental bodies. To ensure that these decisions and allocations are made wisely, it is essential to understand the moral foundations for such actions.

The Examples of Mental Retardation and Hypertension

A bill was presented to the New York State Legislature in 1975 for the establishment of community-based homes for the care and education of the mentally retarded at a cost of $70 million annually. Those who spoke against the bill, although concerned about the care of the retarded, argued that these clients equalled only one-tenth of one percent of the state's population, and that the money could buy hot lunches for all the state's school children, or provide job training for productive members of society. Others argued that the money could be used more efficiently in providing health care for normal children, for those engaged in productive labor, and for pregnant women. One physician showed that much mental retardation can be eliminated through prenatal diagnosis, which he estimated to cost $200 per case for Down's syndrome compared to $60,000 for each institutionalized child. Who has first claim on health care resources? It is very difficult to rank many social goods, such as health care, education, and the environment. The greater good of the greater number seems to be the ethical standard of lawmakers and public servants in a democratic society, since sacrificing the many for the few would only hurt the majority without substantially helping the unfortunate few.

Another example illustrating ethical issues in allocating resources is the case of hypertension. Hypertension is one of America's foremost health problems. It affects about twenty-five million Americans—both men and women—and is the single most important risk factor for cardiovascular disease, which kills and cripples more people than any other. The higher the blood pressure, the greater the risk of strokes, heart attacks, and other disabling or fatal events.

Despite the importance of hypertension and the presumed efficacy of antihypertensive treatment, 30 to 50 percent of American hypertensives are not aware that they have high blood pressure; half of those who know they have it are not under treatment; and of those who are being treated, only half have brought their blood pressures under control.[11]

From a public policy standpoint, it can be argued that a major national effort should be undertaken to provide treatment to as many of the untreated hypertensives as possible. Some advocate mass public screening programs. On the other hand, treatment is costly, accompanied by side effects, and many who are found to be hypertensive do not achieve blood pressure control because they drop out of treatment or because they fail to adhere to treatment regimens, or because their providers fail to prescribe effective treatment.

But hypertension detection and treatment must compete for resources with other programs and activities both within and outside of health care. More hypertension treatment might mean fewer nutrition programs or fewer coronary care units. Moreover, the limited resources available for hypertension must be allocated in the best possible way, consistent with societal goals and principles. How should hypertension treatment resources be allocated—by blood pressure level, age, sex, or other criteria? Considering that many patients do not adhere to medical regimens, is treatment of hypertension nevertheless a wise use of resources? Are public screening programs an appropriate use of resources? Under what conditions? For what target populations? Generally, how should resources be divided among screening for unaware hypertensives, treatment of known hypertensives, and interventions to promote adherence to medical regimens among those under treatment?

An analysis of policy toward hypertension and a systematic effort to clarify the issues that bear most heavily on such questions of resource allocation as well as suggested answers are available for the interested reader.[12]

Many other examples could be cited. Enormous resources of personnel, equipment, time, blood and blood products, and physical and emotional effort are expended on the care of a relatively small number of patients in intensive care units. In one American study, 54 percent of such patients had died by one month and 73 percent within twelve months.[13] Providing intensive care to one group of patients has secondary effects on others in that resources are diverted from a large number of moderately sick patients to a few very sick patients. The most critically ill patients should derive sufficient benefit to justify the expenditures and allocations of personnel and equipment. A similar plea comes from England for health authorities to make wise but difficult decisions, within a finite cash limit, for the allocation of funds to high-technology medicine, such as coronary-artery bypass surgery and renal transplantation.[14]

The problem of the allocation of scarce medical resources has been succinctly summarized as follows:

> Medical science has recently developed a number of complex and expensive treatments capable of saving life. Because it is not yet possible to make these treatments available to all in need, it is necessary to decide to whom the treatment will be given. Sometimes a large number of patients could all receive substantially equal medical benefit from the treatment. In this situation, doctors have wondered whether they should attempt to save the patient of greater value to society. Those who think they should, have considered age, family, and potential social contribution in

making allocation decisions. Since others think that social worth is relevant but insist that the factor is not one for a doctor to evaluate, hospitals have occasionally delegated allocation decisions to committees drawn from the community or from the community and the hospital staff. A third group maintains that social worth is not a proper consideration in allocating scarce resources. They apply a random or first-come rule of selection. These doctors, however, are willing to eliminate from consideration patients who are deemed unsuitable for treatment. It appears that when a resource is scarce, this finding of unsuitability may in part reflect notions of social worth.[15]

The Jewish View

In Jewish tradition a physician is given specific Divine license to practice medicine. According to Maimonides and other codifiers of Jewish law, it is in fact an obligation upon the physician to use his medical skills to heal the sick. Not only is the physician permitted and even obligated to minister to the sick but the patient is also obligated to care for his health and life. Man does not have full title over his life or body. He is charged with preserving, dignifying, and hallowing that life. He must eat and drink to sustain himself. He must seek healing when he is ill.

Another cardinal principle in Judaism is that human life is of infinite value. The preservation of human life takes precedence over all biblical commandments, with three exceptions: idolatry, murder, and incest. Life's value is absolute and supreme. Thus, an old man or woman, a mentally retarded person, a deformed baby, a dying cancer patient, and the like, all have the same right to life as you or I. In order to preserve a human life, the Sabbath and even the Day of Atonement may be desecrated and all other rules and laws, save the above three, are suspended for the overriding consideration of saving a human life.

The corollary of this principle is that one is prohibited from doing anything that might shorten a life even for a very brief time, since every moment of human life is also of infinite value. How does Judaism resolve the dilemma of two patients dying of kidney failure and only one available dialysis machine? Who takes precedence? How does one decide? Is one not condemning one patient to death by offering the dialysis machine to the other patient?

The classic source in Judaism which discusses priorities is the talmudic passage which states that a man takes precedence over a woman in matters concerning the saving of life (because he has more biblical commandments to fulfill) and the restoration of lost property, but a woman takes precedence over a man in respect of clothing (because a woman's shame from wearing shabby clothes is greater than that of a man) and ransom from captivity (because she may be raped by her captors).[16] When both are exposed to immoral degradation in their captivity, the man's ransom takes precedence over that of the woman (to spare him the indignity of pederasty).

The Talmud continues:

> If a man and his father and his teacher were in captivity, he takes precedence [in procuring his ransom] over his teacher, and the latter takes precedence over his father, while his mother takes precedence over all of them [because her dignity is at stake]. A scholar takes precedence over a king of Israel, for if a scholar dies, there is none to replace him, while if a king of Israel dies, all Israel are eligible for kingship. A king takes precedence over a high priest. . . . a high priest takes precedence over a prophet . . .[17]

Finally the Talmud concludes:

> A priest takes precedence over a Levite, a Levite over an Israelite, an Israelite over a bastard, a bastard over a *nathin* [i.e., a descendant of the Gibeonites whom Joshua made into Temple slaves; see Joshua 9:27], a *nathin* over a proselyte, and a proselyte over an emancipated slave. This order of precedence applies only when all these are in other respects equal. If the bastard, however, was a scholar and the high priest an ignoramus, the learned bastard takes precedence over the ignorant high priest.[18]

It thus seems that Judaism considers religious status, personal dignity, and social worth as determining factors in the allocation of limited ransom money to redeem captives from their captors. Would Judaism view differently the situation where someone's life, rather than personal dignity, is at stake?

It is a cardinal principle of Judaism that one may not sacrifice one life to preserve another. In his classic code, Moses Maimonides states that "logic dictates that in regard to taking the life of an Israelite to cure another individual or to rescue a person from one who threatens violence, one may not destroy one human life to save another human life."[19] The reason cited in the Talmud is that the blood of one person is no redder than the blood of another.[20]

The classic example is cited by Maimonides as follows: "If heathens said to Israelites: 'Surrender one of your number to us, that we may kill him; otherwise, we will kill all of you,' they should all let themselves be killed rather than surrender a single Israelite to them."[21]

When a physician chooses one patient over another to provide a scarce or limited type of treatment such as dialysis, he is not actively killing the other patient. However, if six patients occupy six intensive care beds and another patient arrives, should the physician transfer one of the six patients out to make room for the new person? Does such an act constitute an act of murder if the patient transferred out of the intensive care unit dies? Certainly not! The transfer had to be made. But what criteria does Judaism require to make the determination to transfer one patient to make room for another if "one person's blood is no redder than that of another"? The case of the two dialysis patients is different, since the physician is only initiating treatment for one of them and since no dialysis machine is available for the other. In the intensive care unit, however, the physician is actively removing the patient from the intensive care unit and relegating him to receive less than intensive care.

Another classic Jewish source relating to the allocation of scarce resources is the case cited in the Talmud of two people in the desert and one has a pitcher of water.[22] If both drink, they will both die, but if only one drinks, he can reach civilization. One sage rules that it is better that both should drink and die than that one should behold his companion's death. But Rabbi Akiba rules that only the one who owns the pitcher drinks, because "thy life takes precedence over his life," i.e., do not sacrifice your life to save another, since "his blood is no redder than yours." Some commentaries assert that if neither owned the pitcher both should drink because of the principle "one may not sacrifice one life to preserve another." This case seems to be somewhat analogous to the lifeboat ethics situation. If the lifeboat is about to capsize because of excessive weight, should one or more people be thrown overboard to save the others, or should everyone remain on board and all will drown? There are no easy answers.

The hierarchy of precedences in Judaism enumerated above seems to contradict the rule that "one may not sacrifice one life to preserve another." How can these two approaches be reconciled? The precedences seem to suggest that qualitative distinctions can be made on the basis of social worth or personal dignity or religious status. The rule that "one may not sacrifice one life to preserve another" seems to imply that no qualitative distinctions should be allowed. A person can will his organs for transplantation to save the lives of others after he dies. He cannot, however, say: kill me and transplant my organs to preserve others, because "his blood is no redder than theirs." Therefore, in the allocation of scarce medical resources, perhaps a lottery system or a first come–first served approach or pure medical criteria might be preferable in Judaism.

An approach based on medical criteria is suggested by Rabbi Eliezer Yehuda Waldenberg, who states that a patient with a potential for cure takes precedence in the allocation of scarce medical resources over a patient whose illness would at best be only temporarily controlled.[23] This rule, however, applies only when the incurable patient is passively neglected in favor of the curable patient. To terminate the therapy of the incurable patient, continues Waldenberg, so that the curable patient can be given those resources, is forbidden. The same author rules that if there is only sufficient medication for one of two patients, the critically ill patient takes precedence over the less seriously ill patient.[24] If the medication, however, belongs to the less seriously ill patient, he is not obligated to give it to the critically ill patient because "thy life takes precedence over his life." If both patients are dangerously ill and the medicine belongs to neither, one should divide the medication equally, thereby providing each patient with a one- or two-day extension of life. In the meantime, either Divine intervention may heal them or additional medication may be found.

In addition to the axiom that "thy life takes precedence over his life," Judaism subscribes to a specific sequence of priority in regard to assisting one's fellowman in that *thou shalt open thine hand unto thy brother, to thy needy, and to thy poor, in thy land.*[25] Does this sequence also apply to matters of life and death and to allocation of scarce medical resources? Would Judaism require that a Jew receive precedence over a non-Jew or that a religious Jew receive precedence over a non-religious Jew in the decision about who is to be dialyzed if only one machine is available or who is to receive the intensive care bed if only one is available? Certainly not!

The infinite worth of man, a Judaic axiom already cited, is compromised by limited or finite resources. Why should a resident physician have to decide which patient gets the intensive care bed? Why not create more intensive care beds rather than support museums? Why not build more dialysis machines rather than buy more tanks or battleships? These are societal decisions, and one may legitimately ask whether allocation decisions and axioms affecting individuals apply equally to societal or institutional problems. Is society a separate being and more than the sum of its component parts? According to Rabbi Moshe David Tendler, the answer is strongly affirmative.[26] Societal ethics are indeed different than individual ethics. Society or government, according to Tendler, is needed to prevent man from destroying his fellowman. Therefore, society is not bound by the same ethical principles that bind individuals, such as the infinite worth of man. Support for this view can be found in several Jewish writings.

The Talmud asserts that captives should not be redeemed for more than their value, to prevent abuses.[27] The reason for this rule, according to the commentator Rabbi Ovadiah of Bertinoro, is so that captors should not be encouraged to seize more captives and make excessive ransom demands. The Talmud then raises the question:

> Does this prevention of abuses relate to the burden on the community [to redeem the captives] or the possibility that the bandits will be encouraged to increase their activities? Come and hear: Levi ben Darga ransomed his daughter for 13,000 denarii of gold [showing that if an individual is willing to pay more he may do so, and the reason is because of the financial burden imposed on the community]. Said Abaye: But are you sure that he acted with the consent of the sages? Perhaps he acted contrary to the will of the sages.[28]

Thus, two reasons are given why it is forbidden to pay an exorbitant amount of money to ransom anyone: to discourage kidnappers and to prevent society from becoming impoverished by having to divert its resources to the ransoming of captives. Society would thus be unable to provide for the needs of all the people which it serves. The codes of Jewish law rule in accordance with the Talmud that society may not expend excess money to redeem captives. However, a husband may ransom his wife for any amount, and a father may ransom his son or daughter for any amount, as did Levi ben Darga. Thus, we clearly see that societal ethics are different than individual ethics.

Tendler cites another source to support his thesis that society is not bound by the same principles as are individuals in the allocation of scarce medical resources. The Talmud describes a situation of a water supply belonging to town A situated on a hill.[29] Town B, situated at the bottom of the hill, cannot obtain water unless the townspeople of town A do not water their flocks and/or launder their clothes. Rabbi Jose rules that the townspeople from town A at the top of the hill take precedence over those of town B. Although the immediate danger is to the people of town B, who have no water at all, the long-term danger from not washing one's body and clothes to the people of town A, who have the water, overrides the immediate needs of the people of town B at the bottom of the hill. The talmudic sage Samuel said that scabs of the head caused by not washing can lead to blindness; scabs arising through the wearing of unclean, i.e., unlaundered, garments can cause madness; scabs due to neglect of the body can cause boils and ulcers.[30]

Thus we have clear evidence that society must be concerned about future generations and for long-range planning. Society must be concerned about the long-range effects of its actions. This is not so for individuals. The doctor in the intensive care unit must make decisions that affect individual patients here and now. The two individuals in the desert with a single pitcher of water should share that water if it belongs to neither one because they have to be concerned with preserving their lives here and now; maybe they will be rescued tomorrow. The allocation of a medicine or treatment to one of two patients if there is not enough for both is a decision needed for the here-and-now care of one or both patients. An individual researcher using radioisotopes is concerned with the immediate safety from radiation of himself and his co-workers. But society has to be concerned about the disposal of nuclear wastes because of the danger to future generations caused by the radioisotopes used today.

One cannot, however, totally divorce individuals from responsibility to consider future generations in the allocation of resources. Perhaps this point is most beautifully depicted in the talmudic story of the righteous Choni the Circle-Drawer, who was journeying on a road and saw a man planting a carob tree; he asked him: "How long does it take for this tree to bear fruit?" The man replied: "Seventy years." Choni then further asked him: "Are you certain that you will live another seventy years?" The man replied: "I found ready-grown carob trees in the world; as my forefathers planted these for me, so I too plant these for my children."[31]

Conclusion

The allocation of scarce resources is a complicated, multifaceted issue associated with many moral and ethical dilemmas. Many systems have been proposed to equitably distribute finite medical resources and to make allocation decisions which are consonant with basic principles of ethics. None are perfect. All have positive and negative attributes. The criteria to be used by an individual or clinic or hospital division or department may differ from those to be used by large institutions or governmental bodies.

Judaism views each human being as being of supreme and infinite value. It is the obligation of both individuals and society in general to preserve, hallow, and dignify human life and to care for the total needs of individual citizens, to enable them to be healthy and productive members of society. This fundamental principle should help guide the physician making life-and-death decisions at the bedside for individual patients, as well as governmental bodies that are responsible for deciding short- and long-term health needs and priorities for the population as a whole.

Notes

1. "Scarce Medical Resources," *Columbia Law Review 1969*, vol. 69, pp. 620–692.
2. Ibid.
3. Ibid.
4. N. Rescher, "The Allocation of Exotic Medical Life-saving Therapy," *Ethics: An International Journal of Social, Political, and Legal Philosophy* 79 (1969): 173–186.
5. J. F. Childress, "Who Shall Live When Not All Can Live," in *Bioethics*, ed. Th. A. Shannon (New York: Paulist Press, 1976), pp. 397–411.
6. G. Outka, "Social Justice and Equal Access to Health Care," in *Bioethics*, ed. Th. A. Shannon (New York: Paulist Press, 1976), pp. 373–395.
7. R. M. Veatch, *Case Studies in Medical Ethics* (Cambridge, Mass.: Harvard University Press 1977), pp. 221–239.
8. Editorial, "Ethics and the Nephrologist," *Lancet* 1 (1981): 594–596; M. A. Somerville, "Ethics and the Nephrologist," ibid., pp. 1109–1110.
9. J. Childress and J. Fletcher, "Who Has First Claim on Health Care Resources?" *Hastings Center Report* 5 (1975): 13–15.
10. "Scarce Medical Resources."
11. M. C. Weinstein and W. B. Stason, "Allocating Resources: The Case of Hypertension," *Hastings Center Report* 7 (1977): 24–29.
12. M. C. Weinstein and W. B. Stason, *Hypertension: A Policy Perspective* (Cambridge, Mass.: Harvard University Press, 1976).
13. D. J. Cullen, L. C. Ferrara, B. A. Briggs, P. F. Walker and J. Gilbert, "Survival, Hospitalization Charges and Follow-Up Results in Critically Ill Patients," *New England Journal of Medicine* 294 (1976): 982–987.
14. A. M. B. Golding and D. Tosey, "The Cost of High-Technology Medicine," *Lancet* 2 (1980): 195–197.
15. "Scarce Medical Resources."
16. Horayot 3:7.
17. Ibid. 13a.
18. Ibid. 3:8.
19. Maimonides, *Mishneh Torah, Hilchot Yesodei Hatorah* 5:7.
20. Pesachim 25b.
21. Maimonides, op. cit. 5:5.
22. Baba Metzia 62a.
23. E. Y. Waldenberg, Responsa *Tzitz Eliezer*, vol. 9, sec. 17, chap. 10:5.
24. Ibid., sec. 28:3.
25. Deuteronomy 15:11.
26. M. D. Tendler, "Rabbinic Comment: Triage of Resources," *Mount Sinai Journal of Medicine* 51 (1984): 106–109.
27. Gittin 3:6.

28. Ibid. 45a.
29. Nedarim 80b.
30. Ibid. 81a.
31. Taanit 23a.

27

Cigarette and Marijuana Smoking

Tobacco was first implicated as a cause of cancer in 1761.[1] There is no longer any doubt that cigarette smoking is a hazard to health. Overwhelming medical evidence has proved that cigarette smoking is associated with a shortened life expectancy. In January 1964, an Advisory Committee appointed by the Surgeon General of the United States Public Health Service issued its report on the relationship between smoking and health.[2] The conclusions of that report were summed up in the sentence: "Cigarette smoking is a health hazard of sufficient importance in the United States to warrant appropriate remedial action."

Nearly four years later, after reviewing more than two thousand research studies published since the 1964 report, the U.S. Public Health Service published its follow-up report.[3] The report concludes that: "epidemiological evidence derived from a number of prospective and retrospective studies, coupled with experimental and pathological evidence, confirms the conclusion that cigarette smoking is the main cause of lung cancer in men." Other findings include the fact that cigarette smoking is the most important cause of chronic obstructive lung disease (emphysema) in the United States. It is also a significant risk factor contributing to the development of coronary heart disease, cancer of the larynx, and probably cancer of the bladder. Pregnant women who smoke have smaller babies and greater fetal complications.

In the United Kingdom, the Royal College of Physicians of London followed its first report on smoking and health with another report restating the medical hazards of smoking.[4] The reports claim that cigarette smoking has become as important a cause of death as the great epidemic diseases, such as typhoid, cholera, and tuberculosis.

The American Medical Association has prepared reading lists, pamphlets, booklets, films, posters, and a variety of other educational materials to publicize the effects of smoking on health, and to help in the campaign to decrease or even eradicate cigarette smoking. Comparable materials are also available from the American Cancer Society, the American Heart Association, the National Tuberculosis Association, and the National Clearinghouse for Smoking and Health. By act of Congress, the following warning appears on every pack of cigarettes manufactured for sale in the United States on or after November 1, 1970: "The Surgeon General Has Determined That Cigarette Smoking is Dangerous to Your Health." Television advertising for cigarettes was abolished by government decree as of January 1, 1971. Complete or partial bans on cigarette advertising are in effect in England, Holland, Norway, Sweden, Italy, Poland, Russia, Switzerland, and probably other countries.[5]

Yet in Brazil, the Secretary of Federal Revenue recently suggested to cigarette companies that they should organize an even more massive sales campaign than previously to increase the income to the Brazilian government from taxation on industrialized products.[6]

The U.S. Public Health Service's fourteenth report on the health consequences of smoking appeared in 1981 and concluded that there is no such thing as a safe cigarette.[7] The report states that "the smokers of lower tar and nicotine cigarettes who compensate by smoking more or by inhaling more deeply might thereby increase their risk of developing obstructive airway disease." In addition, lower-tar cigarettes do not decrease the risks among pregnant women of spontaneous abortion, premature birth, or low-weight babies. Filtered cigarettes are no safer. A new concern relates to the use of new additives for tobacco processing or flavoring, some of which may give rise to carcinogenic substances when burned, thus offsetting the potential benefit from lower tar and/or nicotine content of cigarettes.

There are new alarms for women who smoke. Deaths from lung cancer among women have increased dramatically in the past twenty years and may soon overtake breast cancer as the leading cause of cancer death in women. Also worrisome is the sharp increase in smoking among teenage girls who are entering their childbearing years. Babies of smokers weigh less than those of nonsmokers and show slower rates of physical and mental growth.

Prematurity, miscarriage, and fetal death are also more common in smokers.

An earlier report in 1979 had already emphasized an array of other warnings to smokers:

a. A smoker has a 70 percent greater risk of death in any given year than a nonsmoker. For two-pack-a-day smokers, the risk is 100 percent greater.
b. Smoking poses a major heart-attack risk in both men and women. The danger of heart attack for women who both smoke and take birth-control pills containing estrogen is ten times higher than for other women.
c. Smoking can be especially hazardous to workers in certain occupations, including the asbestos, rubber, textile, uranium, and chemical industries. Substances in smoke may act synergistically with chemicals to greatly increase a smoker's chances of contracting lung cancer.
d. To further emphasize the value of quitting cigarette-smoking, the report noted that after fifteen years, the mortality ratio for former smokers is nearly as low as for people who never smoked.[8]

Yet people continue to smoke. To some people, cigarette smoking is the greatest single public health problem this nation has ever faced. The solution will not be simple nor easy, but steps in the right direction are beginning to show results in a slight decrease in the number of smokers, particularly young smokers. The present essay is an attempt to show that in light of the overwhelming medical evidence proving the causal relationship of cigarette smoking to cancer of the lung, heart disease, and chronic bronchitis, Jewish law absolutely prohibits this practice, notwithstanding several rabbinic opinions to the contrary.

The Torah tells us not to intentionally place ourselves in danger when it states *take heed to thyself, and take care of thy life* and *take good care of your lives.*[9] The avoidance of danger is exemplified throughout the Bible, Talmud, and codes of Jewish law in the positive commandment of making a parapet for one's roof so that no man fall therefrom.[10] Moses Maimonides enumerates a variety of prohibitions, all based upon the consideration of being harmful to life.[11] They are quoted verbatim since they eloquently illustrate the point under discussion.

> It makes no difference whether it be one's roof or anything else that is dangerous and might possibly be a stumbling block to someone and cause his death—for example, if one has a well or a

pit, with or without water, in his yard—the owner is obliged to build an enclosing wall ten handbreadths high, or else to put a cover over it lest someone fall into it and be killed. Similarly, regarding any obstacle which is dangerous to life, there is a positive commandment to remove it and to beware of it, and to be particularly careful in this matter, for Scripture says, *Take heed unto thyself and take care of thy life.*[12] If one does not remove dangerous obstacles and allows them to remain, he disregards a positive commandment and transgresses the prohibition: *Thou bring not blood.*[13]

Many things are forbidden by the sages because they are dangerous to life. If one disregards any of these and says, "If I want to put myself in danger, what concern is it to others?" or "I am not particular about such things," disciplinary flogging is inflicted upon him.

The following are the acts prohibited: One may not put his mouth to a flowing pipe of water and drink from it, or drink at night from rivers or ponds, lest he swallow a leech while unable to see. Nor may one drink water that has been left uncovered, lest he drink it after a snake or other poisonous reptile has drunk from it, and die. . . .

One should not put small change or *denar* into his mouth lest they carry the dried saliva of one who suffers from an infectious skin disease or leprosy, or lest they carry perspiration, since all human perspiration is poisonous except that coming from the face.

Similarly, one should not put the palm of his hand under his arm, for his hand might possibly have touched a leper or some harmful substance, since the hands are constantly in motion. Nor should one put a dish of food under his seat even during a meal, lest something harmful fall into it without his noticing it.

Similarly, one should not stick a knife into a citron or a radish lest someone fall on the point and be killed. Similarly, one should not walk near a leaning wall or over a shaking bridge or enter a ruin or pass through any other such dangerous place.

This quotation from Maimonides certainly emphasizes the point that placing one's health or life into possible danger is absolutely prohibited. Hence, the smoking of cigarettes, which constitutes a definite danger and hazard to life, should *a fortiori* be prohibited. The subterfuge of "it is no concern of others if I endanger myself" is specifically disallowed by Maimonides.

Similar prohibitions against endangering one's life are found in most later codes of Jewish law, including Karo's *Shulchan Aruch.* The latter devotes an entire chapter to "the positive commandment of removing any object or obstacle which constitutes a danger to life."[14] Elsewhere Karo reiterates the prohibitions against drinking water left uncovered, putting money in one's mouth, putting one's hand or a loaf of bread under the armpit, leaving a knife in a fruit, the consumption of unappetizing food, and the use of dirty pots or dishes.[15] He further states that two people should not drink from the same cup,[16] and that one should wait between eating fish and meat because of danger.[17]

Rabbi Moses Isserles, known as *Ramah*, in his gloss on Karo's code concludes:

> . . . one should avoid all things that might lead to danger because a danger to life is stricter than a prohibition. One should be more concerned about a possible danger to life than a possible prohibition. Therefore, the sages prohibited one to walk in a place of danger, such as near a leaning wall [for fear of collapse], or alone at night [for fear of robbers]. They also prohibited drinking water from rivers at night . . . because these things may lead to danger . . . and he who is concerned with his health [lit. watches his soul] avoids them. And it is prohibited to rely on a miracle or to put one's life in danger by any of the aforementioned or the like.[18]

Ramah thus prohibits reliance on miracles when one's health is at stake. The fact that so many Jewish people smoke is no justification for this dangerous and life-threatening practice. If many Jews commit a transgression, others should certainly not follow suit; rather they should try to reach the sinners to make them repent from their evil ways. The "pleasures" of adultery are not condoned by even the most liberal-minded Jew. Why then should the pleasures of smoking, which also involve biblical prohibitions, be relegated to an inferior status, to be treated more leniently?

Not only is the intentional endangerment of one's health or life, such as by smoking, prohibited in Jewish law, but wounding oneself without fatal intent is also disallowed. The Talmud quotes Rabbi Elazar Hakapar Berabbi, who maintains that a man may not injure himself.[19] He learns this point from the scriptural phrase *And make an atonement for him, for that he sinned regarding the soul,*[20] which refers to a Nazarite who is called a sinner because he deprived himself of wine. Certainly, says Rabbi Elazar Hakapar, a person who deprives himself of his health by injuring himself is considered a sinner. One can extend this reasoning to include smoking.

Maimonides states that he who smashes household goods, or destroys articles of food, with destructive intent, transgresses the commandment *Thou shall not destroy.*[21] Our sages deduce from this phrase a prohibition against the wanton destruction of anything useful to man.[22] Rabbi Solomon Luria extends this prohibition to the willful destruction of one's own body.[23] An example of this is described in the Talmud, where a footstool was broken up for Rabbah, whereupon Abaye said to Rabbah: "But are you not infringing on *Thou shalt not destroy?*" He retorted: "*Thou shalt not destroy* in respect of my own body is more important to me."[24]

The prohibition against intentionally wounding oneself is codified by both Maimonides and Karo[25]. Not only can smoking be considered to constitute wounding oneself or intentionally injuring one's health, but it may in fact constitute a slow form of suicide. Suicide itself, whether slow or rapid, is absolutely prohibited in Jewish law, based upon the biblical phrase *And surely your blood, the blood of your lives, will I require.*[26]

Some argue that the following two talmudic principles mitigate against the imposition of a rabbinic ban against cigarette smoking:

a. We must not impose a restrictive decree upon the community unless the majority of the community will be able to endure it.[27]
b. It is better that they should transgress inadvertently rather than be deliberate sinners.[28]

Both arguments can be rejected, since neither is applicable in the face of *pikúach nefesh*, or danger to life.[29] Furthermore, the smoking of cigarettes is not an inadvertent act (although the sin or transgression may be inadvertent), but an intentional practice of oral gratification which can lead to serious illness and even death.

On the other hand, very few rabbis have to this day issued a prohibition against smoking, though most condemn the practice as foolhardy and dangerous. Rabbi Moshe Feinstein[30] asserts that although it is proper not to begin smoking, one cannot say that it is prohibited because of the danger, since many people smoke, and the Talmud states that *The Lord preserveth the simple.*[31] Rabbi Feinstein also points out that many rabbinic scholars from previous generations as well as our own era smoke. Furthermore, even to those who are strict and do not smoke because of their concern about possible danger to health and life, there is no prohibition in lighting the match for those who smoke. Rabbi Feinstein has recently reconfirmed his opinion in writing.[32]

Rabbi J. David Bleich is of the opinion that smoking does not involve an infraction of Jewish law.[33] He explains that certain actions which contain an element of danger, such as crossing the street or riding in an automobile, involve a certain danger yet are certainly permissible because "the multitude has trodden thereon," i.e., these dangers are accepted with equanimity by society at large. Therefore, an individual is granted dispensation to rely upon God, who "preserves the simple." Bleich also quotes Rabbi Jacob Ettlinger, who distinguishes between an immediate danger, which must be eschewed under all circumstances, and a future danger, such as that related to cigarette smoking, which may be assumed if, in the majority of cases, no harm will occur.[34] Two correspondents take strong issue with Bleich's analysis of the Jewish legal permissibility of smoking.[35] The five points in Jewish law raised by these correspondents are rebutted by Bleich.[36] In spite of the technical inability of Bleich and others to promulgate a formal binding prohibition against smoking, he does urge rabbis to use their extensive powers of moral persuasion and exhortation to urge "the eradication of this pernicious and damaging habit."

Dr. Abraham S. Abraham quotes Rabbi Shlomo Zalman Auerbach and Rabbi Ovadiah Yosef as being in agreement with the thesis that smoking cannot be prohibited in Jewish law, for the reasons cited by Feinstein and Bleich.[37] Nevertheless, "one should do one's utmost to avoid smoking, since this has been proven medically to be injurious to well-being, and dangerous to life."

In regard to passive smoking, there is considerable controversy in the medical literature as to whether exhaled smoke is harmful to others in close proximity to the smokers. There is no doubt that maternal smoking affects fetal development, being associated with low birth weight,[38] prematurity,[39] birth defects,[40] increased spontaneous abortions,[41] and long-term growth deficiency in the offspring[42]. Thus, in Jewish law, a pregnant woman should be prohibited from smoking because she is endangering the health and life of her child. The suggestions that healthy adult nonsmokers may be seriously harmed by other people's smoke is based on four studies, summarized in a recent editorial in the prestigious medical publication *Lancet*.[43] Each of the studies can be criticized for a variety of statistical reasons.[44] At present, the state of the art seems to be that, although suggestive, the evidence is not sufficient to definitively conclude that passive or involuntary smoking causes lung cancer in nonsmokers. Passive smoking may have other deleterious effects, such as the development of atherosclerosis or hardening of the arteries.[45]

Rabbi Feinstein rules that if the exhaled smoke is harmful or even only annoying to others, the smokers are obligated to smoke in private or far removed from other people.[46] Similar opinions have been expressed by Rabbi Eliezer Yehudah Waldenberg and Rabbi Ezekiel Grubner.[47]

The subject of smoking on Jewish festivals has recently been exhaustively reviewed by Rabbi Bleich, who concludes that the majority of authorities prohibit smoking on festivals.[48] The major pronouncement was made by Rabbi Nathaniel Weil, known as *Korban Nethanel*, who said:

> I cannot withhold writing down the trap that Jews fall into in smoking [lit. "drinking *tabak*"] on *Yom Tov* [Jewish holidays] in that they are making unnecessary fire. Smoking is not a necessity for *Yom Tov*. I saw in Responsa *Darchei No'am* a lengthy discussion which concludes that it is permissible, but there is no validity to those arguments. Some say that smoking aids in digestion of food and also serves as a laxative; if so, then people who smoke are taking medicine on *Yom Tov*. Some say that it is a common practice . . . smoking to one who is not accustomed thereto can be dangerous and makes him act as if he is drunk. . . . I am critical not of ignoramuses but of intelligent people who make others sin by setting a bad example. They are not careful and extinguish and light [fire] without need. Not only that but some who are not so accustomed and do not smoke on weekdays go for leisurely walks on *Yom Tov* while smoking, and this is a desecration of the *Yom Tov* in full public view. . . . It is, therefore, good for them to abstain from smoking for one or two days in honor of God and His Torah.[49]

In regard to marijuana smoking, mounting scientific evidence shows that it is a threat to brain function as well as a respiratory hazard.[50] Acute intoxication impairs learning, memory, intellectual performance, and driving ability.[51] Marijuana also has adverse effects on the body's immune, endocrine, and reproductive systems.

Because of the above considerations, Rabbi Feinstein prohibits the smoking of marijuana by stating the following:[52] Firstly, marijuana is harmful to the body. Even those people who suffer no physical damage may suffer mental harm in that marijuana confuses the mind and distorts one's abilities of reasoning and comprehension. Such a person is thereby not only preventing himself from studying Torah but also from performing other precepts. Marijuana use, continues Feinstein, can also bring on extreme and uncontrollable lusts and desires. Furthermore, since the parents of marijuana users are usually opposed to its use, the users violate the biblical commandment of honoring one's father and mother. Other prohibitions may also be involved in marijuana use, and therefore, concludes Feinstein, one must use all one's energies to uproot and eliminate this pernicious habit.

Other rabbis also consider marijuana smoking to be prohibited in Jewish law,[53] but very few prohibit cigarette smoking. An occasional rabbi is finally speaking out on the evils of cigarette smoking and the possible prohibitions involved. Rabbi Moses Aberbach writes that

> the medical and statistical evidence demonstrates that smoking is hazardous to health, and can lead to fatal diseases. The idea that smoking is liable to shorten a person's life is virtually undisputed. It follows, therefore, that the numerous *halakhic* rules prohibiting dangerous activities should be extended to include smoking. This extension should be enacted by the leading rabbinic authorities of our times, preferably acting jointly, and with due publicity. A general rabbinic injunction against smoking has every chance of being gradually accepted, at least in strictly Orthodox circles. Thus, many Jewish lives would be saved, and the health of our people would substantially improve. Finally, not the least fringe benefit would be a demonstration of the relevance of Judaism—and especially *halakhic* Judiasm—to our own times.[54]

Rabbi Nathan Drazin asks, "why, indeed, have the great *halakhic* authorities of our generation been silent concerning the prohibitions of Jewish law in regard to cigarette smoking?"[55] Citing a variety of biblical and talmudic sources, Drazin concludes that it is, therefore, high time, before more irreparable damage is done, that the great *halakhic* authorities of our time come out openly and declare that the use of narcotic drugs and even cigarette smoking are evil practices that are certainly forbidden by Jewish law."

In 1976, the Sephardic Chief Rabbi of Tel Aviv, Rabbi Chaim David Halevy, declared cigarette smoking to be a violation of Jewish law. His prohibition on smoking was widely publicized in the press and was published in his second volume of responsa.[56] Rabbi Levy's discussion concludes with the statement that "it is, therefore, perfectly clear, in my opinion, that it is prohibited to smoke and it is the obligation of every person who cares for his health in order to serve the Lord with all his energies, to refrain from smoking." Rabbi Waldenberg also rules that it is prohibited to smoke because it may be dangerous to one's health.[57]

It is my fervent hope that more rabbis will follow this example and ban smoking. Physicians should urge their patients to stop smoking. Rabbis should deliver sermons urging their congregants to stop smoking, or for nonsmokers not to begin this evil practice. Physicians and rabbis must themselves give up smoking in order to practice what they preach and teach by example. Leading rabbinic authorities should speak out on this subject without timidity. The Jewish community of this nation must marshal its forces in an attack on the promotional activities of the tobacco industry. Judaism must appeal to its people and educate them in the ways of our Torah, which regards life and health to be sacred and their preservation a Divine commandment.

Notes

1. D. E. Redmond, Jr., "Tobacco and Cancer: The First Clinical Report, 1761." *New England Journal of Medicine* 282 (1970): 18–23.

2. *Smoking and Health: Report of the Advisory Committee to the Surgeon General of the Public Health Health Service* (Washington, D.C.: U.S. Government Printing Office, 1964).

3. *The Health Consequences of Smoking: A Public Health Service Review;* 1967 (Washington, D.C.: U.S. Government Printing Office, 1968).

4. Royal College of Physicians, *Smoking and Health* (London: Pitman Medical Publishing Co., 1962); *Smoking and Health Now: A Report of the Royal College of Physicians* (London: Pitman Medical Publishing Co., 1971).

5. E. W. R. Best, A *Canadian Study of Smoking and Health* (Ottawa: Department of National Health and Welfare, 1966).

6. F. C. Barros, "A Government That Encourages Smoking," *Lancet* 2 (1981): 366.

7. *The Health Consequences of Smoking: The Changing Cigarette*, Report of the Surgeon General, Public Health Service (Dept. of Health and Human Services) (Washington, D.C.: U.S. Government Printing Office, 1981).

18. M. Clark and M. Hager, "Slow-Motion Suicide," *Newsweek*, January 22, 1979, pp. 83–84.

9. Deuteronomy 4:9, 4:15.

10. Ibid. 22:8.

11. Maimonides, M. *Mishneh Torah, Hilchot Rotze'ach* 11:4 ff.

12. Deuteronomy 4:9.

13. Ibid. 22:8.

14. Karo, *Shulchan Aruch, Choshen Mishpat* no. 427.

15. Ibid., *Yoreh Deah* no. 116.

16. Ibid., *Orach Chayim* no. 170:16.

17. Ibid. 173:2.

18. Ibid., *Yoreh Deah* no. 116:5.

19. Baba Kamma 91b.

20. Numbers 6:11.

21. Maimonides, *Mishneh Torah, Hilchot Melachim* 6:10, citing Deuteronomy 20:19.

22. Shabbat 140b.

23. S. Luria, *Yam Shel Shlomoh* commentary on Baba Kamma 8:59.

24. Shabbat 129a.

25. Maimonides, *Mishneh Torah, Hilchot Chovel Umazik* 5:1; Karo, *Shulchan Aruch, Choshen Mishpat* 420:31 and *Orach Chayim* 571.

26. Genesis 9:5. For further discussion, see above chap. 17.

27. Baba Kama 79b.

28. Shabbat 148b.

29. M. Aberbach, "Smoking and the Halakhah," *Tradition* 10 (1969): 49–60.

30. M. Feinstein, *Responsa Iggrot Moshe, Yoreh Deah*, sec. 2, no. 49.

31. Shabbat 219b and Niddah 31a, citing Psalms 116:6.

32. M. Feinstein, *Responsa Iggrot Moshe, Choshen Mishpat*, sect. 2, no. 76.

33. J. D. Bleich, "Survey of Recent Halakhic Periodical Literature: Smoking,"*Tradition* 16 (1977): 121–123.

34. J. Ettlinger, Responsa *Binyan Zion*, no. 137.

35. R. J. Hendel and Z. I. Weiss, "Smoking," *Tradition* 17 (1978): 137–140.

36. Bleich, op. cit., pp. 140–142.

37. A. S. Abraham, *Medical Halachah for Everyone* (Jerusalem and New York: Feldheim, 1980), p. 6.

38. G. W. Comstock, F. K. Shah, M. B. Meyer, and H. Abbey, "Low Birthweight and Neonatal Mortality Rates Related to Maternal Smoking and Socioeconomic Status," *American Journal of Obstetrics and Gynecology* 111 (1971): 53–59; D. P. Davies, O. P. Gray, P. C. Ellwood and M. Abernethy, "Cigarette smoking in Pregnancy: Association with Maternal Weight Gain and Fetal Growth," *Lancet* 1 (1976): 385–387.

39. M. B. Meyer and J. A. Tonascia, "Maternal Smoking, Pregnancy Complications, and Perinatal Mortality," *American Journal of Obstetrics and Gynecology* 128 (1977): 494–502.

40. J. Andrews, and J. M. McGarry, "A Community Study of Smoking in Pregnancy," *Journal of Obstetrics and Gynecology of the British Commonwealth* 78 (1972): 1057.

41. J. Kline, Z. A. Stein, M. Susser, and D. Warburton, "Smoking: A Risk Factor for Spontaneous Abortion," *New England Journal of Medicine* 297 (1977): 793–796.

42. N. R. Butler, and H. Goldstein, "Smoking in Pregnancy and Subsequent Child Development," *British Journal of Obstetrics and Gynecology* 4 (1973): 573–575.

43. Editorial, "Passive Smoking: Forest, Gasp, and Facts," *Lancet* 1 (1982): 548–549.

44. P. N. Lee, "Passive Smoking," *Lancet* 1 (1982): 791.

45. H. Sinzinger and A. Kefalides, "Passive Smoking Severely Decreases Platelet Sensitivity to Antiaggregatory Prostaglandins," *Lancet* 2 (1982): 392–393.

46. M. Feinstein, "Concerning the Smoking of Cigarettes in the House of Study," *Noam* 24 (1983): 206–208.

47. E. Y. Waldenberg, "Danger to Health and Smoking in Halachah," *Halachah Veharefuah*, 1983, pp. 320–324; and *Assia* 9, (February 1983): 11–15; E. Grubner, "Is It Permissible to Smoke Among a Group of People Who Object to the Smoke," *Am Hatorah* 2, 3 (5742 [1982]: 92–102.

48. J. D. Bleich, "Survey of Recent Halakhic Periodical Literature: Smoking on *Yom Tov*," *Tradition*, 21 (Summer 1983): 167–178.

49. N. Weil, Commentary of *Korban Nethanel* on Asheri's (Rabbi Asher ben Yechiel, known as *Rosh*) commentary on Betzah 23a.

50. R. L. Dupont, "Marijuana Smoking—A National Epidemic," *American Lung Association Bulletin* 66 (1980): 2–7.

51. R. E. Willette, *Drugs and Driving*, National Institute on Drug Abuse Monograph II, DHEW Pub. No. (ADM) 77-432 (National Institute on Drug Abuse, 1977).

52. M. Feinstein, Responsa *Iggrot Moshe, Yoreh Deah*, sec. 3, no. 35.

53. M. M. Brayer, "Drugs: A Jewish View," in *Jewish Bioethics*, ed. F. Rosner and J. D. Bleich (New York: Hebrew Publishing Co., 1979), pp. 242–250.

54. Aberbach, op. cit.

55. N. Drazin, "Halakhic Attitudes and Conclusions to the Drug Problem and Its Relationship to Cigarette Smoking," in *Judaism and Drugs*, ed. Leo Landman (New York: Federation of Jewish Philanthropies, 1973), pp. 71–81.

56. Ch. D. Levy, *Aseh Lechah Rav* (Tel Aviv, 1978), pt. 2, pp. 9–13.

57. Waldenberg, op. cit.

28

Dental Emergencies on the Sabbath

Introduction

It is axiomatic in Judaism that human life is of infinite value. The preservation of human life takes precedence over all biblical commandments and rabbinic enactments except three: idolatry, murder, and incest.[1] In order to preserve human life, all ritual laws, save the above three, are suspended for the overriding consideration of saving a human life.[2]

How does the practicing dentist apply this basic principle when confronted with an emergency or potential emergency on the Sabbath? What constitutes a dental emergency requiring the dentist to set aside all Sabbath laws to treat his patient? Under what circumstances may the dentist open his office on the Sabbath, turn on the lights, prepare and apply medications, cements, fillings, and the like, use the drill, incise an oral abscess, and perform other therapeutic procedures for his suffering patient?

Abrogation or Suspension of the Sabbath

One of the most renowned halachic controversies concerning medical care on the Sabbath is the question whether danger to life (*piku'ach nefesh*) or potential danger to life completely sets aside the biblical laws and rabbinic rules and regulations pertaining to the Sabbath (*hutra*), or whether this danger only suspends them (*dechuya*). This famous controversy of whether the Sabbath is *hutra* or *dechuya* for *piku'ach nefesh* is more theoretical than practical. Theoretically, if the Sabbath is *hutra*, it is as if the Sabbath does not exist and, therefore, the Jewish dentist may act in accord with standard dental procedures in treating his patient with *piku'ach nefesh* on the Sabbath, similar to that which he would do on a weekday for that patient. (Of course, even if the Sabbath is considered *hutra*, this would apply only to care of the *patient;* it does not mean, for example, that the dentist could smoke a cigarette just because he is taking care of a critically ill person.) If the Sabbath, however, is only *dechuya*—suspended or set aside only for the *piku'ach nefesh* situation—the dentist would have to limit himself to those dental procedures absolutely essential to take care of the dental emergency.

However, it is clear from the codes of Jewish law, including the *Shulchan Aruch*[3] and *Mishneh Torah*,[4] that a physician or dentist must perform all acts required for the care of his patient (*kol tzorchei choleh*) and not limit himself exclusively to those things which would remove the danger to life (*piku'ach nefesh*).[5] The medical or dental practitioner must do everything that he would ordinarily do for his patient on a weekday. Thus, from a practical standpoint, this major distinction between *hutra* and *dechuya* is irrelevant once the patient's condition has been classified as *piku'ach nefesh*.[6]

A second theoretical difference between *hutra* and *dechuya* is in the use of a non-Jewish dentist who is equally competent. If the Sabbath is *hutra* for *piku'ach nefesh;* there is no need to send the patient to the non-Jewish dentist, and the Jewish dentist himself can treat the patient on the Sabbath as if the Sabbath were nonexistent. If, however, the Sabbath is *dechuya*, or only temporarily suspended for *piku'ach nefesh*, there is no need for the Jewish dentist to transgress the Sabbath, and the patient can be cared for by the non-Jewish dentist. However, contrary to this line of reasoning, our sages rule that even if the Sabbath is *dechuya* for *piku'ach nefesh* situations, the most competent Jewish medical or dental practitioners and not a non-Jew should care for the patient. Maimonides clearly states that "when such things have to be done [to save a life on the Sabbath] . . . they should not be left to heathens, minors, slaves, or women, but should be done by adult and scholarly Israelites."[7] Thus, if an illness is classified as *piku'ach nefesh*, it is not proper to refer the patient to a non-Jew. There is no distinction in this regard in practice between *hutra* and *dechuya*. The author of *Mishnah Berurah* concurs that this is the accepted halachic practice.[8]

A real distinction between *hutra* and *dechuya* might be the performance of an act on the Sabbath in an unusual manner (*shinuy*), thereby changing the offense from a biblical to a rabbinic transgression. If the Sabbath is *hutra* for *piku'ach nefesh*, the dentist may perform all acts necessary to treat his patient in the same manner he would perform them on a weekday. If, however, the Sabbath is only temporarily set aside for *piku'ach nefesh*, it would seem preferable to use a *shinuy* to perform all therapeutic acts on the Sabbath in order to lessen the transgression from a biblical to a rabbinic offense.

What is a *shinuy* for a dentist? If a right-handed dentist performs root canal work with his left hand, that might be considered a *shinuy*, but this is obviously highly impractical. The definition of *shinuy* requires that the act be performed in a less competent manner than usual so that either the results of the act are less good or the method is more difficult. Rabbi Abraham Borenstein, known as *Avnei Nezer*, in the introduction to his work *Egley Tal*, specifically states that a *shinuy* is when the outcome of an act is less successful or the method of doing the act is particularly tedious. If neither definition applies, it is not a *shinuy*. Turning the light on with one's elbow or starting the dental drill with one's knee is not a *shinuy*, according to Rabbi Moshe Feinstein,[9] because the *shinuy* of using one's elbow or knee is an act (turning on the light or starting the drill) that does not affect the electrical contact that sets into motion the forbidden activity. It is, therefore, usually not feasible for a dentist to employ a *shinuy* that is halachically valid in the direct care of his patient with *piku'ach nefesh* on the Sabbath.

In practical terms for the dentist, therefore, there is no distinction between *hutra* and *dechuya*. Once a situation has been classified as *piku'ach nefesh*, the Jewish dentist is obligated to do everything necessary to care for his patient on the Sabbath, and that should be his only concern.

Definition of Piku'ach Nefesh

A frequent halachic question in dentistry is whether or not the presence of an abscess is considered to be *piku'ach nefesh* requiring incision and drainage on the Sabbath. The halachic definition of *piku'ach nefesh* is not the same as the medical-dental definition of danger to life. Halachah sets a higher standard of risk-benefit;

i.e., a lower level of risk or danger than that set by medicine is classified as *piku'ach nefesh* by the halachah. Thus, any internal sore from within the lips and mouth, including the teeth, is halachically considered to be a situation of *piku'ach nefesh* if it might lead to an actual or potential danger to life.[11] Our sages were especially cognizant of the fact that any infection in the mouth is potentially dangerous because of the direct circulatory connections between the oral cavity and the brain. The fact that total asepsis in the mouth is nearly impossible to achieve is compensated by God's creation of protective enzymes, antibodies, and other host defense systems which protect the body from sepsis secondary to the bacterial flora of the oral cavity. The fact that any "significant" infection or inflammation or abscess in the mouth can today be treated prophylactically and/or therapeutically with antibiotics in no way eliminates the classification of that abscess or infection as *piku'ach nefesh* requiring the dentist to treat it on the Sabbath. Thus, conditions such as tooth abscesses, jaw swellings, gum infections, and the like, are all defined in the category of internal sore (*makah shel chalal*) for which Sabbath laws must be put aside in favor of the most effective and expeditious dental care.

A canker sore, a broken orthodontist's wire, a mild tooth discomfort, and the like, are not considered to be *piku'ach nefesh*, although one could stretch the above reasoning *ad absurdum* and say that any scratch or pimple in the mouth could lead to infection, abscess formation, and brain infection. What is called *piku'ach nefesh* must be "significant" pathology. Man is mortal, and every human being is subject to an occasional scratch or pimple on his body. "All is by the hand of Heaven except colds and fevers"[12] means that every person can have an occasional cold and/or fever. The norm or baseline is not perfection. A cold or a minor sore is not a pathologic condition to be classified as *piku'ach nefesh*. However, a well-established infection in the mouth is clearly a case of *piku'ach nefesh*.

Categories of Illness Other Than Piku'ach Nefesh

There are four classic halachic categories of illness in relation to the suspension of Sabbath laws: *piku'ach nefesh* (danger or possible danger to life), *choleh she'ayn bo sakanah* (ill person but without danger to life), *meychush be'alma* (minor discomfort), and *chesron eyver* (chance of loss of function of an organ or limb). Elsewhere,[13] Rabbi Moshe Tendler provides an analysis which suggests that there is a fifth category—*choleh she'ayn bo sakanah im tzar gadol* (ill person without danger to life but with great pain or discomfort).[14] This category is tantamount to *chesron eyver* in that it is permissible for such a patient to waive all rabbinic prohibitions in addition to telling a non-Jew to do the act (*amira le'akum*).[15]

Piku'ach nefesh has already been discussed in the previous section of this essay. *Choleh she'ayn bo sakanah*[16] refers to a patient who is suffering from an illness which does not constitute a danger to life or limb but is serious enough or painful enough to make the patient feel that he would rather be in bed (*mutal lemishkav*). A patient with a bad toothache due to an exposed nerve but without infection should be classified in this category. For such a patient to whom there is no danger to life, therapeutic intervention on the Sabbath may only set aside the rabbinic prohibition against telling a non-Jew to do the act (*amira le'akum*). The treatment should, therefore, be provided by a non-Jew.

Meychush be'alma refers to minor discomfort for which the taking of any medication is a rabbinic prohibition. Our sages were concerned that because of discomfort, the person may overact (*bohul al gufoh*) and allow himself some unwarranted leniencies in Sabbath observance.

Chesron eyvor refers not to the loss of an organ or limb but to the loss of normal function of a limb.[17] This category of medical condition is halachically classified in between *piku'ach nefesh* and *choleh she'ayn bo sakanah*. The *Avnei Nezer* exemplifies *chesron eyver* as an orthopedic problem such as a torn ligament or muscle which, if not repaired on the Sabbath, would result in the patient's walking with a limp. *Chesron eyver* does not require actual loss of the limb.

Loss of a Tooth

Is a tooth in the category of *chesron eyver* for which a Jew can set aside all rabbinic prohibitions on the Sabbath? The third opinion in the *Shulchan Aruch* concerning *chesron eyver* is the ruling we follow, namely, a Jew is allowed to waive rabbinic prohibitions in order to preserve a limb or its function.[18] If a patient presents to the dentist on the Sabbath following trauma with two avulsed adult teeth, one could argue that halachah considers this situation as *chesron eyver* requiring the immediate reimplantation of those teeth. Teeth are not cited in the Mishnah in *Oholot* which lists the 248 *eyvorin* (limbs or organs) of the body. However, teeth can be halachically classified as *eyver* based on *Avnei Nezer*'s definition of *chesron eyver* cited above. Less than the normal use of a limb is *chesron eyver.* Since the jaw is an *eyver* and the absence of teeth interferes with its proper functioning, and since the reimplantation of those teeth would restore the proper functioning of the jaw, the traumatic avulsion of teeth represents a situation of *chesron eyver.*

If this analysis is correct, it is permissible to reimplant an adult tooth on the Sabbath provided one does not violate any biblical (*d'oraitha*) prohibitions. A non-Jew is obviously very helpful in this situation because whatever he does for the Jewish dentist on the Sabbath is only rabbinic and not biblical in its implications. In the absence of a non-Jew, is the Jewish dentist permitted to drill, mix paste or cement, cut wires, apply wax, make dental impressions, turn on lights etc., on the Sabbath in order to reimplant a traumatically avulsed tooth? Each of these activities must be evaluated as to whether it involves one or more biblical or rabbinic prohibitions.

A Practical Suggestion

Which activities in the sophisticated modern dentist's office would be classified as rabbinic prohibitions on the Sabbath which may be waived for the sake of *chesron eyver?* Turning on lights on the Sabbath, according to many rabbinic authorities, is a biblical offense. Mixing cement or paste is a biblical offense known as *lishah. Lishah* (kneading) is the mixing of water and fine particles to form a dough or paste. There is no *shinuy* possible with *lishah* since the end result is the same, i.e., the making of a paste or cement. Premade cements in tubes that can be squeezed out, if available, might be acceptable for Sabbath use. Another method is for two people to make the cement together, employing the suggestion of *shenayim she-osu* (see below). Pushing wax into a crevice is a biblical offense known as *memachek* (smoothing or waxing). Cutting a wire with one's left hand if one is right-handed constitutes a *shinuy* but is not practical. Starting the dentist's drill by turning on the motor on the Sabbath may or may not constitute a biblical offense. Most authorities rule that if the motor has no heating element, starting it on the Sabbath would only be classified as a rabbinic prohibition and permissible for a situation of *chesron eyver.* Obviously, it is rather difficult for a dentist to function on the Sabbath by suspending only rabbinic but not biblical prohibitions.

A practical suggestion for dentists who must treat a patient with *chesron eyver* or *choleh she'ayn bo sakanah im tzar gadol* is the intriguing approach of two people performing a single act. *Shen-*

ayim she'osu converts every prohibited act on the Sabbath into a rabbinic prohibition. *Rambam* clearly states that whenever two persons jointly do work that can be done by each one of them alone, they are exempt, and it does not matter if each one does a different part of the work, or whether both do the work together from beginning to end.[19] It is a functional practical solution.[20] *Shenayim she'osu* is like a *shinuy* and considered to be a technical avoidance of a biblical prohibition. If the dentist and an attendant or family member or other bystander simultaneously start the drill, only a rabbinic prohibition is involved, which is waived for *chesron eyver* on the Sabbath. Once the drill is running, the dentist can operate it alone until the procedure is completed.

Some authorities consider starting a dentist's drill to be a rabbinic prohibition if there is no heat or electricity involved in starting the motor, but only if it is an air compressor. However, according to some authorities, starting a motor involves the biblical transgression of converting a useless non-functioning machine into a functioning drill (*metaken manah*). Manipulating or cutting into gums and other soft tissue in reimplanting avulsed teeth is known as *mechatech basar be'alma* and is permitted.

Concerning rabbinic prohibitions (*issurei d'rabbanan*), we have been taught that the rabbis did not enact prohibitions in the face of severe pain (*bemakom tza'ar lo gazru bo rabbanan*). These considerations, combined within the definition of *chesron eyver* cited above, may allow the dentist to function comfortably within halachah to restore the function of a tooth on the Sabbath. This is an often-overlooked category of illness on the Sabbath—no danger of life but great pain. For this category, a Jew may transgress rabbinic but not biblical prohibitions on the Sabbath, as discussed above.[21]

Dental Abscesses

The Talmud considers the piercing of an abscess with a pin to relieve the turgidity and pain and evacuate the pus on the Sabbath (*mapis mursa*) to be a rabbinic prohibition.[22] However, the incision and drainage of an abscess and the insertion of a drain requires the expertise of a physician (*ma'aseh uman*) and is, therefore, classified as a biblical prohibition. Thus, the opening of an abscess to remove pus can be either a rabbinic or a biblical offense if performed on the Sabbath, depending upon how it is done. In dentistry, an oral abscess is nearly always categorized in halachah as *piku'ach nefesh*, and, therefore, all therapeutic measures necessary to treat the abscess must be employed in the most expeditious manner possible.

Although medically the incision and drainage of a dental abscess can be postponed until after the Sabbath and the patient given antibiotics, the difference between the medical and halachic definition of *piku'ach nefesh* is such that once the condition is categorized as *piku'ach nefesh*, definitive treatment must be instituted promptly and not postponed because of the Sabbath.

Dental Anesthesia

The administration of an injection by a physician on the Sabbath might involve the biblical prohibition of "wounding" (*chavalah*) because the physician first aspirates before giving the injection to avoid injecting directly into a blood vessel. If blood is aspirated into the syringe, that would constitute an act of *chavalah*. However, for the dentist, giving an injection of a local anesthetic in the mouth is only a rabbinic act and, therefore, permissible for *chesron eyver* as defined earlier in this essay. In dentistry, injections are mainly for pain relief, and even if they induce some gum bleeding, it is considered unintentional (*davar she'ayn miskaven*) and not in the category of *pesik reysho* (dialectic term for an absolutely unavoidable result of an act). Furthermore, the dentist has no need for the blood; on the contrary, he would prefer that the injection cause no bleeding at all. For all these reasons, the giving of an oral injection of a local anesthetic on the Sabbath by a dentist is considered to involve only a rabbinic prohibition.

Returning Home After a Dental Emergency

When a dentist has completed the treatment of a dental emergency on the Sabbath, he should close his office but not turn off the lights. Shutting off the drill is permitted if otherwise a considerable financial loss might be incurred (*hefsed mamon*) and the dentist might be reluctant to treat another patient on the Sabbath in the future.

If a dentist is called to the hospital on the Sabbath for a dental emergency, the halachic rules of his returning home are the same as for a physician or emergency medical technician returning from a physician emergency. This subject has been described in detail elsewhere.[23] A dentist should not drive his own car home from the scene of a dental emergency (office, hospital, etc.) but should take a taxi or have his car driven by a non-Jewish driver to minimize the Sabbath prohibitions involved.

Miscellaneous Dental-Halachic Issues

DENTAL PROSTHESES, FILLINGS, BRIDGES, AND RITUAL IMMERSION

Dental fillings and all permanent (i.e., functional) dental prostheses are not an impediment or barrier (*chatzitzah*) between a person and the water of a ritual immersion bath (*mikvah*). *Tevilah* (ritual immersion) may be performed without their removal unless they have been improperly placed and must be removed and corrected by the dentist. *Tevilah* must be postponed until such correction is made. For example, a filling that is interfering with chewing and must be corrected by the dentist, or a bridge that is painful because further correction must be made on the device, must be fixed before *tevilah*.[24]

The terms "temporary" and "permanent" are often misinterpreted, since the main halachic criteria relating to *chatzitzah* is whether or not the filling or prosthesis is functional. If a woman has a permanent filling which is too high, and she cannot chew on it because it bothers her and it hurts, she cannot go to *mikvah* until it is ground down. On the other hand, if she has a temporary cement filling which is fully functional, she is allowed to go to the *mikvah*, since it is classified as part of the body. If the filling is not functional, it is considered a *chatzitzah* whether made of gold, cement, or plastic. If it is functional, it is considered as part of the natural growth process of the tooth and is not a *chatzitzah*. Semi-permanent orthopedic dental devices are to be discouraged unless absolutely necessary because of the halachic problems concerning *tevilah* which they raise. Sutures do not hinder *tevilah* by their presence.[25] The question of plastic teeth and *tevilah* is discussed by Rabbi Feinstein.[26]

In summary, permanent bridgework and cemented or wired (i.e., permanent) braces do not constitute an interposing barrier (*chatzitzah*) and therefore do not hinder the regular process of *tevilah*. However, removable dentures, removable braces, removable bridges, and the like, must be removed before *tevilah*. The application of a surgical dressing to the gums during extensive gum work may require a delay in the time of *tevilah*. Rabbinic consultation should be sought in such cases as each case must be adjudicated based upon the particular circumstances of that case.

SEPARATE DENTURES FOR PASSOVER?

Separate dentures are not required for Passover or for *milchig* ("milk foods") and *fleishig* ("meat foods"). Since food that is eaten does not usually reach a degree of temperature or heat that surpasses the pain threshold, no absorption of food by the teeth is considered to occur. Therefore, separate dentures for "meat" and "milk" foods are not required. It is recommended, however, that someone with false dentures should not chew hard *chametz* on the day before Passover eve because of a legal rabbinical technicality based upon the effect of pressure in causing absorption.[27] Because of the unusual severity of Passover law, the false-denture-user is advised not to chew hard *chametz* from noon of the day before Passover eve onwards. He does not, however, have to procure a separate set of dentures for the Passover holiday. If dentures or bridges are removable, they should be soaked for a twenty-four-hour period prior to the holiday after careful brushing to remove all particulate matters.[28]

KOHEN STUDYING DENTISTRY

Under the usual academic conditions, a *kohen* (priest) is not permitted to study dentistry. Because of the requirement in United States medical schools that students take anatomy and pathology courses, it is impossible for a *kohen* to attend medical or dental school. Even if the assumption is made that most, if not all, cadavers are non-Jewish, ritual defilement of a *kohen* still occurs upon contact (*maga*) or by carrying (*massa*) of any dead body. The halachic distinction between Jew and Gentile concerns ritual defilement on being present in the same room with a cadaver (*tumat ohel*).

The same objections expressed concerning medical school apply to dental school. The latter curriculum also includes anatomical dissection, which is forbidden to a *kohen*, irrespective of whether the cadaver is Jewish or non-Jewish. If, however, the dental student can avoid actual dissection and attend only as an observer, and if his early dentistry training does not include a human skull with its dentition, then there may be dispensation for a *kohen* studying dentistry. This possible restricted permissibility rests upon the fact that in the present era we follow the lenient halachic ruling that a non-Jewish corpse does not convey ritual defilement to people in the same room who do not have direct contact with it. Unlike the physician, the dentist is not usually involved with dying patients, death certificates, the mortuary, etc., which pose seemingly insoluble problems to a physician who is a *kohen*.[29]

TRAINING IN HOSPITALS WITH SABBATH OBLIGATIONS

Is a physician or dentist obligated to seek training or employment or attending physician status at a hospital where there is minimum or no conflict between hospital policy and Sabbath observance? The answer is that a physician or dentist must seek association with the most reputable and prestigious hospital possible to ensure excellent training and continuing education. Jewish law requires that the physician or dentist acquire maximum skill and competence to practice his chosen profession. Therefore, he should forgo personal comfort and the convenience of training in a hospital that is sympathetic to his religious needs in favor of a hospital that will provide him with the best possible training, provided that he is certain of his fortitude in maintaining all halachic requirements despite the less favorable environment. However, if the superior training is to be acquired at the price of Sabbath desecration, even of rabbinic ordinances only, the physician or dentist must forgo the educational advantages of the prestigious hospital.[30]

Conclusion

The classic codes of Jewish law rule that "for any internal sore (*makah shel challal*) that is from the lip or teeth inward, and the teeth themselves are included, one must desecrate the Sabbath." Thus, conditions such as tooth abscesses, jaw swelling, gum infections, and the like, are all classified in the category of "internal sore." In such cases, the Sabbath laws must be put aside in favor of the most effective and expeditious dental care. Oral surgery requiring postoperative care is certainly classified as a danger-to-life situation (*piku'ach nefesh*) for which the Sabbath must be desecrated. However, if the patient suffering from a dental condition has only a mild discomfort without much associated pain, no Sabbath law may be desecrated. If there is danger of loss of function (*chesron eyver*), rabbinic but not biblical prohibitions may be transgressed. If there is moderate pain but no real danger, only the prohibition of telling a non-Jew to act (*amira le'akum*) is suspended. In cases of extreme pain, the same rules that govern *chesron eyver* apply. The dentist has all the obligations of a medical practitioner in cases classified as *piku'ach nefesh.*

Notes

1. Maimonides, *Mishneh Torah, Hilchot Yesodei Hatorah* 5:2.
2. Ibid. *Hilchot Shabbat* 2:1.
3. *Shulchan Aruch, Orach Chayim* 328:4.
4. *Mishneh Torah, Hilchot Shabbat* 2:1.
5. *Mishnah Berurah* 328:14 and the commentaries of *Biur Halachah* and *Be'er Hetev* there, where the question is discussed as to whether or not the Sabbath should be desecrated for something whose omission would not constitute a danger to life. Authorities supporting both opposing viewpoints are cited.
6. Although *Rambam* (*Hilchot Shabbat* 2:1) rules that the Sabbath is only suspended (*dechuya*) and not completely set aside (*hutra*) if human life is in danger, he nevertheless clearly states that whatever a skilled physician considers necessary should be done for the patient on the Sabbath. Rabbis Joseph Karo (*Keseph Mishneh*), Nisson Girondi (*Ran*), and Solomon ben Adret (*Rashba*) are also of the opinion that the Sabbath is only suspended (*dechuya*) for danger to life. However, Rabbi Moshe Isserles (*Ramo*) in his Responsa, no. 76, states that the Sabbath is completely set aside (*hutra*) if human life is in danger.
7. *Mishneh Torah, Hilchot Shabbat* 2:3.
8. *Mishnah Berurah* 328:37.
9. Personal communication.
10. *Mishneh Torah, Hilchot Shabbat* 2:5.
11. *Shulchan Aruch, Orach Chayim* 328.
12. Ketubot 30a.
13. M. D. Tendler, *Bet Yitzchak* (Yeshiva University Press, 1987).
14. (a) The Talmud (*Ketubot* 6b) states that he who pierces an abscess on the Sabbath—if in order to cause the pus to come out of it—is free from punishment (and it is permitted). See also the commentary of *Tosafot* there, s.v. *ve'im lehatzi*, which states that the Talmud is certainly concerned with a patient in pain but where there is no danger to life; nevertheless, the rabbis did not enact a preventive measure to prohibit rabbinic "work" on the Sabbath even if performed by a Jew. See also *Shabbat* 107a.

(b) The Talmud (*Ketubot* 60a) states that a man suffering from pain in the chest (lit. groaning) may suck (goat's) milk (directly from the goat) on the Sabbath (even though the release of milk from the animal's udder resembles the plucking of a plant from its root, or the "unloading" of a burden, which is ordinarily forbidden on the Sabbath). What is the reason?—continues the Talmud—because sucking is an "unusual" method of "unloading" against which, where pain is involved, no preventive measure was enacted by the rabbis (even though the Jewish patient himself sucks the milk and does not ask a non-Jew to secure the milk for him).

(c) *Shulchan Aruch, Orach Chayim* 328:28, also rules that it is permitted to pierce a boil on the Sabbath to express the pus therefrom. *Mishnah*

Berurah 328:28 cites the opinion of *Tosafot* that the permissive ruling is due to the fact that where pain is involved, the rabbis did not enact a preventive measure.

(d) *Shulchan Aruch, Orach Chayim* 328:33, also rules that a person suffering from pain in the chest is permitted to suck milk directly from a goat on the Sabbath because where pain is involved, the rabbis did not enact a preventive measure. The author of *Mishnah Berurah* (loc. cit.) cites the explanation of Rabbi Nisson Girondi (*Ran*) that "although the rule in regard to patients in whom there is no danger to life is to tell a non-Jew to perform the act, here [in the case of chest pain] it is different because the cure for the patient's ailment is that he suck [the milk] himself." This means that if there is pain and suffering and the relief thereof cannot be provided by an act of a non-Jew, it is permissible for the Jew to do it himself even if there is no danger to life (*piku'ach nefesh*) or danger about the loss of function of an organ or limb (*chesron eyver*).

(e) One should add that on the second day of *Yom Tov* it is permitted for a Jew(ess) to personally apply medication on his (her) eyes even though on the first day of *Yom Tov* this act can only be performed by a non-Jew. Similarly, for all other rabbinic rules, the rabbis allowed such acts to be performed by Jews on the second day of *Yom Tov* (*Shulchan Aruch, Orach Chayim* 496:2).

15. Tosafot on Ketubot 60a and *Shulchan Aruch, Orach Chayim* 328:28.

16. *Shulchan Aruch*, loc. cit.

17. Responsa *Avnei Nezer*, introduction to *Egley Tal.*

18. *Shulchan Aruch*, loc. cit.

19. *Mishneh Torah, Hilchot Shabbat* 1:15.

20. R. Moshe Feinstein used this rationale in dealing with the problem faced by the Israeli army concerning the intermittent running of the tank air-conditioner on Shabbat.

21. See n. 14.

22. Ketubot 6b, Shabbat 3a and 107a.

23. Responsa *Iggrot Moshe, Orach Chayim*, pt. 4, no. 80; F. Rosner and W. Wolfson, "Returning on the Sabbath from a Life-Saving Mission," *Journal of Halacha and Contemporary Society* 9 (Spring 1985): 53–67.

24. Responsa *Iggrot Moshe, Yoreh Deah*, no. 97.

25. Ibid., pt. 2, no. 87.

26. Ibid. no. 88.

27. Rabbi Aron Felder in *Oholei Yeshurun* (p. 82, par. 33, n. 200). See also *Tzitz Eliezer* 9:25.

28. F. Rosner and M. D. Tendler, *Practical Medical Halachah* (New York: Feldheim, 1980), p. 86.

29. *Shulchan Aruch, Yoreh Deah* 369, 371 and 372:2 and the commentary *Dagul Mir'vavah* on 372:2.

30. Rosner and Tendler, op. cit., p. 116.

29

Unconventional Therapies

Introduction

More and more patients who traditionally sought healing from conventional physicians are seeking out alternative therapies or more natural forms of therapy. Such unorthodox therapies may include naturopathy, acupuncture, homeopathy, chiropractic, herbal remedies, metabolic therapies, and vitamin and mineral therapies. More controversial treatments include nutrition pharmacology, which involves using nutrients to treat illness; chelation therapy, which supposedly draws harmful metals and excess calcium out of arterial walls in order to slow down free-radical damage and plaque formation; clinical ecology, or the treatment of food and environmental sensitivities; and candidology, which involves diagnosing and treating systemic yeast infections.[1]

Alternative and unorthodox medicine has a long history, particularly in relation to cancer prevention and treatment.[2] Unproven or questionable dietary and nutritional methods in cancer prevention are those which have not "been responsibly, objectively, reproducibly, and reliably demonstrated in humans" to be efficacious and safe.[3] Products promoted for profit to the public without passing such efficacy and safety standards are nearly always ineffective, often harmful, and sometimes lethal.[4]

Despite progress in cancer therapy, unorthodox treatments continue to hold a fascination for cancer patients. More than 50 percent of patients undergoing conventional cancer therapy simultaneously pursue unorthodox programs, often from an early stage of their illness. A substantial proportion of such patients ultimately reject conventional treatments.[5] Such widespread use by patients of unorthodox or unproven cancer treatments represents an important social, economic, and clinical problem. The public spends billions of dollars annually on unproven cancer cures labeled as metabolic (e.g., laetrile or hydrazine), dietary (e.g., grape diet or macrobiotic diet), immunologic (e.g., fetal vaccines), megavitamin (e.g., high-dose vitamin C), and imagery (e.g., Simonton technique).[6]

Contrary to stereotypes, patients who seek unproven methods tend to be well-educated, upper middle class, and not necessarily terminal or even beyond hope of cure or remission by conventional treatments.[7] Many practitioners of unorthodox cancer care are licensed physicians who specialize in homeopathic or naturopathic medicine.

Why do people seek out alternative therapies? They may be discouraged and despair about the realities of conventional cancer treatment. Fear, side-effects, previous negative experiences, and a desire by the patient for more supportive care are other reasons. People are unhappy with the "disease oriented technologic authoritarian health care system."[8] People may reject conventional care because they are attracted to the ideology which includes "an emphasis on self-care, a systemic rather than a localized view of pathology and of health, and belief in the fundamental importance of nutrition and whole-body fitness."[9]

Today's physician is many times more able than his predecessors of previous generations, but his practice has changed from intensely personal service to an objective and highly intellectualized approach. "The quack may return in the role of comforter—the provider of hope at small cost, and of death in natural dignity."[10]

Health quackery has been the subject of feature articles in the state medical journals in Arkansas, Florida, Ohio, Minnesota, New York, Rhode Island, Tennessee, and Wisconsin, as well as in nursing, pharmacy, dentistry, and dietetic journals.[11] The American Medical Association, the Food and Drug Administration, and other health groups are valiantly, but mostly unsuccessfully, trying to combat quackery by public-awareness campaigns about health fraud.

In addition to operating in areas of legitimate medical practice, unorthodox therapies involve irregular practitioners and medical sects, including homeopaths, Thomsonians, hydropaths, and numerous other sects and groups all engaged in medical practice. The legal struggles to establish the legitimacy of these nonorthodox practices form a fascinating chapter in medical history.[12] In 1987, the American Medical Association, the American College of Radiology, and the American College of Surgeons were found guilty of antitrust violations in a suit brought against them by American chiropractors. This case, which has been before the courts for twelve years, is currently under appeal.[13]

How does Judaism view alternative or unorthodox therapies? How does Judaism view the practices of chiropractic, homeopathy, naturopathy, and similar medical sects? Even if these are acceptable as alternative or additional or supplementary methods of healing, how does Judaism view health quackery? Are faith healing or spiritual healing acceptable modes of therapy in Judaism? In Judaic teaching, can amulets, incantations, and/or prayers be substituted for conventional medical therapy?

Biblical license is given to a human physician to heal, and biblical mandate is given the patient to seek healing from a human healer. Does this mandate also include alternative therapies, or does it specifically exclude unconventional or unorthodox therapies? Is a patient allowed to supplement standard medical treatment with holistic or spiritual healing? Is quackery condoned in Judaism?

Prayer and Faith Healing

The tradition of healing which combines elements of religion or spiritual healing with classical scientific medicine has probably always existed. In some parts of the world, such techniques range from religious faith healing to nutritional faddism, witchcraft, and ceremonies of the occult. All these treatment forms rely to a considerable extent on the faith and belief of the patient in the practitioner. Faith healing includes those healing efforts for which there is no scientific evidence to support purported "cures." The scientific community, including the medical profession, tends to dismiss such healing as quackery. To true believers in faith healing, the explanation is simple—it is a miracle.

Recourse to prayer in Judaism during pain or illness is not necessarily an indication of despair in the efficacy of traditional medicine. In fact, the majority of mankind prays for the sick at one time or another. The prayers may differ in content, in the manner in which they are offered, or in the person or deity to whom they are addressed, but both religious and nonreligious people offer prayers for recovery when they are sick.[14]

The Patriarch Abraham prayed for the recovery of Abimelech (Genesis 20:17), and God healed him. David prayed for the recovery of his son (II Samuel 12:16), but his son died. Elisha prayed for the recovery of the Shunamite woman's son (II Kings 4:33), and the boy recovered. King Hezekiah prayed for his own recovery (II Chronicles 32:24), and God added fifteen years to his life. These incidents are anecdotal and hence do not constitute "scientific, statistical proof" of the efficacy of prayer, but they are certainly worthy of mention.

The Bible is replete with descriptive prayers (Psalms 6:32, 30:13, 38:1–10, 102:4–6, 107:6), figurative prayers (Psalms 13:4, 34:21, 147:1), philosophic prayers (Psalms 39:5), prayers of youth (Psalms 102:24), and prayers of old age (Psalms 71:9). The shortest prayer on record is the famous one uttered by Moses for the recovery of his sister Miriam, who was afflicted with leprosy. Said Moses: *El na r'fa na la* ("O God, heal her, I beseech Thee"), and she recovered.

The homiletical commentary on the Pentateuch called the *Midrash Rabbah*, in its interpretation of the biblical phrase *whensoever we call upon Him* (Deuteronomy 4:7), describes the rapidity with which prayers can be answered as follows:

> The rabbis said: A prayer can be answered after forty days, as can be learnt from Moses, as it is written, *And I fell down before the Lord . . . forty days* (Deuteronomy 9:18); it can be answered after twenty days, as can be learnt from Daniel, as it written, *I ate no pleasant bread . . . till three whole weeks were fulfilled* (Daniel 10:3), and after this he prayed, *O Lord, hear; O Lord, forgive* (9:19); and it can be answered after three days, as can be learnt from Jonah, as it written, *And Jonah was in the belly of the fish three days and three nights* (Jonah 1:17), and after that [Scripture says], *Then Jonah prayed unto the Lord his God out of the fish's belly* (2:1); it can be answered after one day, as can be learnt from Elijah, as it is written, *And it came to pass at the time of the offering of the evening sacrifice, that Elijah the prophet came near, and said* (I Kings 18:36); and it can also be answered at its time of utterance, as can be learnt from David, as it is written, *But as for me, let my prayer be unto Thee, O Lord, in an acceptable time* (Psalms 69:13); while sometimes God answers a prayer even before it is uttered, as it is said, *And it shall come to pass that, before they call, I will answer* (Isaiah 65:24).

The Talmud describes private prayers (Shabbat 30b, Abodah Zarah 4b and 7b) and public prayers (Berachot 8a, Baba Batra 91a), morning prayers (Berachot 6b) and afternoon prayers (ibid.), prayers to be recited on entering a house of worship (Berachot 28b) and on leaving a house of worship (ibid.), on going to the privy (ibid. 60b) and on entering a bathhouse (ibid. 60a), on going to bed (ibid. 60b), upon arising in the morning (ibid. 28b), and on passing through a city (ibid. 54a and 60a). The Talmud further discusses the prayer shawl (Chagigah 14b), the time for prayer (Shabbat 118b, Berachot 28b, 29b, and 31a), the language of prayer (Shabbat 12b), the place for prayer (Berachot 8a, 10b, and 34b; Shabbat 10a), the position for prayer (Berachot 5b, 6b, 10b, 28b, and 39a), preparation for prayer (ibid. 32b, Shabbat 10a), washing before praying (Berachot 15a and 22a), and sacrifices that accompany prayers (Pesachim 82a, Taanit 27b, Megillah 3a).

Regarding the specific question of the efficacy of prayer in the Talmud, one may cite the following (Berachot 32b):

> Rabbi Eleazer said: Prayer is more efficacious even than good deeds, for there was no one greater in good deeds than Moses our teacher, and yet he was answered only after prayer. . . . Rabbi Eleazar also said: Prayer is more efficacious than offerings.

Another circumstance in which prayers are said to be efficacious is the need of the community for the sick person. Thus the Talmud states (Erubin 29b):

> . . . it once happened that Rabbi Chanina ate half an onion and half of its poisonous fluid and became so ill that he was on the point of dying. His colleagues, however, begged for heavenly mercy, and he recovered because his contemporaries needed him.

One should never be discouraged from praying even under the most difficult and troublesome conditions. The Talmud says that "even if a sharp sword rests upon a man's neck, we should not desist from prayer" (Berachot 10a). On the other hand a person should never stand in a place of danger and say that a miracle will be wrought for him (Shabbat 32a). One should not count on being cured by direct intervention by God without the patient having a hand therein in seeking healing from traditional human medical practitioners.

The relevant references to prayer in the codes of Jewish law are cited by Jakobovits, who concludes:

> These laws indicate unmistakably that while every encouragement was given for the sick to exploit their adversity for moral and religious ends and to strengthen their faith in recovery by prayer, confidence in the healing powers of God was never allowed to usurp the essential functions of the physician and of medical science.[15]

Amulets

From the earliest times people have attempted to ward off misfortune, sickness, or "evil spirits" by wearing on their person pieces of paper, parchment, or metal discs inscribed with various formulae which would protect or heal the bearers. Such artifacts, known as amulets or talismans, are frequently mentioned in talmudic literature. To the Jews, the amulet is called *kemiya* and consists either of a written parchment or of roots (*Tosefta* Shabbat 4:9) or herbs (Jerushalmi Shabbat 8b). It is worn on a small chain, or in a signet ring or in a tube. A *kemiya* is considered to be of proven efficacy if it cures a sick person on three different occasions or if it cures three different patients (Shabbat 60a). An assurance by a physician who prescribed or wrote such an amulet is accepted as credible without question, for in antiquity amulets were considered part of the legitimate therapeutic armamentarium of the physician.[16]

There is no objection in Jewish religious law to the use of amulets for healing purposes. Amulets are apparently deeply rooted in popular belief. Although a long list of acts falling in the category of idolatrous customs is found in the Talmud (*Tosefta* Shabbat, chapts. 7 and 8), anything done for the sake of healing is specifically excluded. Hence, it is permitted even on the Sabbath "to carry as amulets the egg of a certain species of locust [against ear-ache], the tooth of a fox [against insomnia or drowsiness], or a nail from the gallows [against swelling]."[17]

The rabbinic responsa literature of the past several hundred years is replete with references to amulets as preventives to keep off the "evil eye," to avert demons, to prevent abortion, as well as to cure a variety of diseases, such as epilepsy, lunacy, fever, poisoning, hysteria, jaundice, and colic.[18] A distinction is made in Jewish law between the prophylactic and therapeutic use of amulets as follows:

> It is permitted to heal with amulets, even if they contain [Divine] names; similarly it is allowed to wear amulets containing scriptural verses, but only if they serve to protect the wearer from

> becoming ill, but not to heal him if he is afflicted with a wound or a disease. But it is forbidden to write scriptural verses in amulets.[19]

Amulets were usually pendants worn by the user at all times to prevent or to cure certain ailments. Talismans did not have to be carried or worn at all times. Other objects are also cited in Jewish sources as efficacious against specific complaints. A coin tied to the sole of the foot was worn to prevent or heal bruises.[20] A preserving stone is mentioned in the Talmud (Shabbat 66b) and was widely believed in ancient times to protect the wearer against a miscarriage. In his *Mishneh Torah*, Maimonides discusses the subject of amulets and preserving stones that were worn for medical purposes and were thought to be efficacious.

> One may also go out with a garlic skin, an onion skin, or a bandage over a wound—it is also permissible to tie or untie the bandage on the Sabbath—or with a plaster, a poultice, or a compress over a wound, or with a coin or a callus, or wearing a locust's egg, a fox's tooth, a nail from the gallows of an impaled convict, or any other article suspended on the body for medical reasons, provided that physicians say that it is medically effective (Shabbat 19:13).
>
> A woman may go out wearing a preserving stone—or its counterweight which has been weighed accurately for medical use. Not only a woman already pregnant may wear such a stone, but any other woman also may do so as a preventive of miscarriage in the event of pregnancy.
>
> One may also wear a tested amulet—that is, an amulet which has already cured three patients, or was made by someone who had previously cured three patients with other amulets. If one goes out into a public domain wearing an untested amulet, he is exempt, because he is deemed to have worn it as apparel when transferring it from one domain to the other (Shabbat 19:14).

Perhaps amulets and the like were efficacious because of their placebo effect. Patient attitude toward the physician and patient confidence in the treatment being used certainly play a role in the psychological if not physiological well-being of the patient.

Astrology

The work of astrologers was not confined to predicting the future from the stars. They claimed to be able to influence the future by changing misfortune into good fortune. They applied the occult virtues of heavenly bodies to earthly objects. The medicine was an image made by human art with due reference to the constellation. On this principle is based the method of curing diseases with figures especially made for this purpose. For example, Rabbi Solomon ben Abraham Adret, known as *Rashba,* writes that to cure pains in the loins or in the kidneys, people used to engrave the image of a tongueless lion on a plate of silver or gold.[21]

The generally prevalent belief in astrology during the Middle Ages was fully shared by the Jews, many of whom were convinced of the fundamental truth of the power of celestial bodies to influence human destiny. Moses Maimonides was one of the few who not only dared raises his voice against this almost universally held belief, but even branded it as a superstition akin to idolatry. He unequivocally prohibited anyone to influence his actions by astrology, as an offense punishable by disciplinary flogging. In his treatise on idolatry and heathen ordinances, he categorically rejects astrology and other superstitious practices and beliefs.[22]

In his famous *Letter to Yemen,* Maimonides denounces astrology as a fallacy and delusion.[23] In his psychological and ethical treatise entitled *The Eight Chapters* (*Shemonah Perakim*), Maimonides again sharply inveighs against astrology, denouncing it as a deception that is subversive to the faith and teachings of Judaism: "I have entered into this subject so thou mayest not believe the absurd ideas of astrologers, who falsely assert that the constellation at the time of one's birth determines whether one is to be virtuous or vicious."[24]

In his *Letter on Astrology,* in answer to an inquiry from Jewish scholars of southern France, Maimonides exposes the foibles and fallacies of astrology.[25] Noteworthy in this letter is the oft-quoted comment that the Second Temple was destroyed and national independence forfeited because the Jews were occupied with astrology. Maimonides told his correspondents that he did not take the matter lightly, but had studied it thoroughly and had come to the conclusion that astrology was an irrational illusion of fools who mistake vanity for wisdom and superstition for knowledge.

Medical Charms and Incantations

The medical effectiveness of incantations in classic Jewish sources was never in doubt. Incantations to heal a scorpion's bite are permitted even on the Sabbath, as are snake or scorpion charming to prevent injury or harm by them.[26] Maimonides points out that such incantations are absolutely useless but are permitted because of the patient's dangerous condition, so that he not become distraught.[27] Karo is of the same opinion.[28] One whispered a spell to heal eye illnesses (*Tosefta* Shabbat 7:23). Rabbi Chanina healed Rabbi Yochanan by uttering an incantation (Song of Songs Rabbath 2:16). A bone stuck in the throat can be dislodged by an incantation (Shabbat 67a).

The main question concerning the permissibility of incantations in Judaism is whether or not they represent a form of forbidden heathen practice, in that Jews are commanded not to go in the ways of the Amorites (Leviticus 18:3). Some talmudic sages declare that if one whispers a spell over a bodily illness, one is deprived of everlasting bliss, i.e., the world-to-come. These sages further prohibit a person from calling another to recite a biblical verse to calm a frightened child (Jerushalmi Shabbat 6:8b).

On the other hand, the Talmud clearly states that whatever is used for healing purposes is not forbidden on account of the ways of the Amorites (Shabbat 67a). This rule is codified by Asher ben Yechiel, known as *Rosh*, who states that charms used for the promotion of health are covered by the exemption of "anything done for the sake of healing."[29] *Rashba* states that the prohibition on account of the ways of the Amorites is limited to those practices specifically enumerated in the Talmud (*Tosefta* Shabbat, chapts. 7 and 8).

Zimmels lists a variety of diseases cured by charms as found in the responsa literature, including certain eye diseases, headache, infertility, and epilepsy.[30] He also describes the custom of transference, whereby an illness can be transferred to an animal or a plant by a certain procedure, with or without the recitation of an incantation.[31] For example, patients with jaundice were told to put live fish under their soles to transfer the jaundice to the fish. In more recent times, pigeons were placed on the abdomen of the jaundiced patient to transfer the illness to the pigeons.

Sorcery and Witchcraft

Judaism categorically prohibits sorcery as the first and foremost abhorrent practice of the nations. These practices include augury, soothsaying, divining, sorcery, casting spells, consulting ghosts or familiar spirits, and inquiring of the dead. *Anyone who does such things is abhorrent to the Lord* (Deuteronomy 18:9–14). Witchcraft in general is also outlawed: *Thou shalt not suffer a witch to live* (Exodus 22:17). Crimes of sorcery are considered tantamount to the idolatrous crimes of human sacrifices (Deuteronomy 18:10). The various forms of sorcery are defined in detail in the Talmud (Sanhedrin 65a).

Whether the use of sorcery for medical or healing purposes was exempted from the prohibition was a much-debated question in the writings of medieval Jewish authorities.[32] One view is that the practices prevalent in the Middle Ages were not of the idolatrous type prohibited in the Bible as sorcery.[33] Another view is that the prohibition of sorcery can be waived in cases of grave danger to life.[34] Yet another view is that sorcery or witchcraft may be resorted to but only for conditions thought to have been caused or induced by sorcery or witchcraft.[35]

The related topics of exorcism of demons, the "evil spirit" and the "evil eye," the "dreck-apotheke," and other superstitions, occult, and scatological cures are discussed by Jakobovits and Zimmels.[36]

Quacks and Quackery

Judaism has always held the physician in high esteem. Ancient and medieval Jewish writings are replete with expressions of admiration and praise for the "faithful physician." Therefore, it is not surprising that the derogatory talmudic statement "the best of physicians is destined for Gehenna" (Kiddushin 4:14) generated extensive discussion and commentary throughout the centuries.[37]

The Hebrew epigram *tov sheberofim legehinnom* is variously translated as "the best among physicians is destined to Gehinnom,"[38] "the best among physicians is destined for Gehenna,"[39] "the best of physicians is fit for Gehenna,"[40] "the best among doctors is for Gehenna,"[41] "the best of doctors are destined for Gehenna,"[42] "to hell with the best of the physicians,"[43] and "the best physician is destined to go to hell."[44]

According to Kalonymus ben Kalonymus, a Provençal writer and philosopher, in his ethical treatise *Even Bochan* (*The Touchstone*), the epigram "physicians are fit only for Gehenna" refers not to genuine physicians but to quacks, because "their art is lying and deception; all their boasting is empty falsehood; their hearts are turned away from God and their hands are covered with blood."[45]

Based on many interpretations, Jakobovits concludes that "to hell with the best of the physicians" was never understood as a denunciation of the conscientious practitioner. Physicians are among a group of communal servants who have heavy public responsibilities and are warned against the danger of negligence or error. The talmudic epigram with its curse is thus limited to physicians who are overly confident in their craft, or are guilty of commercializing their profession, or lie and deceive as do quacks, or who fail to acknowledge God as the true Healer of the sick, or who fail to consult with colleagues or medical texts when appropriate, or who perform surgery without heeding proper advice from diagnosticians, or who fail to heal the poor and thus indirectly cause their death, or who fail to try hard enough to heal their patients, or who consider themselves to be the best in their field, or who otherwise fail to conduct themselves in an ethical and professional manner.

Jewish law requires a physician to be skilled and well-educated. If he heals without being properly licensed, he is liable for any bad outcome. If he is an expert physician and fully licensed but errs and thereby harms the patient, he is exempt from payment of damages "because of the public good" (*Tosefta* Gittin 4:6). The divine arrangement of the world requires and presupposes the existence of physicians. If one were to hold the physician liable for every error, very few people would practice medicine. The physician, however, is still liable in the eyes of Heaven.[46]

If a physician caused an injury deliberately or acted without a proper license, he can be sued for damages no matter how competent he is (*Tosefta* Gittin 3:13). A physician who kills a patient and realizes that he was in error is exiled to the cities of refuge just like anyone else who kills another person through error (Numbers 35:11 and Deuteronomy 19:3).

Blamelessness in case of error only applies to a *rophe umman* who is an expert or well-trained physician and who heals "at the request of the authorities," that is to say, a licensed physician. A nonlicensed physician is subject to the general law and can be sued and must pay for damages he inflicts. Error and ignorance are used as excuses by quacks whom Judaism looks upon with disdain.

Summary and Conclusion

Judaism considers a human life to have infinite value. Therefore, physicians and other health-care givers are obligated to heal the sick and prolong life. Physicians are not only given Divine license to practice medicine, but are also mandated to use their skills to heal the sick. Failure or refusal to do so, with resultant negative impact on the patient, constitutes a transgression on the part of the physician. Physicians must be well-trained in traditional medicine and licensed by the authorities.

Patients are duty bound to seek healing from a physician when they are ill and not to rely solely on Divine intervention or faith healing. Patients are charged with preserving their health and restoring it when ailing in order to be able to serve the Lord in a state of good health. Quackery is not condoned in Judaism whether or not it is practiced by physicians. Those who deceive patients into accepting quack remedies "are destined for Gehenna."

On the other hand, Judaism seems to sanction certain alternative therapies, such as prayers, faith healing, amulets, incantations, and the like, when used as a supplement to traditional medical therapy. However, the substitution of prayer for rational healing is condemned. Quackery, superstition, sorcery, and witchcraft are abhorrent practices in Judaism, but confidence in the healing powers of God through prayer and contrition is encouraged and has its place of honor alongside traditional scientific medicine.

Notes

1. A. Sobkowski, "Alternative Medicine: Tales of Hoffman," *New York Doctor*, June 26, 1989, pp. 10–12.

2. See R. Cooter, ed., *Studies in the History of Alternative Medicine* (New York: St. Martin's Press, 1989; N. Gevitz, ed., *Other Healers: Unorthodox Medicine in America* (Baltimore: Johns Hopkins University Press, 1988).

3. V. Herbert, "Unproven (Questionable) Dietary and Nutritional Methods in Cancer Prevention and Treatment," *Cancer* 58 (1986): 1930–1941.

4. Ibid.

5. M. L. Brigden, "Unorthodox Therapy and Your Cancer Patient," *Postgraduate Medicine* 81 (1987): 271–280.

6. U.S., Congress, House, Select Committee on Aging, *Quackery: A $10 Billion Scandal*, 98th Congress, 2nd sess., 1984 (U.S. Government Printing Office, Comm. Pub. No. 98-43s).

7. B. R. Cassileth, "Unorthodox Cancer Medicine," *Cancer Investigation* 4 (1986): 591–598.

8. Ibid.

9. Ibid.

10. J. L. Dusseau, "Quack-Quack-Quack: Donald Duck Dissents," *Perspectives in Biology and Medicine* 30 (1987): 345–354.

11. B. N. Saltzman, "Unproven Methods of Cancer Management," *Journal of the Arkansas Medical Society* 83 (1986): 95–99; M. R. Montgomery, "Advances in Medical Fraud: Chelation Therapy Replaces Laetrile," *Journal of the Florida Medical Association* 73 (1986): 681–685; S. Porter, "Health Fraud—When Magic Replaces Medicine," *Ohio State Medical Journal* 82 (1986): 801–805; J. Duffy, "Quackery in Arthritis," *Minnesota Medicine* 70 (1987): 700; J. M. Norses, J. M. Remy, A. D. Nenna, and P. Reygagne, "Malpractice by Nonphysician Healers, *New York State Journal of Medicine* 87 (1987): 473–474; A. B. Lasswell and T. Leddy, "Nutrition Misinformation: How to Protect Your Patients," *Rhode Island Medical Journal* 69 (1986): 263–268; S. Stokes, "Cancer Quackery: A Continuing Problem," *Journal of the Tennessee Medical Association* 78 (1986): 415–421; Anonymous. "Quacks Sell Hope, Not Health Care," *Wisconsin Medical Journal* 87 (1988): 25–26; J. Filicetti, "Unproven Methods of Cancer Treatment," *AAOHN Journal* 35 (1987): 153–158; K. A. Kill, "Unproven Cancer Therapies," *American Pharmacy*, n.s. 28 (1988): 82–86; Anonymous. "Questionable Care: What Can Be Done About Dental Quackery?" *Journal of the American Dental Association* 115 (1987): 679–685; J. M. Ashley and R. Alfin-Slater, *Position of the American Dietetic Association*, 88 (1988): 1589–1591.

12. L. King, "Quackery," *Journal of the American Medical Association* 261 (1989): 1979–1980.

13. N. Gevitz, "The Chiropractors and the AMA: Reflections on the His-

tory of the Consultation Clause," *Perspectives in Biology and Medicine* 32 (1989): 281–299.

14. F. Rosner, "The Efficacy of Prayer: Scientific versus Religious Evidence," *Journal of Religion and Health* 14 (1975): 294–298.
15. I. Jakobovits, *Jewish Medical Ethics* (New York: Bloch, 1975), pp. 15–23.
16. J. Preuss, *Biblical and Talmudic Medicine* (New York: Hebrew Publishing Co., 1978), pp. 146–149.
17. Jakobovits, op. cit., pp. 24–44.
18. H. J. Zimmels, *Magicians, Theologians and Doctors: Studies in Folk Medicine and Folklore as Reflected in the Rabbinical Responsa (12–19th Centuries)* (London: E Goldston & Sons, 1952), pp. 135–137.
19. J. Karo, *Shulchan Aruch, Yoreh Deah* 179:12.
20. Ibid., *Orach Chayim* 301:28, based on Shabbat 65a.
21. S. Adret, Responsa *Rashba*, pt. 1, no. 167.
22. M. Maimonides, *Mishneh Torah, Avodat Kochavim* 11:16.
23. A. S. Halkin, *Moses Maimonides' Epistle to Yemen* (New York: American Academy for Jewish Research, 1952).
24. J. L. Garfinkle, *The Eight Chapters of Maimonides on Ethics* (New York: AMS Press, 1966).
25. A. Marx "The Correspondence Between the Rabbis of Southern France and Maimonides About Astrology," *Hebrew Union College Annual.* 3 (1926): 311–358 and 4 (1927): 493–494.
26. Karo, *Shulchan Aruch, Yoreh Deah* 179:6–7.
27. Maimonides, *Mishneh Torah, Avodat Kochavim* 11:11.
28. Karo, loc. cit.
29. Commentary of *Rosh* on Shabbat 6:19.
30. Zimmels, op. cit., pp. 140–141.
31. Ibid. pp. 141–142.
32. Ibid., p. 221, n. 90.
33. S. Habir, Responsa *Nachalat Shiva*, no. 76.
34. J. Ettlinger, Responsa *Binyan Zion*, no. 67.
35. S. Luria, Responsa *Maharshal*, no. 3.
36. Jakobovits, op. cit., pp. 135–149; Zimmels, op. cit., pp. 135–149.
37. See above, chap. 3.
38. Zimmels, op. cit., p. 170.
39. H. Danby, *The Mishnah* (London: Oxford University Press, 1933).
40. H. Friedenwald, *The Jews and Medicine* (Baltimore: Johns Hopkins Press, 1944), vol. 1, pp. 11–13.
41. P. Blackman, *Order Nashim*, in *Mishnayoth*, 3rd ed. (New York: Judaica Press, 1965), vol. 3, p. 482.
42. I. Epstein, ed., *The Babylonian Talmud: Seder Nashim, Tractate Kiddushin* trans. H. Feldman (London: Soncino Press, 1936), vol. 4, p. 423.
43. Jakobovits, op. cit., pp. 202–203.
44. Preuss, op. cit., p. 26.
45. Friedenwald, op. cit., vol. 1, p. 74.
46. Karo, *Shulchan Aruch, Yoreh Deah* 336:1.

30

Creation versus Evolution

Introduction

The controversy about the teaching of creation as an alternative to or in addition to the teaching of evolution is again in the public press and mass media. The controversy began with the publication of Charles Darwin's *The Origin of Species* on November 24, 1859. Darwin's theory of evolution is taught in almost every country throughout the world and is nearly universally accepted. No textbook on biology, at high school, college or graduate school level is devoid of Darwinism.

The argument of creation versus evolution is only a small part of the larger question of religion versus science. One might ask: is the religious belief in creation right and the scientific theory of evolution wrong? Or is science right and religion wrong? I offer the thesis that both science and religion are correct and that both creation and evolution are true. This approach is an attempt to rationalize the two seemingly opposing viewpoints.

Science and Religion

To avoid the controversy of creation versus evolution, it would be easy to say that science and religion deal with totally different aspects of the same subject and, therefore, cannot conflict. For example, if one analyzed New York City from social, political and economic viewpoints, one would arrive at three different, not necessarily contradictory, analyses of the same subject. Similarly, religion and science may look at the same subject but on separate, not necessarily contradictory, levels.

Such an approach is depicted by Spero[1] who quotes Rabbi Abba Hillel Silver sho said: "The conflict between religion and science is more apparent than real. There is no fundamental issue between them . . . As soon as religion and science discover their legitimate sphere, the conflict ceases . . . "Science investigates, religion interprets. One seeks causes, the other ends." Sol Roth also challenges the fundamental assumptions on which the conflict between science and religion is based.[2] He posits that science and religion "belong to different universes of discourse precluding the possibility of contradiction." He further charges that the centuries-old conflict between religion and science is fictitious and based on misunderstanding.

A more erudite enunciation of this point of view is that of Kasher, who states:

> The whole problem of conflicts between religion and science is a pseudo-problem. The various disciplines, through their differing methodologies, construct systems of acceptable, established propositions and theories. There can be no contradiction between the affirmation of a particular proposition within the context of one discipline and the negation of the same proposition within the context of another discipline since what we are really confronted with here are two totally different concepts of truth—the one defined by the methodology of the one discipline, the other defined by the methodology of the other.[3]

Kasher thus describes not the content of discussions about science and religion but methodology of the discussions.

A similar approach is to look at science and religion as converging on a common goal from opposite directions. The religious Jew conforms to the pronouncement *we will obey first and then we will listen.*[4] That is, explanations for the things we do and the rituals we perform are sought after first complying with them. For some biblical precepts (*chukim*), no logical explanations will ever be found. For others (*mishpatim*), continuing education and learning and study of Torah provides insights into the whys and wherefores of those precepts. On the other hand, a scientist seeks explanations in advance before he accepts the scientific truths he discovers.

Thus, if he cannot smell, touch, feel, see, or hear something, it does not exist. This oversimplified contrast between the scientist and the religious person is perhaps fallacious in that both approaches are really based on unprovable axioms or assumptions. The religious person believes on faith, for he cannot prove that his beliefs are true. Similarly, the scientist begins with unprovable axioms, such as "matter cannot be destroyed or created."

Berkovits expresses this thought more vividly:

> A scientific world-view is not science, but the *leap of faith* undertaken by the scientist who ventures to interpret the whole of reality on the basis of the exact knowledge gained from the scientific investigation of a relatively small segment of the whole. Neither is a religious world-view religion. It, too, is a *leap of faith* which attempts to grasp the essential nature of the whole in the light of a necessarily-limited experience and a specific insight.[5]

Berkovits thus indicates that both science and religion are based on unprovable axioms and assumptions, i.e., faith. Therefore, it is not at all unreasonable to espouse the thesis that since the basic assumptions of both religion and science cannot be proven, they may both be compatible and not necessarily contradictory.

Many of today's Jewish scientists espouse this viewpoint in addition to myself. Psychologist Boris Levinson states that

> the domains of science and religion are in no way antagonistic to each other even though the individual functions are entirely different. The purpose of science is to learn facts and data. . . . the purpose of religion is to develop the ideals, the consciences and aspirations of mankind. . . . Far from being antagonistic, science and religion can be mutually supplementary. . . . it was not a rare occurrence that good teachers of Judaism were at the same time well at home in the sciences of their age.[6]

Radiologist Melvin Zelefsky asserts that "faith does not falter before the scientific advance. Scientific information transforms faith into a more deep and profound religious experience. Science expands religion, it does not contain it."[7]

Not all Jewish scientists subscribe to the blending and harmony of science and religion. Some propound the thesis that science and religion conflict. Physicist Alvin Radkowsky states that "it is acknowledged today by philosophers of both science and religion that the controversy arising out of conflict between these two types of knowledge . . . is not a thing of the past. . . . The claims of secularism which challenge the intellectual integrity of the Jewish faith . . . are fallacious."[8]

Let me illustrate, using three examples, the synthesis of religion and science, and the lack of contradiction and antagonism in spite of much controversy. Most Jews believe in the many miracles wrought by God for the Israelites during their Exodus from Egypt several thousand years ago. Immanuel Velikowsky, in his book *Worlds in Collision*, explains every miracle of the Exodus from Egypt as a natural phenomenon. Even the splitting of the Red Sea is described by Velikowsky as having transpired due to a unique occurrence of a complex constellation of astronomical events. Certainly, no religious Jew accepts such an interpretation of the historical events described in the Book of Exodus. It is conceivable, however, that God wrought all the miracles of that era through natural means.

A second example is the story of the prophet Elisha and the Shunammite woman's son who "died" of sunstroke. The child's revival by Elisha is described as follows: *And he went up and lay upon the child, and put his mouth upon his mouth, and his eyes upon his eyes, and his hands upon his hands; and he crouched over him; and the child sneezed seven times and the child opened his eyes.*[9] Some interpret this incident as of purely miraculous connotation. *Radak* (R. David Kimchi, 1160–1235), however, states that Elisha attempted to breathe on the child in order to provide warmth from the natural body heat which emanated from his mouth and eyes. *Radak* further states that most miracles are performed with direction and guidance from worldly and natural actions. *Metzudat David* (R. David Altschul, 17th cent.) states that Elisha tried to pour some of the life of his own body into the limbs of the child. *Ralbag* (R. Levi ben Gerson, 1288–1344) gives an identical interpretation but adds that "he [Elisha] did this after he prayed." *Ralbag* and *Radak* thus seem to consider a combination of natural and miraculous events as having contributed to the child's revival. Another nearly identical incident relates to the revival by Elijah of the son of the widow of Zarephat.[10] The commentaries there offer similar interpretations to those cited in regard to Elisha's revival of the Shunammite woman's son.

A third example concerns the wars between Israel and her Arab adversaries. Describing the Six Day War of 1967, parasitologist Morris Goldman states:

> For millions of Jews, myself included, the sequence and confluence of events . . . which led finally to the recovery of Old Jerusalem, were so improbable and had such apocalyptic overtones, that they could only be viewed as the clearest demonstration of Divine intervention that we could expect to see in our lifetime. And yet all took place between men of flesh and blood wielding tangible fire and steel, all is describable at a secularist level, and all is no doubt so entombed in State Department memoranda.[11]

Once again, it is conceivable and even plausible that Divine intervention was effected by natural means, i.e., the tools of war and the spirit of the Israeli soldiers.

Creation and/or Evolution

We cannot ignore the theory of evolution, because of its wide acceptance throughout the world, and must, therefore, make attempts to cope with it. Evolution was and still is called the *theory* of evolution because it began as a theory, not as a fact. The hypothesis was formulated and facts were sought to support or reject it. There are still gaps in the theory of evolution. Some facts support evolution (e.g., mutations occur), but even these facts are open to varying interpretations. The theory of evolution is a satisfactory explanation of *some* of the evidence. All living forms, however, cannot be explained by evolution.

Kerkut states that one should not become encased in scientific dogmatism but from time to time stop to think things out for oneself.[12] Over eight centuries ago Moses Maimonides attempted to eradicate preconceived medical notions and dictated dogmas.[13] He encouraged people to observe and experiment for themselves and to develop an attitude of keen criticism and skepticism toward accepted traditions and teachings even if these originate from as renowned an authority as Galen. Using this Maimonidean approach of applying a critical approach to the question of evolution versus creation, I have personally concluded, as did the late Chief Rabbi of the Britist Commonwealth, Joseph H. Hertz, that both creation and evolution are correct. Hertz asserts that even if one accepts the fundamental dogma of Judaism that the "world was called into existence at the will of the One, Almighty and All-good God, . . . there is nothing inherently un-Jewish in the evolutionary conception of the origin and growth of forms of existence from the simple to the complex, and from the lowest to the highest."[14]

One of the basic assumptions of the theory of evolution which is not capable of experimental verification is that a certain series of events occurred in the past. Even if one could today change a reptile into a mammal, it would not prove that this is the way it happened in the past. How did the world originate? Some scientists invoke the "primeval-atom theory," which says that a burst of radioactivity which began life occurred ten billion years ago. After the burst, natural laws took over. Others subscribe to the "steady-state hypothesis," which says that there never was a creation. The Jewish view is enunciated by Maimonides in his thirteen principles of faith: "I firmly believe that the Creator, blessed be His name, is both Creator and Guide of all created beings and that He alone has made, does make, and will make all things." This belief, of course, is based on the first chapter in Genesis. None of these points of view is provable, and thus the evolutionist-scientist stands on no firmer ground than the believer in Divine creation in regard to the origin of life.

A second basic assumption in the theory of evolution holds that life was formed (or created) only once. If living material had developed on several occasions, one would expect a large number of distinct unrelated groups of animals. Yet, another basic assumption says that all living things are related in that the "higher forms evolved from the lower forms." Once again, one theorizes in an area that is not subject to experimental verification. One writer succinctly characterizes the evolution or creation of living beings as "past events which can never be subjected to direct observation."[15]

How Old is the World?

Is the world as we know it 5746 years old, or is it ten billion years old? How can one tell? Is one to accept the Jewish calender, which uses the lower number? Or should one adhere to the higher number propounded by most scientists? Is 5746 reconcilable with ten billion? Are these two necessarily contradictory? I say no.

Let us briefly examine the ten billion figure. There are two major scientific approaches to dating the age of the world, the radioactive decay method and the stratigraphical method. In the radioactive decay approach, one measures the amount of radiation of certain isotopes, such as carbon, potassium, and uranium, in rocks and plants and back-calculates the duration of time the element must have been present using the concept of half-time decay, that is, the duration of time it takes for the radioactivity to halve. The major fallacy in this method is that it is based on the assumption that the rate of radioactivie decay has remained constant over many centuries and eons. This may or may not be true. There are conflicting reports even in the scientific literature concerning deviations in radioactive decay rates, particularly of carbon 14. Furthermore, using different radioactive isotopes one obtains results for the age of the world that differ widely. Finally, when samples of the same rock are given to several laboratories for carbon dating, differences of many thousands of years are reported by the individual laboratories.

The stratigraphical or geological method of estimating the age of the world measures the thickness of each layer or stratum of rock and earth. From the known rate of deposition and erosion of layers, one calculates the age of the earth. This method is also crude, no more than an estimate, and also assumes that no sudden changes occurred. The few centuries where man has been observing nature form too brief an interval by which to measure geological action in all past time. Rabbi Dr. Elie Munk specifically asserts that changes in natural phenomena did in fact take place, and that when man left paradise he succumbed to the forces of nature with a progressive decline in physical strength.[16] Nature also progressively weakened. As evidence Rabbi Munk cites the dinosaur skeletons, which he interprets as extinct supercreatures, perhaps the giants or *bnei anakim* of the Pentateuch. Therefore, concludes Rabbi Munk, since nature changed, one cannot calculate the age of the world from natural phenomena.

Although the scientific methods of estimating the age of the world can be criticized as above, is it not possible that the 5746 and the ten billion figures are both correct? One explanation is that each of the seven days of creation as described in the first chapter of Genesis represented a thousand or a million years. Such an opinion is enunciated by Rabbi Menachem Kasher, who explains the phrase *and there was evening and there was morning, the sixth day*[17] to mean that our system of time reckoning begins after the creation of heaven, earth, and planets was finished, that is, on the seventh day.[18] The system of time measurement for the six days of creation was a separate and relative time for each day.

Another possible way of reconciling the 5746 and the ten billion figures for the age of the world is the midrashic passage which says that the Holy One, blessed be He, created worlds and destroyed them again.[19] That is, prior to the existence of the present universe, which is presumably 5746 years old, certain "formless worlds issued . . .

and then vanished, like sparks which fly from a red-hot iron beaten by a hammer, that are extinguished as they separate themselves from the burning mass. . . . ours is the best of all possible worlds."[20] Thus the total duration of the "Fountain of Existence," including all the previous worlds which God created and destroyed, is perhaps several billion years.

Maimonides denies the concept of earlier worlds being formed and annihilated.[21] He asserts that time itself is one of the things created by Almighty God and that

> the world has not been created in a temporal beginning . . . because time belongs to the created things . . . On the other hand the statement, which you find formulated by some of the Sages, that affirms that time existed before the creation of the world is very difficult. For that is the opinion of Aristotle, which I have explained to you: he holds that time cannot be conceived to have a beginning, which is incongruous. Those who made this statement were conducted to it by their finding in Scripture the terms: *one day*,[22] *a second day*.[23] He who made this statement understood these terms according to the external sense and as follows: Inasmuch as a rotating sphere and a sun did not yet exist, whereby was *the first day* measured? They express their opinion in the following text: "The first day—Rabbi Judah, son of Rabbi Simon, said: Hence we learn that there existed before that an order of time. Rabbi Abuha said: Hence we learn that the Holy One may His name be blessed, used to create worlds and to destroy them again."[24] This second opinion is even more incongruous than the first. Consider what was the difficulty for these two Sages. It was the notion that time existed prior to the existence of this sun. . . . To sum up, you should not, in considering these points, take into account the statements made by this or that one. I have already made it known to you that the foundation of the whole law is the view that God had brought the world into being out of nothing without there having been a temporal beginning. For time is created, being consequent upon the motion of the sphere which is created.

The Origin of Man

For evolutionists, a major and seemingly insurmountable problem is to explain how life began. The concept of creation implies *yesh may-ayin*, or creating something from nothing. No acceptable alternative has yet been offered by evolutionists, although the primeval-atom theory and the steady-state hypothesis cited earlier are attempts to account for the origin of life. Nor can spontaneous generation be proved. Even Darwin, in the last paragraph of his *Origin of Species*, seems to believe in a Creator when he says that "there is grandeur in this view of life, with its several powers, having been originally breathed by the Creator into a few forms or into one."

The biblical account of the origin of life, although not subject to scientific verification, is certainly reasonable and in harmony with the facts as we know them today. How logical and orderly the process of creation revealed in Genesis! First heaven and earth *(domem)*, then plant life *(tzomeach)*, then creatures of the sea and sky and then land animals *(chai)*, and finally man *(medaber)*. Evolution cannot explain the creation of the world, nor does the belief in the Creator of the world negate the possibility that evolution exists and occurs. Each created species is endowed with the ability to produce only its kind and no other kind. A dog cannot produce a kitten, nor can an apple seed produce an orange tree. Within each species, however, evolution may take place. Thus, the scientifically proven facts concerning evolution (e.g., mutations) can be readily explained and need not be refuted as untrue.

In regard to the origin of man, the same question arises as with the origin of the world. Evolutionists assert that humans have lived on earth for hundreds of thousands of years, but history offers no support for such a theory. The earliest records we have of human history, i.e., civilization in Mesopotamia, go back only about five thousand years. The early stages of man's evolutionary progress along his individual line remain a total mystery. It is perfectly reasonable to consider the creation of Adam and Eve by God to have been followed by "evolution" of man into the form we know today. Perhaps Adam was a Neanderthal man. What is unacceptable to me and others is that man may have evolved from monkeys. No fossils have yet been found to prove that man evolved from apes.

Conclusion

I have put forward the thesis that a traditional Jew who believes in Divine creation of the world and of man can also accept the doctrine of evolution on a limited basis. Obviously, such a Jew cannot accept all that is propounded by strict evolutionists, but the concept of evolution with some factual support does not negate belief in the

Creator. This view is most eloquently and forcefully enunciated by Hertz:

> Now, while the *fact* of creation has to this day remained the first of the articles of the Jewish Creed, there is no uniform and binding belief as to the *manner* of creation, *i.e.* as to the process whereby the universe came into existence. The manner of the Divine creative activity is presented in varying forms and under differing metaphors by Prophet, Psalmist and Sage; by the Rabbis in Talmudic times, as well as by our medieval Jewish thinkers. . . .
>
> In face of this great diversity of views as to the *manner* of creation, there is, therefore, nothing inherently un-Jewish in the evolutionary conception of the origin and growth of forms of existence from the simple to the complex, and from the lowest to the highest. The Biblical account itself gives expression to the same general truth of gradual ascent from amorphous chaos to order, from inorganic to organic, from lifeless matter to vegetable, animal and man; *insisting, however, that each stage is no product of chance, but is an act of Divine will,* realizing the Divine purpose, and receiving the seal of the Divine approval. Such, likewise, is in effect the evolutionary position. Behind the orderly development of the universe there must be a Cause, at once controlling and permeating the process. Allowing for all the evidence in favor of interpreting existence in terms of the evolutionary doctrine, there still remain facts—tremendous facts—to be explained; *viz.* the origin of life, mind, conscience, human personality. For each of these, we must look back to the Creative Omnipotence of the Eternal Spirit. . . .
>
> . . .*MAN IS THE GOAL AND CROWN OF CREATION*—he is fundamentally distinguished from the lower creation, and is akin to the Divine. Man, modern scientists declare, is cousin to the anthropoid ape. But it is not so much the descent, as the *ascent* of man, which is decisive. Furthermore, it is not the resemblance, but the *differences* between man and the ape, that are of infinite importance. . . .
>
> Nor is the Biblical account of the creation of man irreconcilable with the view that certain forms of organized being have been endowed with the capacity of developing, in God's good time and under the action of suitable environment, the attributes distinctive of man. "God formed man of the dust of the ground" (Gen. II, 7). Whence that dust was taken is not, and

cannot be, of fundamental importance. Science holds that man was formed from the lower animals; are they not too "dust of the ground"? "And God said, Let the earth bring forth the living creature—this command, says the Midrash, includes Adam as well, תוצא הארץ נפש חיה — זו רוחו של אדם הראשון The thing that eternally matters is the breath of Divine and everlasting life that He breathed into the being coming from the dust. By virtue of that Divine impact, a new and distinctive creature made its appearance—man, dowered with an immortal soul. . . .

God the Creator and Lord of the Universe, which is the work of His goodness and wisdom; and Man, made in His image, who is to hallow his week-day labours by the blessedness of Sabbath-rest—such are the teachings of the Creation chapter. Its purpose is to reveal these teachings to the children of men—and not to serve as a textbook of astronomy, geology or anthropology. Its object is not to teach scientific facts; but to proclaim highest religious truths respecting God, Man, and the Universe. The "conflict" between the fundamental realities of Religion and the established facts of Science is seen to be unreal as soon as Religion and Science each recognizes the true borders of its dominion.[25]

Notes

1. S. Spero, "Does the Science-Religion Conflict Rest on a Mistake?" *Tradition* 9 (1978): 119–130.
2. S. Roth, *Science and Religion*, Studies in Torah Judaism (New York: Yeshiva University Press, 1966).
3. A. Kasher, "Fundamental Assumptions for Discussion on Religion and Science," *Tradition* 10 (1968): 87–99.
4. Exodus 24:7.
5. E. Berkovits, "The Scientific and the Religious World View," *Intercom* 6 (1965): 6–12.
6. T. Levitan, "The Scientist and Religion," *Synagogue Light* 35 (1969): 5–7.
7. Ibid. 36 (1970): 5–6.
8. Ibid. 35 (1969): 5–6.
9. II Kings 4:34–35.
10. I Kings 17:17–22.
11. M. Goldman, "Man's Place in Nature," *Tradition* 10 (1968): 101.
12. G. A. Kerkut, *Implications of Evolution* (New York: Pergamom Press, 1960), chap. 2, pp. 6–17.
13. F. Rosner, and S. Muntner, *The Medical Aphorisms of Moses Maimonides* (New York: Bloch, for Yeshiva University Press, 1973), vol. 2, pp. 171–202.
14. J. H. Hertz, "Additional Notes to Genesis," in *The Pentateuch and Haftorahs*, 2nd ed., (London: Soncino Press, 1960), pp. 193–202.
15. W. E. Le Cros Clark, "The Crucial Evidence for Human Evolution," *Proceedings of the American Philosophical Society*, 103 (1959): 159–172.
16. E. Munk, *Das Licht der Ewigkeit* (1935), p. 115.
17. Genesis 1:31.
18. M. Kasher, *Encyclopedia of Biblical Interpretation* (1953), Genesis, 1.
19. Genesis Rabbah 3:7.
20. Hertz, op. cit., pp. 193–194.
21. Maimonides, *Guide for the Perplexed* 2: 30; trans. Shlomo Pines (Chicago: University of Chicago Press, 1963), p. 349.
22. Genesis 1:5.
23. Ibid. 1:8.
24. Genesis Rabbah III.
25. Hertz, *op. cit.*, pp. 193–195.

Index

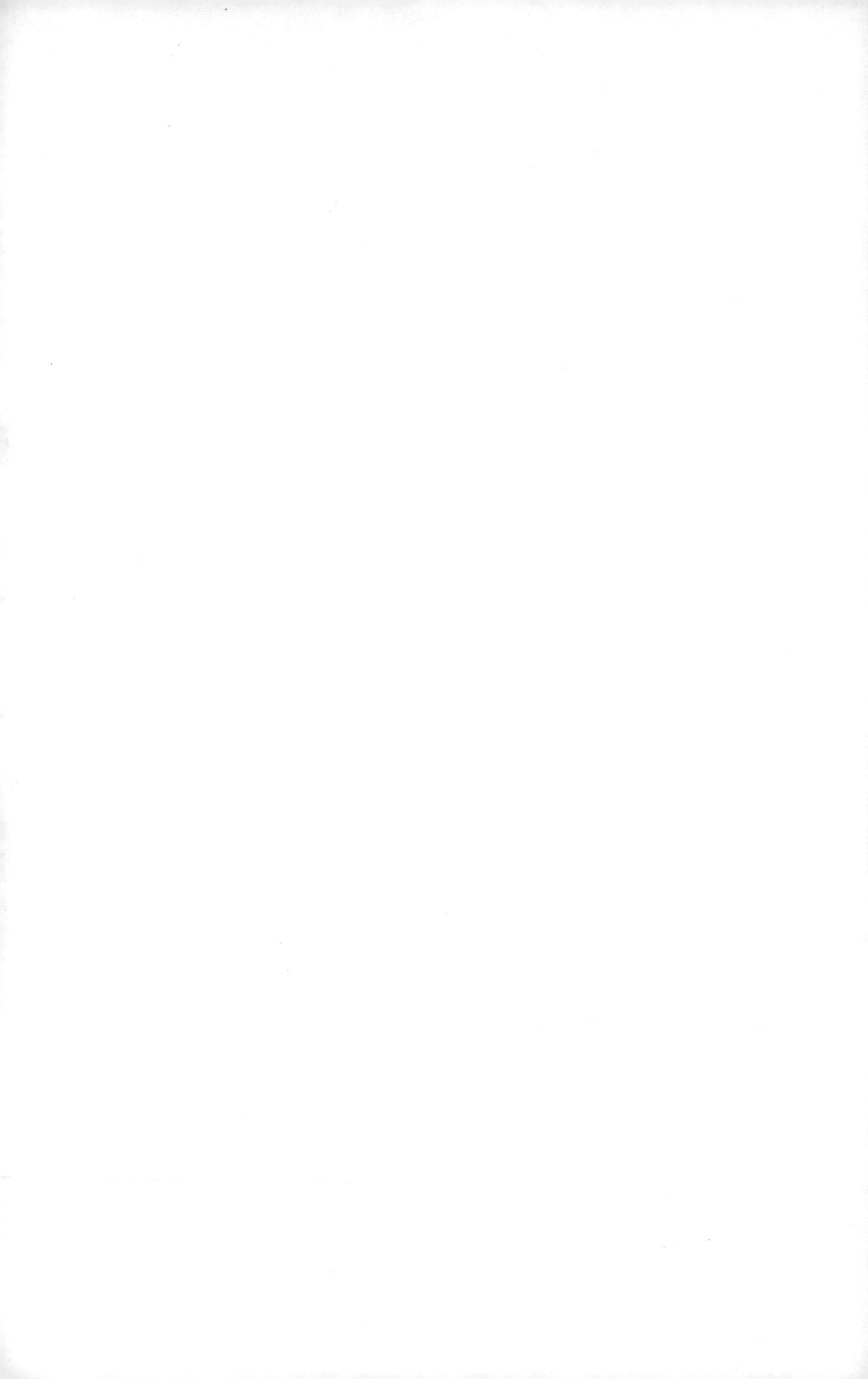